THE UNCONSCIOUS

Psychoanalysis and Psychological Science

Elliot Jurist, *Series Editor*

Books in this series aim to bridge the work of researchers and the work of clinicians. They reflect the current empirical findings and state of the art in psychoanalysis and psychodynamic treatment. They are written to be practical and relevant to clinicians.

Attachment and Psychoanalysis:
Theory, Research, and Clinical Implications
Morris N. Eagle

Minding Emotions:
Cultivating Mentalization in Psychotherapy
Elliot Jurist

The Unconscious:
Theory, Research, and Clinical Implications
Joel Weinberger and Valentina Stoycheva

The
UNCONSCIOUS

THEORY, RESEARCH, AND CLINICAL IMPLICATIONS

Joel Weinberger
Valentina Stoycheva

Series Editor's Note by Elliot Jurist

gp

THE GUILFORD PRESS
New York   London

The authors have checked with sources believed to be reliable in their
efforts to provide information that is complete and generally in accord
with the standards of practice that are accepted at the time of publication.
However, in view of the possibility of human error or changes in
behavioral, mental health, or medical sciences, neither the authors, nor
the editor and publisher, nor any other party who has been involved in
the preparation or publication of this work warrants that the information
contained herein is in every respect accurate or complete, and they are
not responsible for any errors or omissions or the results obtained from
the use of such information. Readers are encouraged to confirm the
information contained in this book with other sources.

Library of Congress Cataloging-in-Publication Data

Names: Weinberger, Joel L., author. | Stoycheva, Valentina, author.
Title: The unconscious : theory, research, and clinical implications / Joel
    Weinberger, Valentina Stoycheva.
Description: New York : The Guilford Press, 2020. | Series: Psychoanalysis
    and psychological science | Includes bibliographical references and
    index.
Identifiers: LCCN 2019025679 | ISBN 9781462541058 (hardcover)
Subjects: LCSH: Subconsciousness. | Cognitive neuroscience.
Classification: LCC BF315 .W295 2019 | DDC 154.2—dc23
LC record available at *https://lccn.loc.gov/2019025679*

About the Authors

Joel Weinberger, PhD, is Professor in the Derner School of Psychology at Adelphi University. He is a Fellow of the Association for Psychological Science and of the American Psychological Association. His research on unconscious processes has been recognized with the Ulf Kragh Award from the University of Lundh, Sweden. Author or coauthor of approximately 100 publications, Dr. Weinberger is a founder of Implicit Strategies, which consults for political campaigns, nonprofits, and businesses. His political and business commentaries have appeared in the national media. He is also a practicing clinical psychologist.

Valentina Stoycheva, PhD, is a staff psychologist at Northwell Health in Bay Shore, New York, where she works with military service members, veterans, and their families. She is also a cofounder and director of Stress and Trauma Evaluation and Psychological Services (STEPS), a group practice that focuses on the integrative treatment of trauma. Dr. Stoycheva has taught undergraduate- and graduate-level courses and has contributed to over a dozen publications and presentations in the fields of trauma, family dynamics, and the psychotherapy process. In 2018, she was named one of Adelphi University's 10 Under 10 outstanding young alumni.

Series Editor's Note

Across all domains of psychology, there is an appreciation of the importance of bringing research into closer proximity to practice. The language that is often and typically used is to seek to "apply" research to practice.

The Psychoanalysis and Psychological Science series embraces that aim and hopes to substantiate it. However, in order for research to be applied well to practice, it first must be interpreted and translated. Indeed, a strong motivation for this series is to demonstrate that research, which is informed by and responsive to theory, offers the most stimulating and optimal path for helping clinicians to be able to improve their work. I wish to affirm a positive connotation of the term "philosophical" precisely because it uses a less contested language that can foster communication between researchers and clinicians, at once providing a bridge to the past in psychology and a way forward.

It is a pleasure, therefore, to introduce into this series Weinberger and Stoycheva's *The Unconscious.* This book reflects three decades of Joel Weinberger's accomplished work in the field. It draws on several branches of psychology and is attentive to arguments pro and con for whatever point of view is under consideration. For example, the authors introduce and discuss a wide range of contemporary theories and research about the unconscious from cognitive psychology and neuroscience. Part of their aim is to emphasize what has become displaced from psychoanalytic thinking about the unconscious. They argue as well that clinicians, psychodynamic as well as others, have failed to integrate this contemporary thinking and research in their work.

There is a genuine seeking for truth here, a balance that stands out against the clamor of assertions that "we are decisively right and you are utterly wrong." The authors weigh arguments carefully and thoughtfully and are less concerned with defending a particular point of view than with suggesting fruitful lines of ongoing work and valuable insights for practitioners to take up and develop further. Yet, they do not shy away from clarifying where they believe the evidence points—such as defending the notion that the unconscious is normative and not the source of psychopathology, or that competing computational models, such as massive modularity, parallel distributed processing, and neural reuse, can be integrated. It is worth stressing how practical the authors' conclusions are: I have had success in encouraging a patient to open up about bizarre associations, overcoming the fear of feeling too vulnerable, by encouraging an appreciation that this was simply how the mind works.

Given how ambitious the book is in terms of its breadth, readers from across the field are certain to learn new things, be they forgotten paths of research or the latest computational models. The book is especially valuable to clinicians who realize that in order to help their patients, they must become more knowledgeable about how the human mind functions and inspire patients in facing that there is much that they do not know about themselves. Bravely, Weinberger and Stoycheva are prepared to argue that recognizing unconscious processes as part of psychotherapy ensures, rather than diminishes, its future.

ELLIOT JURIST

Preface

This is both an ambitious and a modest book. It arose out of our years-long efforts to understand unconscious processes empirically as well as our dedication to helping people whose quality of life is not what they wish it to be.

The goal of this book is to come to an understanding of unconscious processes. This goal is much simpler to state than to achieve, as the field of study of unconscious processes is not a unified one. Rather, it is often messy, controversial, and maze-like. Nonetheless, learning about it was tremendously rewarding. We hope the reader will feel similarly after reading our state-of-the-art review. But we are also clinicians and want to apply what we have learned about unconscious processes to psychotherapy. And we want the book to be accessible to researchers, clinicians, and curious educated laymen. To achieve these goals, we have adopted a comprehensive approach: we cover history, philosophy, research, clinical theory, and computational models of the mind. The breadth of knowledge in these areas helps us understand how we got to where we are, what we now know, and what kind of theory could encompass it all. We then take it one step further by applying it to psychotherapy and sketching a theory for that endeavor.

Parts I and II cover the history of addressing or denying unconscious processes. We discuss philosophy, beginning with Descartes, and we discuss medical approaches, beginning with Mesmer. We review the early history of psychology and how the pioneers of the field came to grips (or failed to come to grips) with the phenomenon of unconscious processes. We also review early empirical approaches to unconscious processes, highlighted by the New Look. We show how and why these largely failed. Early attention theories, on the other hand, succeeded. They eventuated into the cognitive revolution, in turn resulting in the acceptance of unconscious processes. After this early history, we discuss the one discipline that engaged in a sustained effort to understand unconscious processes: psychoanalysis. Our focus here is on the main models of psychoanalysis and their understanding of unconscious processes, but we also address the historical, theoretical, and psychotherapeutic implications of this work.

In Part III, we discuss more early as well as recent empirical work, setting the stage for what we term the "normative unconscious." Drawing from research in social, clinical, experimental, and cognitive psychology, we offer our best understanding of the work and controversies relating to the following normative unconscious processes: heuristics, implicit memory, implicit learning, attribution theory, implicit motivation, automaticity, affective versus cognitive salience, and embodied cognition.

Following this, in Part IV, we review three computational models of the mind/brain (massive modularity, parallel distributed processing, and neural reuse) that we believe could allow for models that encompass all of the previously reviewed work. And throughout we discuss the psychotherapeutic implications of all of these areas. We try to make sense of it all so as to come up with an integrated model that can handle most of the empirical findings and provide a scaffolding for future research and theorizing. In the end, we propose a modified neural reuse model. We believe that this kind of model offers the most empirically supported understanding of unconscious processes, given current knowledge. We then offer a model of psychotherapy, normative implicit psychotherapy (NIP), that we believe is in line with the empirical findings we report and with the model we offer. We suggest that this could put the theory and practice of psychotherapy on more solid footing.

The modest aspect of the book is that, in addition to communicating what we do know, we also discuss what we do not know, what scholars disagree about, and what these disputants are saying to support their assertions. We readily admit that our conclusions and interpretations are tentative and could easily, and probably will, be overtaken by time. We do not really know enough yet to come to a comprehensive and empirically supported model of unconscious processes. Nor do we yet know enough about how psychotherapy works to offer a definitive model of treatment. But we think there is enough out there to make an educated guess, and suggest that the time is right to begin a discussion that we hope will become ongoing. So we offer our take on how this all looks now and we hope it generates some enthusiasm and even some efforts at refutation so that the enterprise can move forward.

We had some concern that the diverse audience we are hoping to reach might be unfamiliar with some of the terms we use, as they originate in subdisciplines not their own. We also created or made new use of some terms in our efforts to integrate the findings and theoretical writings across these subdisciplines. These terms are defined (and <u>underlined</u>) in the book, but we thought that some orientation to them, outside of the main text, might be beneficial to the reader. In order to facilitate such an orientation, we offer a Glossary that consists of general terms that we believe are central to an understanding of the issues we address. More specialized terms are not included in this Glossary. These terms are defined in the body of the book.

Acknowledgments

Acknowledgments for Joel Weinberger: The list of people I would like to thank is a long one and I'm sure I missed someone (or two). Many people helped to make this book possible. Of course, my coauthor, Valentina Stoycheva, was indispensable. Beyond the book, the collaboration was rewarding and worth it in its own right. I also want to thank my family. My sons, Liam and Aiden, bring joy into my life as they grow into wonderful young men. They had to put up with "not now" when their father was working at home and could not interact with them. They did so with very little complaint. Thanks guys. I love you. May your baseball careers blossom. My wife, Debbie Heiser, provided unending support and encouragement and critically read parts of the manuscript. I could not have done this without you. I love you more than I can say. My mentors Lloyd Silverman and David McClelland believed in me when few others did. They taught me the importance and value of unconscious processes and I am forever grateful to them. I wish they were here so I could tell them personally. Larry Hjelle encouraged me when I was a struggling and insecure master's student. Nathan Brody took on my dissertation when no one at my graduate school would. Thanks for your belief in me. I hope you see this. Sorry I lost touch. Robert Prince encouraged me to write this book when I was ambivalent. I might not have taken it on were it not for his encouragement. Thank you. I hope your faith was not misplaced. Jim Nageotte, Senior Editor at The Guilford Press, tolerated my delays and made many valuable suggestions. I hope you think it was worth it. Series Editor Elliot Jurist read the many iterations of the chapters and offered invaluable advice and support. Thanks for your patience and sage advice. All of these people deserve credit for any contributions this book may make. I take responsibility for any weaknesses it has.

Acknowledgments for Valentina Stoycheva: There are so many people to thank for supporting, encouraging, and guiding me throughout the years that this page is simply not enough to contain their names, or my gratitude. However, I would like to thank Joel Weinberger for being an instrumental force in the development of my professional and personal identity. His mentorship throughout the last 13 years transcends being a brilliant teacher to becoming a stable force of support and knowledge way beyond the academic. I would also like to thank Series Editor Elliot Jurist for recognizing a book waiting to be written in an article we published some 6 years ago, as well as Senior Editor Jim Nageotte for patiently reading through previous versions of the manuscript. This book would simply not have been published without your feedback and support along the way.

I would also like to dedicate this book to a few people who, at various stages in my life, have been the single most powerful force of positive change:

> To my parents, who taught me that big dreams are only as important as the amount of hard work and perseverance one is willing to put into achieving them.
>
> To my brother—my first and forever role model. To him, I owe my curiosity and competitiveness. I hope one day I learn his humility too.
>
> To the best friend anyone could ever hope for, Ally Merchant, for teaching me object permanence in a foreign land.
>
> To Josh, for enduring a thousand and one "Still working on the book" statements and finding a supportive response to each one of them. Your unconditional love is the scaffolding around which I grow and which helps me strive to be a better person every day.
>
> And last but not least, to all my patients, past and present, for the trust you give me. It is the most precious gift.

Contents

THE UNCONSCIOUS

CHAPTER 1

Introduction

The major goal of this book is to communicate what is known about unconscious processes and to demonstrate how central they are to our functioning. We believe this knowledge will have an impact on the work of academic researchers, psychotherapy theorists, and clinical practitioners alike. (We also hope the educated and interested layperson can take something of value from this book.)

The first issue that must be addressed in any book purporting to tackle this area is that no unifying paradigm concerning unconscious processes currently exists. Instead, there exists a welter of work in different areas, often without communication between them. Moreover, each area of research and theory is rife with disagreements. Because of the disjointed and controversial nature of the field, several disparate and unconnected research literatures are examined. We review the differences and commonalities between these seemingly unrelated areas of research and try to make sense of them. We also consider what we believe are the most promising theoretical explanations of unconscious processes, which we identify as emerging from computational neuroscience. We discuss the potential as well as the limitations of these approaches. As with the research we review, we try to find unifying themes in these computational models and attempt their overall integration. And then we try to place the principles we have identified as common to unconscious processes into the unified theoretical account we have suggested.

Another goal of this book is to apply these insights to the theory and practice of psychotherapy. We (the authors) are psychotherapists as well as researchers ourselves. We argue that it is past time to incorporate what we know about unconscious processes into the theory and practice of psychotherapy. Most current psychotherapy models are based on systems of thought and/or research that are decades old. We believe that current work on unconscious processes has to be seriously considered by researchers, theorists, and practitioners in the psychotherapy arena. Some of what this work suggests is in line with mainstream views of psychotherapy, and some is at odds with them. These need to be examined empirically in a psychotherapy context. Empirical research and clinical practice need to adjudicate between these views when they differ and offer support when they agree. And then whatever proves out should be incorporated into constructing new clinical models, which, in turn, should be tested empirically and clinically. We sketch what the first such model might look like.

HISTORY

Before we review current research and theory, we embark on a brief historical journey to provide context and explain how we arrived at our current formulations. This will also help to make sense of some of the controversies that have plagued and continue to plague the study of unconscious processes. We will show that for most of the history of Western thinking, unconscious processes were ignored, minimized, or flat-out denied.

PSYCHOANALYSIS

No review of unconscious processes can ignore the contributions of psychoanalysis. (But see Kihlstrom, 1999, a major influence on the acceptance of unconscious processes, who argues that this contribution was negative.) In contrast to the general neglect of unconscious processes elsewhere, psychoanalytic theory has always placed them front and center. We therefore examine the place of unconscious processes in several psychoanalytic models, including early and later Freud, object relations, self-psychology, the intersubjective approach, and modern relational outlooks.

Although their views of the unconscious, its contents, and how its operations are relevant to clinical work differ in some important ways, the centrality of unconscious processes has always been affirmed by Freudian and post-Freudian psychoanalysts. All agree that unconscious processes are affectively charged, poorly integrated, and more influenced by early than by later experiences. Thus, for all psychoanalytic models, many, if not all, of the roots of our behaviors are unknown to us, affectively based, and poorly integrated into our personality. A major task of psychotherapy, therefore, is to integrate these processes into our personal narrative. Our well-being depends on the success of this integration. Psychoanalytic schools were among the first to insist that unconscious processes can be influenced and integrated through treatment and proposed concrete ways of doing so.

What psychoanalytic thinkers did not generally do was offer empirical data in support of their conceptions. Instead, they preferred to illustrate them with clinical case studies and offered theoretical constructions to make sense of their observations. Thus, psychoanalysis was relatively unaffected by developments in academic research. In turn, researchers were relatively unaffected by the work of psychoanalysts. There were a couple of exceptions to this rule, the most influential of which was a decade-long foray into the study of psychoanalytically inspired unconscious processes, termed the "New Look." There are also two continuing programs of research that study unconscious motivation and subliminal psychodynamic activation. But for the most part, these remain exceptions.

THE NORMATIVE UNCONSCIOUS

With this history and psychoanalysis as context, the next several chapters, constituting the main body of this book, are devoted to continuing areas of research that are centrally concerned with unconscious processes. These include heuristics, implicit memory, implicit learning, implicit motivation, automaticity, affective salience, attribution theory, and embodied cognition. We address the main points of consensus and conflict in each of these literatures and try to determine what (if any) general principles they offer concerning unconscious processes. We also discuss the implications of each of the above areas of research, as well as the general contributions that they offer concerning psychotherapy. Although we firmly believe that much of this work has important psychotherapeutic implications, it is largely unknown to psychotherapists. This is somewhat due to a lack of interest in this work on the part of many clinicians but is also attributable to the fact that most researchers in these areas have not considered the clinical implications of their work. We try to bridge this gap.

We begin with the work on heuristics that made Kahneman and Tversky (deservedly) famous. A heuristic is an unconscious cognitive strategy for making a judgment or solving a problem that does not involve logic or effort. Although these heuristics often work, Kahneman and Tversky showed that the nature of their operation is such that they can lead to predictable erroneous conclusions in certain situations. We tend to be unaware that we have made these mistakes unless they are explicitly pointed out to us (and sometimes not even then). Finally, unlike the dynamic unconscious of psychoanalysis, this kind of unconscious processing is not attributable to conflict, defense, relational needs, or psychopathology. That is, it is not motivated. Rather, these heuristics are normative and simply represent the structure of our cognitive architecture. So, *much of our thinking is normatively arational, unconscious, and can be flawed without our realizing it.*

We then review implicit memory. Implicit memory is inferred from behavior rather than assessed through conscious recollection or recognition. It is said to be present when a person performs an action, voices an attitude, or in some other way appears to have been influenced by a prior event even though she denies any memory of that event. That is, there is a measurable effect of past experiences that the person does not consciously recall.

We next discuss implicit learning, which refers to learning that takes place outside of awareness, such that the person does not realize what he has learned. The trajectory of the study of implicit learning paralleled that of implicit memory, which is not surprising, given that implicit learning is just the other side of the coin of implicit memory. Since one cannot learn what one does not remember and one cannot remember what one has not learned, we are talking of similar if not identical processes. The two areas are separated in the literature because they emerged from different research traditions. The study of implicit memory developed largely through examination of brain-damaged individuals. Only later did it transition to examining people without such damage. Research into implicit learning, in contrast, focused on unimpaired children and adults early on. Some studies, even earlier in the history of psychology, focused on animals (Tolman, 1949).

Like implicit memory, implicit learning is ubiquitous and unconscious. It turns out that we humans are exceptionally well equipped to recognize and pick up patterns in our environment. We learn all sorts of things without realizing what we have learned, or even that we have learned anything at all.

The next unconscious process we review, automaticity, has assumed huge importance in the field, especially in social psychology, probably because of John Bargh's (e.g., Bargh & Ferguson, 2000) work in this area. Automaticity was important to the history of unconscious processes, beginning with James's (1890/1950) understanding of habit and culminating in Shiffrin and Schneider's work on the development of automaticity in a simple learning task. Until Bargh's innovative work in the area changed it, our understanding of automaticity was that it was an either-or phenomenon. Either a process was automatic, in which case it was characterized by certain properties, or it was controlled, and therefore characterized by the obverse of these properties. In contrast to this view, Bargh argued that the relevant properties of automatic and controlled functioning could be separated and could manifest in any combination. Moreover, although conscious practice or repetition could result in automatic behavior, this was not necessary to the development of automaticity; it could develop completely outside of awareness (i.e., unconsciously).

Attribution, the next area of interest, refers to the tendency, nay compulsion, people feel to explain their experiences, which includes events taking place in the world, the actions of others, and their own behaviors. Although this was initially considered a conscious process, we now know that it occurs outside of awareness and has some biases built into it (as do heuristics).

Affective primacy is next. The issues addressed here include: Are emotion and cognition served by two separate systems? Is one of these types of processing primary? And, which of the two is faster? Zajonc's (1980, 1984, 2000; Murphy & Zajonc, 1993) response to the above questions was that there are separate cognitive and affective systems in the brain/mind, and that affect was both primary and faster. That is, affectively charged information is processed separately from, as well as more readily and more quickly than is cognitive information. Lazarus (1984) had exactly the opposite point of view and argued for cognitive primacy. After a review of more recent literature on the subject, we conclude that, as with automatic and controlled processing, these are distinct questions that ought to be considered separately rather than together. And the answer to each depends upon specific factors in the situation being studied.

Embodied cognition refers to the idea that our thought parallels and is based on the physical body, largely sensory and motor functioning. We can see this operating in metaphors, which invariably refer to such parallels. We review a large body of research that shows how metaphors are literally true. For example, we like someone (i.e., perceive them as a warmer person) more when we experience physical warmth and we see the physical environment as warmer when we like someone. And, of course, all of this occurs outside of awareness.

COMPUTATIONAL NEUROSCIENCE MODELS OF THE BRAIN/MIND

Lastly, we review modern computational neuroscience models of the brain/mind. The models we discuss are massive modularity, connectionism (as instantiated by <u>parallel distributed processing</u> [PDP]), and <u>neural reuse</u>. Each has submodels within it. We discuss each model in a bit of detail and then compare them to one another. Although there are important differences between them, most critically in terms of the a priori organization of the brain/mind each proposes, they all have certain characteristics in common as well. All posit parallel processing, and all take unconscious processes as a given. In fact, such processes are held to be central to mental/brain functioning. And all have important implications for psychotherapy. These models can be used to tie together many of the empirical findings and clinical implications we have discussed and that have thus far remained unconnected in the literature. We then attempt to integrate the models and hypothesize an overarching model to account for most of the findings and therapeutic implications we discussed.

WHAT DO WE KNOW AND WHAT DOES IT MEAN?

We close the book by summarizing what we believe we know about unconscious processes and how that knowledge can relate to a general theory of the brain/mind. We also show how the data and models we have reviewed can be applied to the theory and practice of psychotherapy. Finally, we place what we have gleaned about psychotherapy into the overall computational neuroscience model we have sketched. This chapter is necessarily speculative given the paucity of our current knowledge.

PART I

EARLY HISTORY
OF THE UNCONSCIOUS

To explore the unconscious, to work in the subterranean
of the mind with especially adequate methods, this will be
the main task of psychology in the opening century. I do
not doubt that fine discoveries will follow, as important
perhaps as have been in the preceding centuries those of
physical and natural sciences.
—BERGSON (1901, quoted in Ellenberger, 1970, p. 321)

Was Henri Bergson right? Did we develop sophisticated methods
of exploring the "subterranean of the mind" in the 20th century? In
a word, no. Not only did advances in understanding unconscious processing not match the revolutionary growth of the physical and natural
sciences of Bergson's time, the 20th century did not offer a unified (let
alone accepted) view of unconscious events. In fact, the importance (e.g.,
Greenwald, 1992) and even the existence (e.g., Brody, 1972; Goldiamond, 1958; Hollender, 1986) of unconscious processes continued to be
questioned well into the 20th century.[1]

But Bergson was not wrong, it's just that his timing was off by
about a century. Psychologists, neuroscientists, and cognitive scientists
have begun to investigate unconscious processes in a somewhat systematic manner in this, the 21st, not the 20th century. At first blush, this
delay seems strange. The lay public has accepted and been interested
in the notion of unconscious events for generations. Why has academic

psychology only recently discovered them? Why has the discipline ostensibly devoted to studying human functioning ignored this crucial aspect of it for so long? Why did it, in fact, shun it? The answers to these questions provide the context for the research and theoretical endeavors reviewed in this book. They also highlight the assumptions that have not been acknowledged and continue to drive work in the field, even by many who accept the reality of unconscious processes. They will also help to explain why, despite the current respectability of studying unconscious processes, there remains powerful resistance to it.

The contemporary state of affairs in studying unconscious processes becomes more easily comprehensible when we examine the development of philosophical precursors as well as prescientific work in the area. When these are clarified, the welter of contradictory and apparently counterintuitive positions concerning the unconscious makes sense. This overview does not pretend to be comprehensive. Moreover, the positions reviewed are limited to those aspects bearing on notions of unconscious processing. In this sense, they will be somewhat skewed; those aspects regarding unconscious processes will be emphasized to the relative neglect of the rest of the systems.

We will show that the very existence of unconscious processes was largely denied in mainstream Western thinking for centuries, beginning with Descartes, and explain why (cf. Whyte, 1960). Romantic philosophy and the treatment of those suffering from emotional disorders (dynamic psychiatry; Ellenberger, 1970) provided counterweights to this rejection, but these represented a secondary movement in Western thought. Psychoanalysis was the primary exception to this zeitgeist. We therefore review its tenets on unconscious processes in some detail—bearing in mind that its lack of empirical emphasis and separation from the academy weakened its influence.

Once this philosophical, medical, and psychoanalytical journey is completed, we review some early 20th-century psychology (influenced by these philosophical and "dynamic psychiatry" positions), as it bore on the study of unconscious processes. We show that investigating unconscious events was actually prohibited by the academic pioneers in the field but taken up by the medical profession. We then argue that even these early academically oriented schools of psychology had to find a place for unconscious processes. That is, once they began to actually investigate human functioning, it proved to be impossible to construct a model of psychological functioning that did not include unconscious processes. Often these were unacknowledged or given different, more palatable names. This includes systems that claimed to explicitly abjure such processes. It even includes a system that excluded (rejected) the whole concept of mind (i.e., behaviorism). The structure and function of these constructs vary, often radically, from system to system but they are invariably present. We try to demonstrate that no effort to understand human functioning can succeed without including some conception of unconscious processing.

NOTE

1. Some still question it (e.g., Lahteenmaki, Hyona, Koivisto, & Nummenmaa, 2015).

CHAPTER 2

Philosophical Precursors

RENÉ DESCARTES AND THE CARTESIAN MIND

Problems with unconscious processes began with Descartes (1596–1650), who sought to found a wholly new system of philosophy that reconciled Christianity with the newly developing and productive sciences (Whyte, 1960). In his *Discourse on Method* (1637/2017) and his *Meditations* (1642/2013), Descartes began by doubting everything that he could. (This state of being has been termed "Cartesian doubt"; Broughton, 2002.) That which he could not doubt must perforce be true, and what was true could then serve as the basis of his own and every other ensuing system of philosophy. Using this rationalist technique, he found that he could doubt his senses, arithmetic, geometry, and even his own body. But he could not doubt that he thought, that he was aware. That is, in order to doubt, there has to be a self-aware doubter. The person consciously thinking and doubting had to exist. This led to the famous dictum "cogito ergo sum" (I think, therefore I am), which could just as readily have been stated as "I am aware, therefore I am," and constituted the first principle of Cartesian philosophy.[1]

Descartes went on to conclude that the soul (or mind), whose essence is self-aware thinking, is wholly distinct from the material body. The material world, on the other hand, takes up space and has parts that can be differentiated through their movement (extension in motion). Mathematical calculation can determine all that will happen in this physical world. Having brilliantly reconciled the Catholic Church and science by assigning the soul to the former and the material world to the latter, Descartes left his successors with the thorny issue that has come to be termed the "mind–body problem" (see Young, 1990). This creation of two separate realms of mind and body constitutes the beginning of the problem of unconscious events. The problem is this: There are only two substances, mind and body. The defining characteristic of the mind, according to Cartesian thought, is awareness; anything not of the mind has to be of the body, whose essence is extension in motion. So anything a person is not aware of cannot be of the mind; it must be physical. This meant that unconscious mental processes were ruled out of court. They constituted a threat to Cartesian dualism. The Cartesian system would have to be discarded if something could not be characterized by either awareness or extension. And this is precisely the case for unconscious processes. After all, one could hardly say, "I think, although I am unaware of doing so, therefore I am."

Jackson (1958) made exactly the same above anti-unconscious argument. He averred that if consciousness is lost, so is mind, so that unconscious states of mind involve a contradiction in terms. Klein (1977) later endorsed a similar view. Still later, the argument became that unconscious events do exist but are primitive and really do not reflect thought; they are automatisms and reflect very rudimentary and inflexible information processing. That is, they are machine-like (see, e.g., Greenwald, 1992).

ROUSSEAU AND ROMANTICISM

Over a century later, an influential challenge to the primacy of the conscious intellect rose to prominence. Rousseau (1712–1788) is generally credited with launching this "Romantic" movement through the publication of his novel *La Nouvelle Héloise* (1761), although Spinoza's (1632–1677) and Boehme's (1575–1642) identification of God and nature (pantheism), as well as Pascal's (1623–1662) emphasis on unconscious emotional wisdom, were also counterpoints to Cartesian dualism and influenced Romantic thought. Romantic-like notions have remained influential ever since, with their influence waxing and waning in counterpoint with empirical, rational, and analytic points of view. As Rousseau and the Romantics saw it, people's inner, natural selves were their emotional natures. If left to their own devices, people would rely on this inner nature, which would result in moral and productive behavior. It is society that corrupts humankind and leads to all evil.[2]

KANT, GERMAN IDEALISM, AND BEYOND

The next most influential philosopher after Descartes was Immanuel Kant (1724–1804). Like Descartes, he altered the nature of philosophical debate and influenced philosophical discourse from his time onward. Kant argued that perceptions are not accurate copies of reality.[3] Instead, what appears in perception are "phenomena," which are composed of two parts: that due to the object or thing-in-itself (Kant calls this the "sensation") and that due to inborn (a priori) systems that cause the sensation to be ordered according to space, time, and several other categories. Kant's views led to two movements. The first accepted Kant's conclusions that ultimate reality was unknowable and that only experience could be examined; it therefore advocated a radical empiricism. This point of view developed into positivism as advocated by Comte (1798–1857) and, later, after an intermediate stage embodied in the phenomenalist work of Mach (1838–1916), into the logical positivism of the Vienna circle. It led to abjuring of the study of unconscious (and later even conscious) phenomena. The other movement would not accept the idea that the thing-in-itself could not be known and set about trying to know it. This led to German idealism as exemplified in the work of Fichte (1762–1814), Schelling (1775–1854), and Hegel (1775–1831), as well as to the philosophy of nature of Schopenhauer (1788–1860) and von Hartmann (1842–1906). We will also include here the work of Nietzsche (1844–1900), even though he despised Kant (he despised a lot of people), because he considered himself (with some justification; see Janaway, 2002) Schopenhauer's successor.

German idealists believed that all of reality could be reduced to the mind and its ideas. Reality was seen as unitary and intelligible through reason (Widgery, 1950), and people's unconscious minds (Fichte, 1802/1982, was the first philosopher to conceive of dynamic unconscious processes underlying conscious processes) were seen to be part of a universal mind to which said people had no conscious access (see Neuhouser, 1990). Like the idealists, the philosophers of nature (e.g., Schopenhauer and von Hartmann) also could not accept Kant's conclusion that ultimate reality is unknowable. Unlike the idealists, however, they did accept the limits he set on reason. Schopenhauer devalued reason, much like the Romantics, and posited the existence of a blind driving force ("will") that controls the behavior of each person as well as all of the rest of nature. This will is largely unavailable to awareness (its immediate ends may be perceived, but its ultimate goal is unknowable) and it is certainly not amenable to reason. In fact, it bends reason to serve its ends so that the veracity of reason is not to be trusted. Regardless of why a person thinks he is doing something, behind it lies the will, which has its own purposes (usually procreation).

Schopenhauer's work, combined with Romanticism, and especially Carus (1770–1807) and Hegel, significantly influenced von Hartmann, who further developed the ideas of a driving force outside of awareness. His book *Philosophy of the Unconscious* (1884) was very popular in late-19th-century Europe. Like Schopenhauer, he described a purposive but blind force underlying the universe, which he called the "unconscious," and posited three levels of it: the absolute unconscious, the physiological unconscious, and the psychological unconscious. The latter is the source of the individual's mental unconscious life and is the aspect of this system most relevant to the aims of this book. All states of consciousness, all awareness, were held to depend on this level of the unconscious. Thus, von Hartmann saw consciousness, that is, perceptions, emotions, and social relationships, as secondary to or dependent upon unconscious processes.

Nietzsche, while denying being influenced by the above philosophers, also offered a complex and sophisticated vision of unconscious functioning. He agreed with Schopenhauer that the will underlay everything, but he identified it with power rather than with procreation. He also, similarly to von Hartmann, argued that the unconscious part of the mind is far more important and central to an individual's life than is consciousness. For Nietzsche, the mind is a system of drives and emotions made up of unconscious representations and states of the will. These drives can and do come into conflict with one another, but they can also cooperate and even fuse. So the mind is a seething cauldron of contradictory and complementary urges, an arena of confused thoughts, emotions, and instincts. It is the realm of wild, brutal instincts derived from the early stages of individual and species development.

The urges in Nietzsche's unconscious are charged with psychic energy seeking discharge. Nietzsche describes the many, often circuitous, routes the drives can take to achieve this discharge, as well as efforts to prevent discharge from taking place. These include blocking the drive (inhibition), turning the impulse against the self, displacing it onto a secondary object, sublimating it into acceptable channels, and even the possibility (remote and only for a select few) of putting it under conscious and voluntary control. The activity of the unconscious can be seen most clearly in the disorder and incoherence of dreams, as well as in passionate actions and mental illness. Nietzsche coined the term "the it" (*das es*) to signify this central aspect of mental functioning. Freud (1933) took over the term (at the suggestion of Groddeck, 1923) to denote his conception of an impersonal irrational unconscious. (It is now called the id, possibly because of a mistranslation; see Bettelheim, 1983).

Although Nietzsche would disagree, his notions are closely related to those of the Romantics. His aversion to Romantic ethics differentiates him from them, but his conception of the unconscious binds him to them. Like the Romantics, Nietzsche sees unconscious processing as primary and rationality as untrustworthy. He sees value in unbridled emotionality. And finally, he avers that conscious and unconscious processes follow qualitatively different rules.

POSITIVISM AND LOGICAL POSITIVISM

Unlike the German idealists and the philosophers of nature, the positivists accepted Kant's dictum that the thing-in-itself was unknowable. They argued that inquiry should be restricted to questions amenable to fairly definite answers, thus limiting themselves to what Kant had termed the "world of phenomena"—that which is directly experienced. They became radical empiricists and refused to speculate upon ultimate reality or causes. Comte (1830/1988), the founder of positivism, even suggested elimination of the term "cause." This is reinforced by Kant's view (based on Hume [1711–1776]) that causality has no actual existence but is a construction of the mind, an a priori category. Comte argued that merely knowing the regular sequences followed by phenomena was sufficient to allow for prediction and control, which he saw as the sole goals of science (see Frankel, 1950). This meant restricting the quest for knowledge to immediate experiences, which were termed "facts." Moreover, these facts were not to be interpreted. In their zeal to clear science of any hint of theology or metaphysics, the positivists expelled the soul from the study of psychology and vitalism from the study of biology. This paralleled the earlier elimination of animism from physics by Galileo and Newton. Physical-chemical forces were sufficient to explain organic functioning, just as they were sufficient to account for inorganic systems. Mental processes were held to be reducible to brain structures or even physical and chemical processes (see Ellenberger, 1970).

Positivism prospered and came to dominate 19th-century thought. This was aided and abetted by the spectacular and continuous advances made by science during that time period. One unfortunate outcome of this kind of thinking was the development of a belief system—termed "scientism"—positing that knowledge of the world could *only* be acquired through science. Scientism became somewhat of a quasi-religion throughout the later decades of the 19th century and dominated Western thought by 1880 (see Ellenberger, 1970). This is exceedingly important because the first efforts to found psychology as a science took place at around that time. According to most official versions of the history of psychology, the first psychological laboratory was founded by Wilhelm Wundt (1832–1920) in 1879 (although it is probably more accurate to say that William James [1842–1910] began lab work in psychology a few years earlier, in 1875; see Heidbreder, 1933). Historical priority aside, the important point is that psychology's attempt to become an academic scientific discipline began during positivism's heyday. Its pioneers therefore had a positivistic and scientistic view of their task (which continued long after 1880). As we shall see, this strongly affected their dealings (actually, the lack thereof) with unconsciousness.

Logical positivists also had a strong negative effect on efforts to uncover unconscious processes. This is a more recent philosophical position than is positivism (early 20th century) and as such served to reinforce already existing tendencies. Like positivism more generally, logical positivism was more a movement than a school. Logical positivism developed in two major locations: the Cambridge school of analysis in England (during the 1930s) and the so-called Vienna circle (roughly 1922–1938). The Vienna circle had particularly extreme views, holding that the meaningful core of all philosophical questions could be completely answered through the operational analysis of science. By that, they meant (see Bridgman, 1938) translating all terms into something measurable so that any term is defined by how it is measured (e.g., someone's intelligence is the score they achieve on an IQ test). So they denied the status of empirical fact to phenomenally given data (Bergmann, 1950/1978). They maintained that since no two observers could agree on what was occurring in the mind, there could be no truth of agreement on such matters. This meant that mental events are unobservable and scientifically untenable. Examination of such events should therefore be abandoned.

The same criticisms, leveled earlier against positivism (see Singer, 1959), are equally (if not more) valid for logical positivism: it was scientistic and restrictive. Not only did logical positivism eliminate the unconscious, as did positivism, it also eliminated consciousness. It argued that no mental operations should or could be studied scientifically. As we shall see, the founders of psychology embraced positivism and so refused to allow unconsciousness into the scientific (scientistic) pantheon. Behaviorists and logical positivists conducted a mutual love affair and eliminated all mental phenomena from scientific consideration. This further hampered efforts to understand unconscious processes. Small wonder, then, that the study of unconscious processes (and even conscious processes during the dominance of behaviorism) began so late in psychology.

JOHANN HERBART

Herbart (1786–1841; 1824, 1834/1850), unlike his contemporaries the positivists, accorded a central place to unconsciousness in human functioning. Although Herbart was Kant's successor at Konigsberg University in Germany, he does not seem to have been directly influenced by Kant. His system is not at all concerned with the thing-in-itself or with reason. Instead, Herbart was strongly influenced by both Leibniz (1646–1716) and the British associationists, but it is the Leibnizian influence that is more relevant to his notions of the unconscious.

Leibniz's (1704/1896, 1714/1989) ideas are somewhat complex, but, in essence, he tried to solve the Cartesian mind–body problem by positing only one substance, the mind. In his view, all material objects could be reduced to mind or ideas. So Leibniz was (as was Berkeley [1685–1753] later) an idealist. (The interested reader can examine Savile, 2000, who both translates Liebniz and offers a scholarly review of his work.) What is extremely relevant to Herbart's system is Leibniz's assertion that the visible, physical universe can be reduced to an infinite number of invisible elements that he termed "monads," and conscious perception can be reduced to an infinite number of unconscious elements he termed *"petites perceps."* The person is not aware of individual petite perceps; they must summate to produce conscious perception. Leibniz termed this summation to awareness "apperception." There are always more petite perceps below the threshold than there are apperceived conscious percepts. Consciousness therefore represents a very small percentage of the sensory stimuli impinging upon the sense organs at any time.

Instead of neutral percepts, however, Herbart focused on interacting and conflictual ideas. According to Herbart, all mental phenomena, of whatever complexity, are attributable to the actions and interactions of simple ideas. Each idea possesses a certain degree of force, which it uses in an effort to achieve consciousness. It then tries to remain conscious and to drive ideas with which it is incompatible off of the conscious stage. Some ideas are stronger than others and force incompatible weaker ones out of consciousness. If the weaker idea is compatible with the stronger one, however, it can be assimilated to it. Herbart employs the Leibnizian term apperception to describe this assimilatory process. A group of assimilated ideas is termed an "apperceptive mass."

Uncongenial weaker ideas that are forced out of consciousness do not cease to exist nor do they become inert. They are merely thrust below the conscious threshold where they continually try to force their way back into consciousness. There is therefore constant competition at the threshold, as those ideas holding the field seek to keep antithetical ideas from supplanting them, while ideas below the threshold seek to drive their way past the threshold and into consciousness. Like conscious ideas, ideas below the threshold can be assimilated to one another (apperceived). They then form an unconscious apperceptive mass. If this mass becomes strong enough, it can force its way into consciousness and replace the previously conscious set of ideas. The originally conscious apperceptive mass is then forced below the threshold and into unconsciousness, where it strives to regain its conscious status.

As new ideas and percepts enter the mind, they join forces with one or another already existing apperceptive mass or form a wholly new such mass. They then enter the struggle to achieve consciousness. Sometimes there is no clear victor, and consciousness may reflect a blend of incompatible sets of ideas. Alternatively, a set of ideas may not be able to completely force its way into consciousness but is strong enough to indirectly affect it. This competition is unending and constitutes the dynamics of the mind as conceptualized by Herbart—a mind that operates through the dual mechanisms of inhibition and association. Mental life largely consists of a struggle between associated sets of ideas, with each set trying to attain an exclusive hold on consciousness. This struggle never ends; victorious and vanquished ideas alternate, fuse, compromise, and change their character with the entry of new information. This somehow does not usually lead to paralysis or chaos but to relatively adaptive functioning. That is, the struggle of ideas reflects the person's progressive adaptation to personal and social situations.

Herbart's system cannot be said to belong to either positivism or Romanticism. It partakes of both and contains aspects antithetical to each. Its characteristics are probably best understood as a throwback to associationist doctrines and Leibnizian dynamics. Whatever its classification, it was popular in its time and had enormous influence on beginning conceptions of the unconscious. It is fair to say that its influence on the study of the unconscious was commensurate with that of positivism. The latter had an inhibitory effect, however, whereas Herbart's work led to an acceptance of and actual efforts to examine unconscious processes. And, like positivism, it was in the air in late-19th-century Europe and was known to Janet (1823–1899) and Freud, whom it certainly influenced.

FECHNER AND THE BEGINNING OF EXPERIMENTAL PSYCHOLOGY

The philosophical doctrines described thus far were not based on any systematically collected data. But one philosopher, Fechner (1811–1887), developed an empirical methodology and collected large amounts of data. Fechner is now best known as a progenitor of experimental psychology and the inventor of psychophysical methodology. Interestingly, he did so as a Romantic, not as a positivist. Fechner sought a scientific, mathematically calculable way of assessing the relationship between the physical and the spiritual (psychological) worlds (Ellenberger, 1970). The outline of such a law occurred to him in 1850 when he noted that there might be an observable and measurable relationship between a physical stimulus and the sensation it elicited. Fechner's insight was that sensation may increase arithmetically as stimulus value increases geometrically. As he began to test this hypothesis, he came across the work of Weber (1795–1878), who had reported that the perception of a difference in the weight or length of two objects did not depend upon their absolute weight or length difference. Rather, it depended on the ratio of the two measurements (Heidbredder, 1933).[4] Fechner attached enormous philosophical significance to Weber's findings and thus dubbed them Weber's Law. He thought he had discovered the *via regia* for connecting the physical and the psychical worlds, spending the rest of his life working out methods for testing this relationship (his work was then continued by Wundt [1832–1920], and many of his methods are still in use). He termed his endeavor psychophysics because he believed that he was connecting the physical and psychological worlds (Ellenberger, 1970).

Fechner's Romantic notions also led to meaningful contributions to understanding unconscious processes (see Heidbredder, 1933), which significantly impacted Freud's thinking and theorizing (Ellenberger, 1970; Gay, 1988). Fechner was the first to argue that behavior was motivated by seeking pleasure and avoiding unpleasure (Fechner, 1846), a notion later adopted by Freud as his famous pleasure principle. Fechner (1873) later argued that organisms seek stability (i.e., quiescence), which is a drive-reduction view of motivation and which may have influenced Freud's positing of a death instinct. The work of those who followed him (e.g., Wundt) ensured that Fechner's thinking about unconscious processes disappeared from academic psychology. But his influence did live on in the work of Freud who took the notions of pleasure–unpleasure, the seeking of stability, and a topographical conception of the mind from Fechner (Ellenberger, 1970; Gay, 1988).

Freud cannot be identified with any of the philosophical positions we have described so far; nor can he be considered an early academic psychologist. He is more accurately described as the most eminent and influential product of what Ellenberger (1970) termed "dynamic psychiatry." So Fechner's influence on notions of the unconscious was on dynamic psychiatry rather than on academic psychology. It is to dynamic psychiatry and its precursors that we now turn in order to trace some other important influences on conceptions of unconscious processing.

NOTES

1. Augustine (2009, Book 11, p. 26) made the same observation a millennium (early fifth century) earlier. But Augustine did not recognize its far-reaching implications. Nor did he place it at the center of his thinking as Descartes did.

2. Carl Rogers (1961) offered a 20th-century version of the inherent goodness of people corrupted by family and society.

3. Augustine (2009, Book 12, p. 15) said this first as well.

4. Later Stevens (1957) substituted a power law for the ratio relationship posited by Weber.

CHAPTER 3

Dynamic Psychiatry
and Early Academic Psychology

Not all early thinking about unconscious processes was philosophically based. There were also early attempts to examine and work directly with unconscious phenomena. Such efforts were largely the work of physicians trying to understand and treat emotionally troubled individuals. Their work resulted in what Ellenberger (1970) termed "dynamic psychiatry." Unlike the philosophically inspired conceptions reviewed thus far, empirical work (in the sense that the conceptions were based on experience) was the rule rather than the exception in dynamic psychiatry. This movement culminated in the clinical and theoretical work of Bernheim (1840–1919), Charcot (1825–1893), Janet (1859–1947), and, most notably, Freud (1856–1939). However, the effects of this work on academic psychology were (and remain) negligible.

THE BEGINNINGS OF DYNAMIC PSYCHIATRY

Dynamic psychiatry began with a clash between supernatural Baroque and rational Enlightenment (also known as "the Age of Reason"; roughly the 18th century) views of mental illness (Ellenberger, 1970). In the Baroque corner stood Johann Joseph Gassner (1727–1789), a priest who treated emotional problems through exorcism. In the Enlightenment corner stood Franz Anton Mesmer (1734–1815), a physician and would-be scientist who saw himself as a disciple of Newton. Mesmer believed that planetary bodies, not demons residing in the body, affected health. The clash took place in 1775 at a meeting of the Bavarian Royal Commission, where Mesmer but not Gassner was called on to testify. Mesmer claimed that both his and Gassner's cures (unbeknownst to Gassner) were due to natural forces. The Enlightenment view won out. Mesmer's views were supported by the commission, and Gassner was ordered to cease his exorcisms.

Mesmer proposed that an invisible fluid, which he termed "animal gravitation," was responsible for gravity and also affected people's bloodstreams and nervous systems. Later, he decided that this fluid was not limited to gravitation but accounted for magnetism, electricity, heat, and light as well. He then changed its name to "animal magnetism," by which it came to be popularly known (see Buranelli, 1975; Kelly, 1955/1991). Mesmer came to believe that bodily conditions could be affected by animal magnetism and that this relationship in turn could result in a new sort of curing. According to him, although everyone possesses animal magnetism, some have more of it than others, and the sick have less than the healthy. Recovery is achieved through the restoration of the proper equilibrium, quality, and strength of animal magnetism. The magnetizer is able to accomplish this feat by establishing a "rapport" and provoking what Mesmer termed "crises" in the sufferer, that is, a controlled production of the disease by the magnetizer. Through this rapport, the magnetizer could transmit his own stronger and qualitatively better fluid to the patient. Health was restored when the fluid in the patient became sufficiently strong and well distributed.

Mesmer's theory had little to say directly about unconscious processes. He saw his technique as involving physical rather than psychological principles. His influence on theorizing about the unconscious lay in the work of his successors and in the co-opting of some of his principles by the Romantics. Puységur (1751–1825), for instance, an early follower of Mesmer, dispensed with Mesmer's notion of a magnetic fluid and physical conductivity. He realized that psychological forces were at work and that the rapport between patient and magnetizer was a psychological phenomenon. He saw this rapport as an unconscious relationship. Puységur also observed that rather than experiencing the dramatic crises reported by Mesmer, his own patients seemed to fall into a kind of sleep (artificial somnambulism) in which they showed a remarkable ability to respond to the magnetizer in a lucid manner. He saw this as evidence for a second, powerful mind, normally hidden from awareness, which had wisdom and knowledge not available to normal consciousness. The idea of two minds and of special powers in the hidden, second one led to a model of the mind termed "dipsychism" (see below).

Animal magnetism and artificial somnambulism soon became connected with Romantic notions of a mystical connection between a hidden emotional mind and nature. As Romanticism and the philosophy of nature gave way to positivism, artificial somnambulism also lost influence. It became so discredited that from 1860 to 1880, it could be ruinous for a scientist or physician to admit to be doing any work in the area. Despite the career threat that such work entailed, a few brave souls continued to study animal magnetism and eventually brought it respectability. Bertrand (1823) and Noizet (1854), for instance, both emphasized the unconscious nature of the phenomena they studied. In 1843, the respected English physician Braid (1843/1976) published a work on animal magnetism. He changed its name to "hypnotism" to accord with its identification with somnambulism (*hypnos* means sleep in Greek). The name stuck but his work did not, because he tried to integrate hypnosis with phrenology.

The physician Liébault (1866) wrote of successfully treating his patients with hypnosis. His book was published during the nadir of belief in hypnotic phenomena. He was vilified when he was not ignored and would have been forgotten altogether if it were not for the notice of a prominent French physician named Bernheim, whose reputation was such that any work he admired had to be taken seriously. Charcot, an even more prominent physician than Bernheim, also helped to revive hypnosis and its acceptance as a treatment method for hysteria. His work and a paper presented to the French Académie des Sciences in 1882 made hypnosis respectable and even mainstream. Charcot's work was to dynamic psychiatry what the opening of Wundt's lab in 1879 was to academic psychology. Both represented official recognition of a fledgling enterprise. In addition, both Charcot and Bernheim were important to the progress of thinking about unconscious processes. This is so for two reasons. First, they directly influenced both Janet (Ellenberger, 1970; Perry & Laurence, 1984) and Freud (Ellenberger, 1970; Aron & Starr, 2013). Second, despite their differences and the ephemeral quality of their eminence, they made respectable a view of unconscious processing and a way of studying it that has remained influential (although not in mainstream academic psychology).

DIPSYCHISM AND POLYPSYCHISM

The major contribution of early dynamic psychiatry, for our purposes, was the two models of the mind it inspired (Ellenberger, 1970), dipsychism and polypsychism. They remain with us and have cropped up in modern conceptions of unconscious processes. Dipsychism grew out of the finding, first reported by Puységur, that a separate consciousness seemed to become manifest during artificial somnambulism. It could only be demonstrated through hypnotism and therefore seemed to be an unconscious mind. This raised the questions of how these two minds coexisted and interacted. Dessoir (1890), for instance, posited two independent layers to the mind (upper and under consciousness), operating according to different principles. Both were made up of complex chains of associations. Upper consciousness was familiar everyday awareness, whereas under consciousness was vaguely manifest in dreams, clearer in spontaneous somnambulism, and clearest under hypnosis. Divisions of the mind into conscious and unconscious or, later, automatic and controlled (e.g., Shiffrin & Schneider, 1977) are offshoots of this type of thinking. Both can be categorized as dual-processing models (Strack & Deutsch, 2015), which are quite popular currently.

The second model of the mind was termed polypsychism (Durand, 1868). Here, the mind is seen as consisting of a cluster of subpersonalities, subject to a central executive personality that contains everyday consciousness. Typically, the person is unaware of these subpersonalities and their functioning. Under hypnosis, however, their connections to central consciousness are temporarily severed. The hypnotist thereby gains direct access to the various subpersonalities. This is essentially a dissociationist view of mental functioning and of hypnosis. Clinically, it can be seen also as a predecessor of Bromberg's (1998, 2006, 2011) theories on dissociation, as well as relational psychoanalysis. Janet was an earlier polypsychist thinker who, however, saw it as pathological. Hilgard (1986, 1992) later developed a similar conception, but saw dissociation as normative. The so-called split brain (Gazzaniga, 1998) and massive modularity (Kurzban, 2010), which are reviewed later in this book, are also examples of polypsychist thinking.

THE BEGINNINGS OF ACADEMIC PSYCHOLOGY

The first efforts to make psychology into a scientific discipline began in the late 1870s and early 1880s, at a time when positivism and scientism were at their apex and Romantic conceptions were at their nadir. Dynamic psychiatry had just started to gain some momentum but was dealing with phenomena that were distrusted by the positivist community. As a consequence, the founders of the field profoundly distrusted the work of their psychiatric colleagues. They believed that psychology had to be built on a laboratory-based, experimental foundation. They felt that they had to isolate the object of their investigation from the mundane concerns of everyday life—needs, desires, and feelings—and their own subjectivity (Hornstein, 1992).

Given their predilections, it is not surprising that psychology's founders rejected the literal meaning of *psychology* as the science of the soul. They could not tolerate any Romantic fancies. They had to ruthlessly expunge these discredited ideas from the field lest they threaten the scientific respectability of their fledgling enterprise. This meant total abolition of the notion of the unconscious, especially as it was embodied in the still popular (and therefore dangerous) works of Schopenhauer and von Hartmann. Thus, the study of unconscious events was ruled out of academic psychology at its inception.

Despite the utter rejection of the possible relevance of unconscious events, they kept creeping into even these initial efforts to construct a scientific psychology. We briefly illustrate this muddle in three major early schools of psychology: structuralism, functionalism, and behaviorism (Boring, 1950), as well as in the theoretical framework of William James (1842–1910). These early schools of psychology either minimized or overtly denied the existence of unconscious processes while covertly (unconsciously?) trying to account for them and thus assigning them great importance. This resulted in a strange kind of split wherein unconscious processes were examined and discussed but still somehow denied.

Structuralism was the earliest movement in academic psychology. Its most authoritative proponents were Wilhelm Wundt (1832–1920), who is usually credited with starting the discipline of psychology in Germany, and his most eminent protégé, Edward B. Titchener (1867–1927), who brought it with him when he emigrated to the United States. Wundt began as a follower of Fechner and taught at the University of Leipzig, just as Fechner did. In fact, they overlapped on the faculty for some 20 years. At first (between 1860 and 1880), Wundt tried to develop Fechner's ideas and accepted many of his views concerning unconsciousness. In 1876, however, he repudiated any notions of unconscious processing (see Klein, 1977). (For a scholarly exposition on Wundt's work as it relates to unconscious processes, see Araujo, 2012.)

With unconsciousness banished, the question arose as to what could be included in the new psychology. Titchener (1929/1972) spelled that out very clearly: psychology is the science of the mind, defined as all mental processes occurring in a person's lifetime. Mental processes occurring at any given moment in time make up consciousness, so the contents of the mind are completely subsumed by consciousness. The structuralists thereby adopted the Cartesian view of mental life. Further, psychology had to be objectively observable in order to be studied. They developed a rigorous and disciplined form of introspection so as to achieve this end. They sought, in this way, to dissect consciousness into its elements. They thought they could develop a kind of "mental chemistry" by beginning with the creation of a periodic table of mental elements. So the structuralists also bought into a scientistic version of positivism. Despite their best efforts, however, unconscious events kept stealing into their introspective investigations. Thus, Marbe (1901) and Watt (1905) independently reported that introspective judgments of weight and word associations, respectively, seemed to take place unconsciously.

Unconscious processes were also evident (if not acknowledged) in the theoretical formulations of the structuralists. Thus, their official position on attention (Titchener, 1908) was that it is essentially a patterning of consciousness into foreground and background (or focus and margin, as Wundt called them). The focus of attention is clear and available to introspection (awareness). The margin of attention, on the other hand, is obscure and relatively unamenable to conscious introspection. This sounds suspiciously as if attention involves unconscious events, although the structuralists never acknowledged this idea. Structuralism died with Titchener, but it had a lasting influence in that it began the practice of excluding unconscious events from meta-theory while surreptitiously making use of them to account for actual psychological phenomena. As we shall see, this became virtually universal in psychology.

Functionalism was interested in how activities contribute to adaptation. As a result, in contrast to structuralists, the functionalists emphasized process over content, and advocated studying psychological processes as they occurred in their natural setting, as opposed to the laboratory (Boring, 1950; Heidbredder, 1933). Functionalism saw consciousness as helping the organism adapt to and survive in novel situations. As the situation recurs and novelty diminishes, consciousness becomes less useful, eventually waning. Habit (automaticity) then takes over.[1] Boring (1950) termed this an "emergency" theory of consciousness. It relegates unconsciousness to a secondary, relatively unimportant role; it is the absence of consciousness. It is rather dumb and inflexible and only operative as long as everything is going smoothly. (This conception has more recent proponents as well—see Greenwald [1992].)

Functionalism as a school has long since ceased to exist. This is largely because it won its battles and has become incorporated into mainstream academic psychological thinking (see Heidbredder, 1933). Its terms have been renamed, but its central doctrines have remained intact. A number of more recent conceptions like automaticity (e.g., Schneider & Shiffrin, 1977; Shiffrin & Schneider, 1977) are simply functionalism in new dress. And, as we shall see when we investigate recent models of automatic processing, functionalist concepts are powerful in today's psychology.

William James's views of unconscious events are especially important because he is erroneously seen as having issued a blanket condemnation against resorting to unconscious processes as an explanatory concept. In fact, James often attributed behavior to unconscious processes and welcomed the work of others who did so as well. (See Weinberger, 2000, for a more detailed exposition.) The source of the misunderstanding comes from an oft-quoted sentence in a section entitled "Can States of Mind Be Unconscious?" in chapter 6 ("The Mind-Stuff Theory") of *The Principles of Psychology* (1890): "It [belief in unconscious mental states] is the sovereign means for believing what one likes in psychology and of turning what might become a science into a tumbling-ground for whimsies" (p. 163). A closer inspection reveals that all is not as it appears, however.

First (and it is surprising that others have not addressed this issue), the book was published in 1890 (after James worked on it for 12 years). What we think of as "unconscious mental states" of mind today were not what James was writing about and disparaging over 125 years ago. In the above quote, James attacked the belief that consciousness in humans presupposes some rudimentary form of consciousness in elementary particles that he called "mind-dust." In essence, he attacked Leibniz's notion of conscious experience being composed of an aggregate of individually imperceptible sensations (petite percepts). He was also concerned with refuting the then relatively recent propositions put forth by von Hartmann and Schopenhauer that lent a mystical aspect to unconsciousness and saw all activity, animate and inanimate, as reflecting unconscious forces.

Far from denying the existence of unconscious processes, James promoted them. Careful reading of his 1890 book reveals that he believed in dissociation and hypnotic phenomena. Additionally, he explained habit in terms of the development of automaticity (a position later adopted by the functionalists). Finally, in his efforts to understand the flow of consciousness, James argued that thoughts do not exist independently but are embedded in contexts made up of experiences associated with those thoughts. James depicts such contexts as a "psychic overtone" or "fringe of relations" that accompanies and influences every mental event. The mental processes and images contained in this "fringe" are not strong enough to be directly translated into consciousness. Instead, they function as an "overtone" and influence other processes, which do result in a conscious idea. In most cases, the person is ignorant of this fringe and of its effect on her thought processes.

James's notion of the "fringe" of relations is closely akin to modern cognitive conceptions of associative networks and schemas made up of various pathways or nodes (see, e.g., Smith & Kosslyn, 2007). Also paralleling James's ideas is the assumption that whenever any aspect of the schema is triggered, the entire schema becomes active (Smith & Kosslyn, 2007). Additionally, in both conceptions, the contents and connections in the network determine the direction cognitive activity takes. And, finally, awareness depends upon strength of activation and nodal distance from the particular aspect of the network most directly activated. This means that not all of the schema enters consciousness. The part (or parts) that does not still influences cognitive activity, however. Thus, James anticipated modern cognitive conceptions of associative networks with remarkable clarity. (For a more detailed view of James's position, see Weinberger, 2000.)

James also wrote favorably on the work of others investigating unconscious processes like Janet's views on subconscious personality structures. To view James as a voice raised against unconscious processes is quite simply wrong. It is based on overemphasizing and misinterpreting a single quotation. As a counterpoint to the anti-unconscious quote so often cited, we offer James's evaluation of the work of Janet and likeminded investigators: "They prove one thing conclusively, namely, that *we must never take a person's testimony, however sincere, that he has felt nothing, as proof positive that no feeling has been there*" (1890/1950, p. 211; italics in original). What could be a stronger endorsement of unconscious states? James was also certainly not advocating an anti-Freudian view either, as the Freudian view did not yet exist. Supporting our understanding of James's views is his famous reaction to hearing Freud's (1910) landmark lectures at Clark University. Freud's disciple Jones reported that James put his arm around Freud and declared that "the future of psychology belongs to your work" (Jones, 1955, p. 57). And we need not rely solely on the testimony of Jones. There is also evidence of James's approval of Freud's work in James's own writing, as cited by Evans and Koelsch (1985). In a letter to Flournoy, James (1920) wrote: "I hope that Freud and his followers push their ideas to their utmost limit so we may learn what they are. They cannot fail to throw light on human nature" (pp. 327–328). As unconscious processes are at the heart of Freud's ideas, James certainly could not have been opposed to them. Moreover, as Mann (1936) pointed out, Freud's ideas bore a strong resemblance to Schopenhauer's, translated from metaphysics to psychology. Since James condemned Schopenhauer in 1890, he either changed his mind or was responding positively to Freud's empirical bent and negatively to Schopenhauer's metaphysical orientation. As he never publicly recanted his position on Schopenhauer, we again are inclined to believe the latter.

Finally, behaviorism was the school of psychology that adopted the most extreme position on unconscious processes. Not only did behaviorists dismiss such processes, as did the structuralists, they also discarded consciousness along with them. In fact, they banished anything having to do with the "mind" from the realm of psychological inquiry.

The two names most closely associated with behaviorism are Watson (1913, 1919), the founder of the movement, and Skinner (1953, 1974), its most prominent modern proponent. Watson's main thesis was that human beings are best understood as stimulus–response mechanisms. Conditioning was said to be able to account for any and all behavior, whereas consciousness and unconsciousness were remnants of medieval superstition and best consigned to the trash heap of history. A scientific psychology must have nothing whatsoever to do with them. In fact, the whole concept of mind must be jettisoned. Despite this radical view of the mind, Watson (1919) somehow felt compelled to address the issues of consciousness and unconsciousness. He, in fact, acknowledged the existence of many of the phenomena described by Freud and his followers, but he offered an alternative interpretation for them, equating conscious and unconscious phenomena with verbalized and unverbalized responses, respectively. That which can be verbalized is perforce conscious; whatever cannot be named is part of the person's unconscious world.

Watson postulated two classes of behavior that tend to remain unverbalized (unconscious): visceral responses, for which verbal labels are regularly absent, and behavior learned in infancy and early childhood, before verbal conditioning begins. As a result, these infantile and emotional responses (including aversions, phobias, preferences, etc.) tend to remain out of the person's and even society's control. Watson conceded that a large proportion of experience is and remains unverbalized, essentially admitting that most behavior goes on unconsciously and is out of the person's control. In Watson's work, even so extreme a strategy as dismissing the entire concept of mind and mental events did not suffice to keep notions of the unconscious out.

Later versions of behaviorism have been no more successful in excluding unconscious processes. Radical behaviorists in the Skinnerian tradition (as opposed to the Watsonian "methodological" behaviorists) kept wondering whether awareness is necessary for operant conditioning to occur. This is an odd concern given the premise that awareness is an unproductive, even nonsensical concept. Behavioral researchers (e.g., Greenspoon, 1955; Hefferline, Keenan, & Harford, 1959; Postman & Sassenrath, 1961) wanted to determine whether conditioning is affected by awareness, even though it should have been theoretically irrelevant to them.

Skinner himself (1974) was concerned with this issue. He insisted that behaviorism deals with unconsciousness while, at the same time, he argued that hundreds of years of speculation about the nature of consciousness had been a waste of time. Skinner identified consciousness with the sensing of bodily conditions, whereas he defined unconsciousness as unanalyzed and/or unobserved contingencies of reinforcement. According to Skinner, when the contingencies are unobserved, the behavior is completely out of awareness. When they are observed but unanalyzed, it is unconscious in a more limited sense. The person knows what she is doing but not why she is doing it. Although he acknowledged the power of unanalyzed and/or unobserved contingencies as controllers of behavior, Skinner strongly rejected the notion of unconsciousness (and consciousness itself for that matter) as a causal agent. Nonetheless, he saw fit to differentiate between awareness and its lack. He even cited Freud approvingly (Skinner, 1953, 1974). Thus, despite his disavowals, even Skinner had to come to grips with unconscious processes.

AND BACK TO DYNAMIC PSYCHIATRY

While academic psychology was denying the existence or importance of unconscious processes, the devotees of dynamic psychiatry made liberal use of conceptions of unconscious processes. The two camps were able to maintain such diametrically opposed views by ignoring one another's work. We now turn to the work of one of the giants of dynamic psychiatry, Pierre Janet.

Janet was a scholar of immense gifts, erudition, and productivity, although his views lost their popularity rapidly. This was probably due to the immense impact of Freud's psychoanalytic theory on all of Western culture and its overshadowing of Janet's writings. (The interested reader is referred to Hilgard [1986, 1992], Kihlstrom [1984], Ellenberger's [1970] scholarly tome, Kihlstrom's [1984] summary, and Perry and Laurence's [1984] lucid account of Janet's work.)

Janet did not follow the predominant lines of thinking about hypnotism of his time (i.e., Charcot or the Nancy school of Liébault and Bernheim). Instead, he developed his own set of ideas. Like Charcot and contrary to the Nancy school, he believed that subconscious (he preferred this term to unconscious) processes were manifestations of pathology. He developed Charcot's notion that unconscious "fixed ideas" lie at the root of many emotional difficulties. But, unlike Charcot and similarly to the Nancy school, he saw and demonstrated the role of suggestion in hypnosis.

Janet believed that the mind was composed of activity, and rather complex activity at that. He labeled these active elements psychological "automatisms" (Kihlstrom, 1984) and endowed them with a rudimentary consciousness (Ellenberger, 1970). Under optimal circumstances, consciousness integrates the aforementioned elements of the mind into the personality. In a properly functioning individual, all mental operations achieve consciousness. With all of this integrated information at his conscious disposal, the individual is in the best possible position to adapt to environmental exigencies. Often, however, circumstances are not ideal. Sometimes psychological events or automatisms bypass consciousness and are therefore not integrated into the personality. This may come about when a person lacks adequate resources for coping with stress. It can be precipitated by a traumatic incident, a chronically demanding environment, or a genetically based weakness in the ability to tolerate stress. Whatever the reason, when a person is under pressure, she must find the resources to deal with it. Sometimes the person frees up energy by constricting consciousness, which becomes unable to perform its integrative function on all stimuli impinging on the organism. When this occurs, experiences that cannot be integrated are said to be split off or dissociated (Janet's term is actually "disaggregated") from the personality. The dissociated automatism then functions outside of awareness and voluntary control. Such an occurrence adversely affects adaptation and produces psychopathology.[2]

In order to treat these difficulties, the split-off or dissociated experiences must be brought back into the domain of consciousness, there to be integrated or synthesized into the personality. The first step is to find out what experiences have been dissociated. The source of the problem, the stressor, has to be identified. Once identified, the automatism's course of development into a subconscious system has to be reconstructed. Then it has to be integrated into the personality via consciousness. It would then cease to exist as an autonomous quasi-conscious entity. To these ends, Janet utilized hypnosis, as well as automatic writing and talking.

Although both began with goal-oriented activity, Janet's view of unconscious processing was 180° different from that of the functionalists. For Janet, everything is initially unconscious but must enter consciousness and be ruled by it. If an experience remains outside of consciousness's purview, it means that something has gone wrong and dire consequences can be expected. To the functionalist, the sequence is exactly the reverse, and the consequences are far from grim. Consciousness is a troubleshooter to be withdrawn when the matter no longer presents a difficulty. It is not only not pathological for behavior to go on automatically and unconsciously, it is the natural state of affairs. If consciousness is present, it is because a behavior remains problematic.

The functionalist conception won the day. Janet's view of automaticity did not survive. In fact, Janet's influence virtually disappeared in his own lifetime. For a while, his ideas were kept alive by the American psychologists Sidis (1902) and Prince (1906), but their influence also soon waned. The whole notion of dissociation gradually disappeared from the literature and has only begun to stage a comeback in the last few decades. This was probably due to the overwhelming impact of psychoanalysis. Janet's conceptions of dissociation and quasi-independent aspects of personality probably would not have survived at all had they not been resurrected in Hilgard's (1986, 1992) neodissociation theory. We next turn to the force that all but eliminated Janet's influence: psychoanalytic theory.

NOTES

1. The first to explicitly discuss automaticity (not his term) was probably von Helmholtz (1859/1962; see Klein, 1977). His unconscious (or "basic process" as he later preferred to call it) was a primitive, inflexible, and altogether limited mechanism.

2. Janet's theory is an early harbinger of more current theories of dissociation (e.g., Bromberg, 1999, 2006, 2011), which, it is important to note, do not see it as inherently pathological.

CHAPTER 4

Psychoanalysis

The driving force behind psychoanalysis was its remarkable founder, Sigmund Freud. It is not an exaggeration to say that Freud changed the course of Western thought through his conceptions of unconscious processes and the importance he attributed to them in human functioning. In fact, he (1926) once identified psychoanalysis with the study of unconscious processes. In 1900, at age 44, Freud published his landmark book *The Interpretation of Dreams,* which launched the psychoanalytic movement and began a period of incredible productivity that lasted for the remainder of his life. Freud's ability to make major contributions was also unaffected by age. He made substantial changes in his model of the mind at age 67 (when he introduced his famous structural model of the id, ego, and superego; Freud, 1923) and at 69 (when he significantly altered his views on anxiety: Freud, 1926). In this chapter, we review the role of unconscious processes in his two major models of the mind, the topographical and structural models, and then introduce post-Freudian developments in psychoanalysis.

FREUD'S TOPOGRAPHICAL MODEL

Freud introduced what he called the topographical model of the mind in his seminal book *The Interpretation of Dreams* (Freud, 1900). It conceptualized mental functioning in terms of accessibility to consciousness. In 1915, Freud published his most complete treatise on the topographical view of unconscious functioning (suitably entitled "The Unconscious"). First, he argued that without the notion of unconscious processes, it would be impossible to understand much of psychological functioning. This is most clear for hypnotic phenomena, which are often completely unavailable to consciousness. It also holds for everyday phenomena like parapraxes (commonly known as slips of the tongue), dreams, and neurotic symptoms. Similarly, people often seem to be visited by ideas apparently unconnected to what they can report thinking about at the time. These inexplicable ideas can even feel alien, as when a poet is visited by her muse. The data provided by consciousness are, at best, limited and incomplete concerning such phenomena. They can be rendered sensible only if we interpolate unconscious events between the experiences we are conscious of.[1]

Once we accept the existence of unconscious processes, we must next attempt to understand their nature and their place in mental functioning. In his topographical model, Freud (1900, 1915) proposed a tripartite division of the mind into conscious, preconscious, and unconscious systems. This division is based on the capacity to be aware of mental contents. Thus, awareness, or the lack thereof, is the central defining feature of mental functioning in the topographical model.

The conscious system simply involves what a person is aware of at any particular moment in time. But a person can only be aware of a very small part of the information potentially available to him. This means that the vast majority of potentially available information remains dormant for lengthy stretches of time and is therefore unconscious by definition. Freud reasoned that this latent information resides in a preconscious system, which consists of mental contents (memories, experiences, etc.) that a person can bring into consciousness when needed but that are not conscious at that moment. Both the conscious and the preconscious systems are organized rationally and linguistically, that is, their contents can be expressed sensibly and in language. The only difference is that of phenomenal awareness controlled by attention. With one important exception, described below, communication between the preconscious and conscious systems is relatively free and easy; all the person has to do to bring preconscious content to awareness is to focus attention on it. As a result, Freud sometimes referred to these two systems as a single system, the "preconscious–conscious" system.[2]

Freud found that there was more to the mind than conscious–preconscious functioning, however. His studies led him to conclude that some processes in the mind operated in ways that were radically and qualitatively different from the operation of the aforementioned conscious–preconscious system. This unconscious system, he argued, is the psychological representative of the inborn drives or instincts of the human species. Drives are more somatic than mental and therefore can never be directly present in the mind in the way conscious/

preconscious content is. They can (and do) have mental representations, however. These take the form of unconscious nonverbal ideas suffused with desire (e.g., a person dying of thirst in a desert may visualize cold, wet, refreshing water), as well as similes, metaphors, and the images of poetry (cf. Schimek, 1975, 2011).[3] In Freud's terminology, they are invested with the energy (cathected) of the instinct. In simple English, they are affectively charged or emotionally meaningful. This explains the incredible power that symbols hold over people, a fact well understood by politicians and advertisers. Early on, Freud (1904) focused on the sexual drive, but later he (1920) added an aggressive drive and assigned it equal importance. Sexual and aggressive symbols therefore hold the most affective punch (are most highly cathected). According to Freud, these passionate unconscious libidinal and, after 1920, aggressive needs and impulses constantly strive for expression in the form of wishes. Some unconscious desires, Freud averred, are in sync with one another, some are orthogonal, and some are mutually contradictory. This has no effect on them or on their striving for expression, however, and neither do reality and its constraints. The unconscious system cares not a whit about the practical aspects or consequences of achieving its aims.

Freud understood the unconscious system's effort at expression of wishes as an attempt to discharge instinctual energy. The buildup of such energy or the prevention of its discharge is experienced as discomfort; its release is experienced as pleasure. Freud, following Fechner (see Chapter 2), termed this the "pleasure principle." In the service of their unremitting pressure for discharge, the needs are not irrevocably tied to any one means of expression. If one avenue does not lead to satisfaction, another will be tried. This phenomenon (i.e., when one means is given up in favor of another) is termed "displacement." So, for example, if you can't be with the one you want, love the one you're with (with apologies to Stephen Stills). Sometimes an avenue of expression can be made to serve several needs. This process, called "condensation," constitutes expanding the use of a successful means so as to allow for expression of several desires. Thus, some people can both love and aggress against an individual they love (e.g., sadomasochistic sex: pleasure is tied to hurting the one you love). When two incompatible wishes strive simultaneously for expression, they may combine to form a compromise or intermediate desire. Freud termed this capacity for the emotional investment (cathexis) of wishes to flow from one conduit of expression to another *primary process*—an unbounded capacity to alter the object of desire. The operation of primary process means that there is an almost infinite number of ways to express a wish.

A problem soon became apparent, however. Unbridled expression of drives would quickly get the person into serious trouble and could even have deadly consequences. A person cannot simply have sex with and/or engage in aggression against anyone she pleases, at any time the mood strikes. Since there is a real world with environmental and social constraints on free and easy expression of desires, the drives of the unconscious system must often be frustrated, either through denying them altogether or by delaying their expression. Something must come between these drives and their enactment, and that something, according to Freud, is the preconscious–conscious system. What this means is that the unconscious and preconscious–conscious system are in almost perpetual conflict. The ways in which they interact and resolve (or fail to resolve) their conflicts are therefore crucial to understanding and evaluating the topographical view of psychological functioning.

The unconscious system communicates with the preconscious–conscious system in one of two ways, depending upon whether mental activity is triggered by external or internal stimulation. External stimulation has relatively ready access to the unconscious system. As a result, the effects of external reality can be used to fulfill unconscious wishes in accord with the pleasure principle. The person comes to value or be affectively stimulated by whatever object in the environment facilitated satisfaction of his unconscious wishes. In this way, many unconscious desires come to revolve around actual people and objects in the real world. For example, the mother, by virtue of satisfying many of her infant's needs and because she is so often present when those needs are met, becomes highly valued and the object of many of the infant's wishes. This leads to unconscious sexually and aggressively tinged desires for and fantasies concerning the mother. In Freud's terminology, she becomes cathected with instinctual energy.

Mental activity that originates internally, in the unconscious system, starts as a wish striving for expression. In order to be granted, this wish must become conscious. But there is a problem. One of the functions of the preconscious system is to monitor unconscious desires and, if necessary, control or censor their access to consciousness. This blocking of conscious access is termed "primal" repression. If an unconscious content passes this censor, it gains access to the preconscious system. There, it comes up against another censor, which represents the one exception to the free and easy interchange between the preconscious and conscious systems. If this second censor rejects the impulse, it tries to thrust it back into the unconscious system. Freud termed this "after-repression." After-repression can also occur when stimulation from outside, that entered the unconscious through the preconscious system, becomes invested with unconscious desires. If, in its new incarnation as an unconsciously invested idea or memory, it is rejected by the conscious–preconscious censor, it is forced into the unconscious system. The person will then have no conscious recollection of that memory. Most repression occurs during early childhood when the psychic apparatus is comparatively weak and the child is relatively helpless and dependent.

The censors are not always completely effective, however. Repression can and often is partly overcome. Freud described the three most common ways for this to occur (cf. Arlow & Brenner, 1964). First, the censor can weaken or the repressed content can gain strength so that some aspect of the wish (termed "a derivative") literally forces its way past the overmatched censor. Typically, this results in distortion of the underlying wish as the censor engages in a kind of rear-guard action against it. The result is usually a neurotic symptom and the person suffers for it. Second, sometimes repression is temporarily removed and then promptly reinstated so as to allow for fleeting expression of a derivative. This permits a relatively harmless letting off of steam, so to speak. Jokes and parapraxes are examples of such events. Finally, the censor can become less repressive when it determines that expression of an unconscious wish is unlikely to pose any danger to the person. This occurs regularly in sleep. Because the person can be allowed freest expression of his desires in sleep, dreams are the least distorted of unconscious representations and so constitute *the royal road* to the unconscious.

Freud claimed to have discovered a way to systematically learn about and even influence unconscious processes, which he termed "psychoanalysis." He encouraged patients to report everything that comes to mind regardless of whatever resistance they may feel regarding doing so. This is termed "free association." Free associating to dreams is especially revealing. Because the censor never completely relaxes and never totally ceases its activity, the analyst *interprets* the patient's utterances. She is also on the lookout for parapraxes and nonverbal behaviors that may have slipped past the censor and betray the patient's true unconscious intent. Once repression is bypassed in these ways, the derivative and, eventually the wish, can achieve consciousness. This, in turn, eliminates the neurotic symptom brought about by the now unnecessary resistance to acknowledging the underlying wish. This is why Freud (1916) described the goal of psychoanalysis as making the unconscious conscious. This is not an easy task. Resistance can be quite powerful and so it may take years of painful and painstaking work before the repressed wish appears in consciousness. Psychoanalytic treatment is therefore very time-consuming (and expensive), taking place several days a week for years.

FREUD'S STRUCTURAL MODEL

The topographical model was conceptually tight, easy to follow, and tied together time-honored philosophical traditions. Preconscious–conscious processing follows the rationalist conceptions of the mind, then represented by the dominant positivistic movement. Unconscious processing seemed to obey the rules elucidated by the still influential Romantics and philosophers of nature. Moreover, the two systems coincided almost exactly with Nietzsche's conceptions of Appolonian (preconscious–conscious) and Dionysian (unconscious) thought (although Freud denied ever being influenced by or, in fact, ever having read Nietzsche's work). Freud had brought together, in a coherent system, two types of functioning that philosophers had been arguing about for centuries. And he claimed to have empirical support for it all. It seemed like a stunning achievement. Alas, it was not to last. To his credit, Freud himself saw flaws in the topographical model and did not hesitate to point them out (e.g., Freud, 1915). He altered his position when he realized that the operation of the censor, which the topographical model placed in the preconscious, was actually unconscious.

Another problem was fantasy. From the beginning of his investigations, Freud uncovered many unconscious, apparently repressed, fantasies with varying levels of narrative coherence and moral concerns (see Abend, 1990; Arlow, 1969; Beres, 1962; and A. Freud, 1992, for more on ego and superego contributions to fantasy). This required preconscious activity. Unconscious fantasies had no home in the topographical model. They belonged to both and neither system (see Arlow, 1969). Efforts to correct these flaws gave birth to a new model of the mind (Freud, 1923). Consciousness and unconsciousness no longer had systemic significance; rather, they were descriptive. This new model was termed the "structural model," although it could more accurately be termed the "functional model."

The three major components of the structural model—the id, the ego, and the superego—displayed varying mixtures of primary and secondary process. Moreover, secondary process itself was not necessarily conscious or preconscious. What had been called the unconscious system—the drives (libidinal and aggressive)—became the id. It was governed by primary process and was said to feel external, even alien to the person, hence its original name, the "it" (*das es*; and, once again, Freud denied having been influenced by Nietzsche). The id is the agency of the drives, the seat of desire. This is little more than a change in terminology. The id is almost exactly like the unconscious system of the topographical model. Real changes are evident in what had once been the preconscious–conscious system(s), which became the ego and was now conceptualized to contain both conscious and unconscious aspects. Id impulses, for instance, are managed through usually unconscious ego functions termed "defenses," which, like unconscious fantasy, fall in the gray area of the ego, between the primary and secondary processes. Clinically, defenses must be brought into awareness before the therapist can get to the unconscious wishes. Freud found that moral thinking also had a strong unconscious component that he termed the superego (because it stood "over" the ego). It develops through the internalization of parental (and, later, other external authority) exhortations, moral injunctions, and prohibitions and directly opposes id wishes. Although the superego was seen to develop out of the ego, its operation more strongly resembles id than ego functioning. That is, it is irrational, cares little for reality considerations, and derives its power from aggressive impulses. Nonetheless, it could not fit into the old unconscious system because it contained moral rather than drive imperatives. As both id and superego demands are unremitting, the ego has to mediate between them.

The structural model is messier, that is, not as conceptually tight as the topographical model. Unconscious processes exist in all agencies of the mind, id, ego, and superego. There is no strict set of rules for all unconscious dynamics. Instead, they exist on a continuum from primary to secondary process (Arlow & Brenner, 1964).[4] Clinically, the task has changed from an exclusive focus on making the unconscious conscious to the more varied goals of uncovering resistances, defenses, and superego injunctions in the service of making them more flexible and rational and then integrating them into the personality.

LATER DEVELOPMENTS IN PSYCHOANALYTIC CONCEPTIONS OF THE UNCONSCIOUS

Psychoanalytic hypotheses about unconscious processes may have begun with Freud, but they did not end with him. Following Freud's death, psychoanalysis may be said to have developed into six major schools: classical psychoanalysis, ego psychology, object relations, self psychology (and the intersubjective model of Atwood and Stolorow), and relational psychoanalysis. Each has its own views on unconscious processing. Ego psychology and classical theory have more or less merged, so we treat them as one. Object relations and interpersonal theory, although distinct in many ways, have such similar views (or lack of views as we shall see) on unconscious processes that we consider them together as well.

Classical and Ego Psychology

Classical psychoanalysis and ego psychology's views are most directly tied to Freud's conceptions. However, they no longer try to explain the origins and goals of wishes by speculating about somatically based sexual and aggressive instincts or principles of nervous system functioning. Instead, they simply describe libidinal and aggressive wishes and their modes of expression, as they see them in the clinical setting (see Schimek, 1975, 2011). The basic features of Freud's structural model have been retained. The mind is still understood in terms of the interacting and often conflicting functions of id (needs), ego (reality), and superego (morality; see Brenner, 1982), but their relationship to one another has been changed somewhat.

Ego psychologists, starting with Hartmann (1939/1958), have extended the power and autonomy of ego functions beyond the limits set by Freud. The overarching function of the ego is conceptualized as organizing and making sense of inner and outer experience (cf. Arlow, 1963; Arlow & Brenner, 1964; Beres, 1962), integrating internal drives (the id) with internalized societal demands (the superego) and the external world (the reality principle of the ego). Its abilities to perceive, think, and remember aid the ego in its organizational task. These abilities are present in rudimentary form from birth and then become increasingly sophisticated over time (Rapaport, 1960). Ego psychological views have pretty much been incorporated into mainstream classical psychoanalysis. The most important work of both traditions for our purposes concerns unconscious fantasies (Arlow, 1953, 1961, 1963, 1969, 1987; Reed, 2017), which are said to originate as wishes. Infants do not differentiate between inner and outer experiences, so when the outer world cannot meet a need, an internal fantasy is conjured up to do just that. The mental image is gratifying and the need is satisfied. This is the so-called hallucinatory wish fulfillment described by Freud (Schimek, 1975, 2011). Such a wish is almost entirely unconscious and operates largely in accord with the rules of primary process. How adaptive an unconscious fantasy is depends upon the level of development of the ego at the time the fantasy is created (cf. Abend, 1990; Arlow, 1969). The less well developed the ego, the poorer the person's understanding of reality and the less able she is to successfully understand and integrate relevant internal and external factors. The poorer this integration, the more primitive and primary-process-like (unconscious) the fantasy will be (Arlow, 1963; Shapiro & Inderbitzin, 1989). As ego functions mature, fantasies become more stable, coherent, and concerned with reality and moral considerations. As a result, they generate less anxiety and defense and are more likely to be conscious (Arlow, 1969).

The well-known Oedipus complex is a prime example of an unconscious fantasy uncovered by psychoanalysis (Beres, 1962). Because Freud postulated that the resolution of the Oedipal complex had lifelong ramifications, he considered it the most crucial psychological event of early life (perhaps in all of life) and so do most classical psychoanalysts (e.g., Brenner, 1982). In fact, classicists use the Oedipal period as a convenient developmental benchmark for categorizing fantasies (see e.g., Inderbitzin

& Levy, 1990). Pre-Oedipal thinking is said to be a preconceptual or relatively primary process, as well as more likely to be defended against. Post-Oedipal thinking is conceptually organized and reflective of secondary process.

Unconscious fantasies provide the mental set in which experiences are perceived, understood, and integrated (see, e.g., Shapiro, 1983). That is, they help organize psychic reality (Arlow, 1969; Inderbitzin & Levy, 1990). Under their sway, the ego is oriented to selectively scan the world for information consonant with them (Linn, 1954). Cognition, memory, and even perception are utilized to these ends. The extent to which unconscious fantasies affect the organization of experience depends upon both internal and external factors. External factors include the ambiguity (Arlow, 1969) and affective charge (Dowling, in Shapiro & Inderbitzin, 1989) of the situation; a critical internal factor is the affective charge (cathexis) of the fantasy itself and the wish at its center.[5] Under some conditions, the fantasy may lead the person to seriously distort reality. This is especially likely when the fantasy originated in early childhood because it already reflects reality poorly. Neuroses, for example, regularly distort reality, which can be traced to the effects of unconscious, defended-against fantasies originally formed in early childhood (Inderbitzin & Levy, 1990).

In psychoanalytic treatment, the ambiguity of the setting, the emotional charge of what is being discussed, and the supposed "tabula rasa" of the classical analyst all encourage the expression of unconscious fantasies. Once activated, they lead the patient to attribute various, often distorted, qualities to the analyst and to the interactions between them. This is termed "transference" and it is central to psychoanalytic treatment. These transference fantasies (as well as any other fantasies that emerge) can then be examined and understood in the relatively safe and controlled setting of the therapeutic situation, which increases the likelihood that they can be made more flexible and adaptively integrated into the personality.

Object Relations Theory

As we travel from the topographical through the structural to ego psychologists' model of the unconscious, unconscious processes are gradually seen as ruled less by primary and more by secondary process. Object relations theorists have gone even further. Although they never seem to acknowledge it, they have virtually eliminated primary process from human functioning, at least in any important way. This follows from the fact that they do not see objects as very variable. Wishes, drives, and desires all are said to present themselves complete with their satisfying objects. Desire, therefore, necessarily implies an object of that desire (Fairbairn, 1952; Isaacs, 1943; Klein, 1952/1975). The a priori connection between object and desire is the starting point and is at the heart of all object relations theories.

Object relations theories vary tremendously but all have certain things in common. First, as stated above, all wishes come complete with their objects. Objects are therefore not very variable. This effectively removes primary process from any significant role in human functioning. Second, objects are always relational. What humans really want, according to object relationalists, are relationships. Therefore, *an object of desire is always a person or an aspect of a person.* This further limits the variability of objects. Finally, object relation theories concern themselves with exploring the dynamic interplay between a person's real-world relationships and his internal representations of those relationships.

Object relations theories almost never discuss the role or manner of functioning of unconscious processes in their systems. They have not only eliminated primary process (virtually limitless variability of objects) without acknowledging it but also failed to replace it with a different set of rules. That the issue seems not to have concerned them is problematic for the purposes of this book. Kernberg (e.g., 1987, 2004) is the only object relations theorist who seems to have given any serious thought to the issue of how unconscious processes operate.

Klein

Consistent throughout Klein's work is her emphasis on the importance and ubiquity of unconscious fantasies (see, e.g., Greenberg & Mitchell, 1983; Isaacs, 1943; and Segal, 1964, for elaborations on this topic) and the objects at their core (Klein, 1952/1975). She believed that all psychological activity is motivated and accompanied by such fantasies. These fantasies begin at birth, if not before, and are often quite elaborate. The bulk of them concern the child's imagined relationship to parts of the mother and later to the mother as a whole person.

The earliest fantasies involve what Klein termed "part objects" because they do not involve a whole person. The child is mostly concerned with the mother's breasts and the inside of her body. The motivation for these fantasies is variously attributed to a libidinal desire to know the mother (Klein, 1926) or to an aggressive desire to possess and control her (Klein, 1930). In either case, the child experiences frustration of these desires and responds with angry destructive fantasies aimed at the offending body parts and aspects of the mother (at the part objects). These then become "bad objects." The satisfying aspects of the mother become "good objects," and they are kept separate from the bad objects in the child's mind. Angry and destructive fantasies are projected out into the world so that the child comes to fear that the mother will retaliate in kind. Elaborate unconscious fantasies of the form this retaliation will take are constructed, all ultimately ending in the child's annihilation. The fear of such annihilation is termed "paranoid anxiety." The stage where all of this occurs is termed by Klein the paranoid or paranoid-schizoid position. The child is not well related at this point. He is only relating to body parts (good or bad part objects), which are imbued with motives and desires. He has no awareness or recognition of how these all cohere.

Soon, however, as early as between 4 and 8 months (Klein, 1935), the child becomes able to relate to the mother as a whole person or, as Klein puts it, "whole object." At this point, the child realizes that her destructive fantasies, if realized, would destroy the good as well as the bad aspects of the mother. After all, both sets of characteristics belong to the same person. A kind of abject horror at this realization ensues, which Klein calls "depressive anxiety." It is accompanied by fantasies of being alone and empty. The child then engages in reparative fantasies to make it up to the mother and prevent her destruction. Klein calls this phase of development the depressive position. Now the child can relate to a person as a whole being and this is reflected in his fantasies.

Klein sees unconscious fantasy as central to human functioning, and all such fantasies center around significant others. Moreover, these fantasies are very highly charged emotionally. In her belief in the centrality of unconscious fantasy, she agrees with (perhaps even surpasses) the classical psychoanalysts and ego psychologists reviewed earlier. There are also serious disagreements, however. One such difference concerns the centrality of relationships in fantasy. Klein (1952/1975), like all object relationalists, says that all fantasies are relational in nature; the classicists say they need not be relational.

The two positions also differ radically on the developmental antecedents of fantasies. Ego psychologists argue that fantasy formation requires organizational abilities that improve with development. Fantasies, then, reflect whatever organizational skills existed at the time of their formation. There is therefore an important cognitive aspect to unconscious fantasy as posited by ego psychologists. Klein, in contrast, argues that little if any development is required.

Fairbairn

The vast bulk of Fairbairn's papers have been collected in a single volume (Fairbairn, 1952). The interested reader can therefore easily peruse his thoughts there.

Fairbairn argued that all impulses are relational and have what he termed "natural" or "primary" objects. He averred that these objects are always other individuals. In his terminology, libido is object seeking, not pleasure seeking as Freud would have it. This is in agreement with all other object relations theorists.

The first and preeminent natural object is the mother. If all goes well, relational development proceeds from dependence on the mother in infancy and childhood to intimacy with significant others at maturity. Unfortunately, all rarely goes well. The mother can be gratifying, enticing, and/or depriving to her child. Anything other than gratification results in negative consequences. Therefore, the child is particularly vulnerable to separation from the mother, who is responsible for early gratification.

In order to compensate for any relational inadequacies, the child establishes internal objects. That is, she creates and then relates to an internal representation of a compensatory, substitute relationship. So what had been a relationship to an external object is replaced with a relationship to an internal one. Later, a similar sequence of events results in a set of object relations centering on the father. The two sets are then combined somehow, and a complex system of pathological fantasized internal relationships is set up.

According to Fairbairn, internal imaginary relationships siphon off psychic resources meant for external, real relationships. This leaves fewer resources to deal with actual, external relationships. The more the person invests these resources in internal relationships, the less she will have available for real relationships. Moreover, internal relationships are often in conflict with one another. This ties up even more of the person's psychic capital. Object representations in Fairbairn's system are therefore inherently maladaptive. They take up libidinal resources better employed elsewhere.

Kernberg

Like all object relations theorists, Kernberg (1976, 1987, 2004) begins with the premise that there are no drives without objects and that objects are always relational. Unlike other object relations theorists, however, Kernberg discusses the implications of this for the structure of the mind as conceived by classical psychoanalysis. Kernberg points out that if relational objects are at the core of psychic functioning, then the id must be more organized than classicists think and must contain repressed representations of drive-infused relationships. He terms these "repressed internalized object relations." That is, if wishes come complete with objects, primary process cannot be as free-ranging as classicists believe. Kernberg's work also makes use of Freud's (1938) observation that sometimes the deepest, most repressed id material achieves consciousness, even in nonpsychotic individuals. To explain this phenomenon, Freud hypothesized a process wherein the structural integrity of the ego could be compromised. Kernberg argued that such "splitting" of the ego indicates that the ego and the id are not as strongly differentiated as Freud thought.[6]

In concert with other object relations theorists, Kernberg believes that mental life begins with inborn propensities to relate and to form representations of relationships (object relations). The form these representations take depends upon the interaction of the person's relational experiences with her maturing organizational capabilities. At first, affectively powerful experiences are most salient to the infant (as opposed to the sensory-motor experiences favored by the classicists). The infant therefore begins his organizational efforts by structuring experiences around affect-laden gratifications and frustrations. Because this organization is affectively and not perceptually based, parallel representations can develop around the same object. As a result, the world becomes divided into two organized sets of representations. One set comes to be based on affectively positive whereas the other comes to be based on affectively negative relational experiences. Since the mother is the source of most important early interactions, these initial representations focus on her. As a result, the infant develops a conception of the "good" mother in parallel to an independent conception of the "bad" mother. At this point in development, the infant is not aware that the object of these feelings is one and the same person. As positive and negative affective experiences accumulate and cognitive skills mature, each set of representations begins to become more completely organized and structured. Gratifying, positive affective experiences, which are largely sensual and sexual, cohere into what classicists term libido. Frustrating, negative affective experiences, which are largely aggressive, cohere into the aggressive drive. Thus, in Kernberg's model, objects and their associated affect precede the development of drives.

As development continues, the child begins to integrate good and bad representations of important individuals. Similarly, greater recognition of what differentiates the self from others begins to develop. This allows for some integration of representations; a rudimentary sense of self (an I) and of others (not-I) begins to manifest itself. This integration of self and object representations constitutes Kernberg's understanding of the ego. The better the integration, the stronger the ego and the more differentiated it is from the less-well-organized id. The superego follows a similar course of development. It integrates idealized and sadistic/persecutory representations of parental figures. The more complete and coherent this integration, the less austere and the more realistic the superego is. At this point, the id is composed of all good and all bad self and object representations that the ego failed to integrate. If the environment provides no basis for integration (e.g., child has dangerous or depriving relational experiences), the individual will be prone to what Kernberg terms "splitting": rapid and profound mood changes that operate independently of one another (a prominent feature of borderline psychopathology). Thus, Kernberg has a unique position vis-à-vis repression, which he sees as a later-arriving defense. It takes place only if good and bad representations have been integrated without splitting.

Self Psychology and the Intersubjective Model of Atwood and Stolorow

Self psychology was the creation of Heinz Kohut (1971, 1977, 1980). His initial objective was to address what he perceived to be an insufficient emphasis on healthy narcissistic needs on the part of classical psychoanalysis (Kohut, 1971). However, he soon created an alternative school of psychoanalysis (Kohut, 1977). While he said virtually nothing about the unconscious, his followers (e.g., Shane & Shane, 1990) did. In addition, the intersubjective model of Stolorow and Atwood (Atwood & Stolorow, 1984; Stolorow & Atwood, 1989; Stolorow, Atwood, & Brandschaft, 1994; Stolorow, Brandschaft, & Atwood, 1987) was derived from self psychology and has a very explicit position on unconscious processes.

According to Kohut (1977), infants are born as psychologically as they are physically helpless. For Kohut, development revolves around the caregiver-assisted construction of a sense of self. The young infant is not yet well differentiated from his surroundings, and significant others are only experienced as objects whose function it is to satisfy and regulate needs (self objects). Responsive and attuned caregiving, characterized by mirroring and mutual idealization, will fulfill this purpose and therefore result in a positive self-image, healthy self-esteem, and thus a healthy self. The functions originally performed by self objects are ultimately internalized so that the child can regulate her own needs and self-esteem. If parents are chronically unempathic (they do not mirror and/or permit idealizations), self-esteem will continue to depend upon the use of external self objects and the self will remain underdeveloped. The result will be a disorder of the self, manifested in a continuing, inappropriate dependency upon need-fulfilling objects rather than intimacy with valued separate individuals. There will be no mutuality in relationships. Treatment of self disorders, then, requires the therapist to serve as a series of empathic self objects for the patient. In essence, the patient is to be re-parented.

Kohut says nothing about what is conscious and what is not, let alone what identifies and/or is unique to either. The closest he comes to any mention of consciousness is in his discussion of vertical versus horizontal splits. A vertical split refers to a mental content that is unconscious. That is, the person has no awareness of it at all. A horizontal split refers to a content that is disavowed. This has been called dissociation in other contexts and can be traced at least as far back as Janet (see Chapter 3). Another more explicit contribution self-psychology may have made to thinking about unconscious processes could be the suggestion that unconscious themes to a person's life are reflected in their fantasies (Shane & Shane, 1990). The person may be aware of these themes but fail to see their relevance in his life (the horizontal split). Importantly, Kohut (along with Sullivan; see, e.g., 1964) influenced Stolorow and Atwood in the development of their model, which has much to say about unconscious processes.

The intersubjective model of Stolorow and Atwood (Atwood & Stolorow, 1984; Stolorow & Atwood, 1989; Stolorow, Atwood, & Brandschaft, 1994; Stolorow, Brandschaft, & Atwood, 1987) avers that all psychological phenomena develop in an interpersonal context they term the "intersubjective matrix." This model postulates three kinds of unconscious processes: the prereflective, the dynamic, and the unvalidated. The prereflective unconscious incorporates the person's socially obtained but unexamined (therefore prereflective) assumptions or axioms concerning the functioning of the world. It constrains and shapes the understanding and interpretations the person makes about his surroundings like a kind of Piagetian meta-schema or an interpersonally based Kantian category. Since all information is open to interpretation, all experiences are affected by the prereflective unconscious. The existence of this type of functioning means that all experiences and perceptions are subjectively shaded and influenced by prevailing biases (a theme that will come up later in this book as we discuss normative unconscious processes). In short, the prereflective unconscious serves an organizing function just as the ego does in the classical and ego psychology views. Unlike any psychological structure posited by classical psychoanalysis or object relations theory, however, there is no conflict or pathology inherent in its functioning.

Although it is not inherently conflictual, the prereflective unconscious influences what can become conflictual. Consistent with Kohut's ideas, the infant's developing consciousness is articulated through the validating responsiveness of the interpersonal environment. The most critical experiences are those laden with affect, whatever their theme, because they are most open to interpretation and reflection (within the constraints of the prereflective unconscious). Failure to validate or affirm the developing child's affective experiences leads to construction of the other two kinds of unconscious. The infant wishes to express and integrate all of her affective experiences; however, when the infant's affective expression is ignored or rejected, the result can be a traumatic fear of severing the tie with a (perceived) disapproving parental figure. To stave this off, affect is severed (split off), and the dynamic unconscious is born. The dynamic unconscious houses these defensively walled-off affect states (as opposed to the drive derivatives and wishful fantasies of the classical ego model or the relationship configurations of object relations theory). Finally, affective expression need not be ignored or rejected to be denied expression. The environment may simply be depriving and not provide any opportunities for affective expression. Under such conditions, expression is not walled off; it simply never becomes articulated at all. Such poorly developed affective expressions comprise the unvalidated unconscious.

Therapeutic technique in this model is designed to affect all three types of unconscious. The prereflective unconscious is the most important, however, because it underlies the others. Most analytic work is therefore directed at illuminating its unquestioned assumptions. The dynamic unconscious is treated through analysis of its resistances, whereas articulation of heretofore undeveloped experiences serves to undo the deficits of the unvalidated unconscious. The boundary between what is conscious and what is unconscious is somewhat fuzzy in this model, depending upon the intersubjective context. Consciousness is a product of important others' responsiveness to and affirmation of different aspects of the person's experiences. Because all of psychological experience is said to take place in the context of and is fostered by interpersonal interaction, the therapist–patient relationship assumes primary importance in treatment.

Relational Psychoanalysis

Relational psychoanalysis also emphasizes relatedness as central to human functioning. All relational theorists (e.g., Aron, 1996; Benjamin, 1995; Hoffman, 1998; Mitchell, 1988, 1998; Stern, 1997) see unconscious processes as emerging from an interpersonal context.[7] Beyond this, relationists hold varying views on the structure and contents of the unconscious (see Bachant, Lynch, & Richards, 1995). The more radical of them (e.g., Mitchell, 1988) believe that no phenomenon—wish, drive, or fantasy—can be intrapsychic. Others (e.g., Greenberg, 1991; Ogden, 1992; Zeddies, 2000) adopt a more integrative approach, allowing for intrapsychic phenomena. But all relational theorists argue that the relational part of the unconscious is more important than any other aspect of the unconscious (or any other aspect of human functioning).

All relationists also stand united behind the idea that interpersonal transactions are necessary to the creation of both unconscious and conscious experience. They view the unconscious as nebulous and inchoate, referring to it as unformulated experience (Stern, 1997). It can take any number of shapes/meanings depending on the interaction in which the person is engaged. Unformulated experience, like the classical unconscious, precedes verbal organization and expression. In contrast to classical views, no features of unformulated experience are distinguishable in the absence of interpersonal interaction. Further, unlike both the classical (and object relational) unconscious, it is not brought to awareness through an interaction with the therapist but is actually created within that interaction (Stern, 1997).

Because the particular ways in which unformulated experience becomes organized are dependent on the interpersonal interaction, the goal of psychotherapy is to help formulate and structure this unconscious so as to integrate experiences, bodily sensations, perceptions, a sense of self, and a sense of others in an adaptive manner (Mitchell, 2000). The nature of this integration is not the logical connections usually associated with conscious thought; rather, it is based on using the interpersonal relationship in psychotherapy to link idiosyncratically organized imperceptible qualities, with no differentiation of or regard to time, place, and person, and bring them into awareness (Newirth, 2003). The idea is to literally construct the experience, thereby helping the unformulated (unconscious) to attain structure and meaning. Because any such interaction is unique, the created meaning is also unique to the interaction. This way of understanding unconscious processes is singular to the relational view.

The relational view of unconscious meaning, arising as a function of intersubjective processes, has major implications for relationists' view of clinical work. Conflict, instead of involving wishes, internalized objects, or self-esteem, is generally between relational configurations. For instance, one may have experiences of unacceptable object-related fantasies/wishes or even incompatible self-experiences with another (i.e., feeling both demeaned and empowered in relation to an abusive caregiver), but conflict is never strictly intrapersonal. This has much in common with the intersubjective and object relations conceptions of the unconscious. The unformulated unconscious departs from the object relations view of the unconscious, however, in that the relational unconscious is vague and amorphous, not an internalized object with an inherent form and meaning.

The relationists also do not strongly differentiate between conscious and unconscious phenomena; they see the boundaries between the two as fluid (Zeddies, 2000). Similarly to the intersubjective model (and unlike classical psychoanalysis), what is conscious and what is unconscious depends upon interpersonal interactions at a particular moment in time. Additionally, to use another favorite relationist term, meaning has to be co-constructed (or co-created; see Aron, 1991; Mitchell, 1988). According to Zeddies, it is the presence of another that makes it possible to turn one's attention to the unformulated and to loosen the boundary between the unconscious and the conscious. Zeddies does not see this boundary as predetermined by early experiences (and defense) but as a fluid process that reflects contingencies in the immediate intersubjective space—the "relational matrix," to use Mitchell's (1988) term. The interactional exchange between patient and therapist determines what unformulated experience will be brought into focus and how it will be imbued with meaning.

The relational view has implications for transference and countertransference as well. No longer is either process seen as a distortion of reality (see Gill, 1982). Since the unformulated relational unconscious is co-constructed, as opposed to given or intrapersonal, it is also co-constructed in therapy between patient and therapist in the here and now. Transference, in the sense that classicists conceive of it, does not exist. If we give shape to unformulated experience in a co-constructing relationship, the patient cannot superimpose ("transfer") already formed unconscious material onto the therapist. Although patient and therapist's perceptions of each other are still considered valuable, they are thought of as a means of examining their mutual impact on each other rather than a one-directional dynamic (Hadley, 2008). The focus is on the dyad, not on the inner workings of each individual within it.

Relationists also provide a novel view of defensive functioning. Stern (1983) challenges the idea that any lack of knowledge or clarity is inherently due to the operation of defense or distortion. Unformulated experience, relationists claim, has never been articulated clearly enough to be defended against in the classical sense. Instead, the relational view of defense involves not attending to the unformulated experience. This line of thinking strongly emphasizes dissociation. Bromberg (1998, 2006, 2011) has written extensively about splitting off experiences, which, due to the impact of early interactions, cannot be integrated into the patient's experience of the self.[8] Classical defenses like repression have not been entirely eliminated (e.g., Zeddies, 2000, talks about repressed material) but, like intrapsychic phenomena, they are not centrally important.

THE PSYCHOANALYTIC MODELS COMPARED

Psychoanalysis offers an embarrassment of riches concerning unconscious processes. Scientific testing of the various psychoanalytic tenets is sorely needed (Grünbaum, 1984).[9] Despite variations, outright disagreements, and a dearth of discriminatory studies, all models converge on certain points (see Westen, 1998). First, all psychoanalytic approaches stress the importance of unconscious processes in human functioning. Next, the unconscious processes of all the models are affectively charged, nonrational, poorly integrated into the personality, and formed under the crucial impact of early experiences. This means that many (perhaps most) of the springs of our behavior are unknown to us. There are also points of convergence concerning fantasy. Classicists, ego psychologists, and object relationists emphasize the central role of unconscious fantasies in the organization of the mind. Fantasies, composed of representations and the connections between them, are the templates through which experiences are understood and organized. Self psychologists, at least as represented by Shane and Shane 1993), have followed suit and added global fantasies, which represent the major themes of our lives. The position of the intersubjective model is unclear on this point but does not seem to contradict it. For the more interpersonal models (as well as less extreme relationists), these fantasies and representations center around relationships. Whatever their theme, fantasies and representations are invariably affectively charged and can bias the interpretation of even perceptual events.

There are also some changes in psychoanalytic precepts, from those originally outlined by Freud, that seem to be accepted today. No one advocates a pure primary process anymore. This is manifested either in the form of a mixture of primary and secondary process or in terms of desires always having objects. Free-floating desire, unorganized, and infinitely malleable, is no more. This is not an innocuous change. It goes to the heart of what it means to be unintegrated and/or poorly organized. Nothing has been substituted for primary process in object relations conceptions. The intersubjective concept of the unvalidated unconscious and the relational concept of unformulated experience represent an effort to replace primary process with an alternative conception: unintegrated material. This retains some of the capacity of primary process to be malleable and capable of taking on multiple forms. It differs in that the form is always relational and so is the means for creating it. However, the qualitative differences between conscious and unconscious remain vague in both conceptions.

Finally, all psychoanalytic models agree on the techniques that therapists should employ to help overcome patients' unconsciously motivated problems (see Josephs, 1995). Empathic understanding and clinical interpretations are emphasized, to various degrees, in all psychoanalytic approaches. The models differ enormously in their emphasis on one or the other, in their understanding of why these methods work, in how to interpret, and in what ought to be interpreted. However, all agree that unconscious processes can be influenced and integrated through these means. All also agree on the importance of the therapeutic relationship, albeit for different reasons.

As stated earlier, psychoanalysts have generally not offered empirical evidence in support of any of their conceptions. Instead, they have presented clinical case studies and have debated their meaning. But they have created a rich body of hypotheses potentially open to test and contrast. Their work can be said to be rich in what Reichenbach (1938/2006) termed the "context of discovery." Some empirical work has tried to test psychoanalytic tenets (Reichenbach's context of justification). Many early studies on unconscious processes focused on psychoanalytic tenets. We now turn to these early studies.

NOTES

1. Interpolating invisible, hypothetical events or hypothesizing unobservable phenomena to serve as explanatory bridges between observable events is a common practice of science. In physics, we read of subatomic particles and that light is both a wave and a particle. No one has ever seen a subatomic particle (or an atom for that matter) or observed a photon. What we do see are effects that can be explained through use of these constructs. Belief in these hypothesized phenomena rests on their explanatory and predictive power. So it is with Freud's (or anyone else's) conceptions of unconscious processes. To the extent that they clarify and are predictive of psychological phenomena, they are useful. To the extent that they fail in these efforts, they ought to be discarded.

2. One way to conceptualize this is to think of the conscious system as the RAM in a computer, what the computer is doing at the moment, and the preconscious as the hard drive, what the computer can call up when needed. This analogy breaks down for the unconscious, however. There is nothing in computer hardware or software that is comparable.

3. Late in this book, we discuss embodied cognition and the work of Lakoff that also understands the mind in terms of metaphor (Lakoff, 2012, 2014; Lakoff & Johnson, 1980a, 1980b).

4. Freud may have been on to something because, as we will later see, social cognitive theorists came to a similar, messy solution by moving away from a simple dichotomy between automatic and controlled processes to conceptualizing many levels of automaticity (Bargh, 1989; Bargh & Ferguson, 2000). The data will also lead us to conclude that all processes are a mix of conscious and unconscious processes.

5. Later in this book, we review a research program innovated by David McClelland (1985) that assesses the centrality of motivated unconscious fantasy on behavior. We also examine a psychoanalytically inspired research program that investigated affectively charged fantasies (Silverman, 1976; Weinberger & Silverman, 1987; Weinberger & Smith, 2011).

6. This idea is central to Kernberg's (1975; Kernberg, Yeomans, Clarkin, & Levy, 2008) understanding and treatment of borderline psychopathology, which probably constitutes his best-known contribution to psychoanalysis and the broader field of clinical psychology.

7. This movement is similar to a much older sociological/social psychological viewpoint, innovated by Charles Horton Cooley (1902) and George Herbert Mead (1934), and which was subsequently termed "symbolic interactionism" (Blumer, 1969). The basic premise, as with relational psychoanalysis, was that the self is a social product and cannot be divorced from social interaction.

8. Janet offered a very similar view. See earlier review of Janet, in Chapter 3.

9. There are many who argue that psychoanalysis is inherently unscientific. Some claim it is hopelessly muddled and unprovable (e.g., Popper, 1962; Eysenck, 1963). If we take this argument seriously, the whole enterprise ought to be dispensed with. And Eysenck said exactly that. Others say psychoanalysis is a hermeneutic discipline to be studied as one studies literature. It cannot (and ought not to) be subjected to scientific scrutiny. Exegesis and narrative coherence are better tools with which to study human experiences in this view (see, e.g., Habermas, 1972; Ricouer, 1970; Schafer, 1980). See Grünbaum (1984) and Eagle (1983) for ripostes to these arguments.

PART II

EMPIRICAL APPROACHES
TO THE UNCONSCIOUS

Part I documented the historical reasons behind the resistance to studying or even admitting to unconscious processes. Exceptions to this denial were the Romantics, the philosophers of nature, and those who practiced dynamic psychiatry. The only sustained effort to study unconscious processes was psychoanalysis, which tended to neglect empirical methods and was not generally included in the academy. So unconscious processes were not held in high regard when psychology, the discipline, began and developed. In this section, we briefly discuss early empirical attempts to actually study unconscious processes. These include the word association test, recovery of unnoticed and subliminal stimuli begun by the Viennese physician Poetzl, and the prescient work of Bartlett on memory. These were generally scattershot.

The mid-20th century saw a decade-long sustained effort to study unconscious processes termed the "New Look" (see Dixon, 1971, 1981). This work began when Bruner and Postman (1947), inspired by Bartlett's work, tried to demonstrate that perception was as affected by internal psychological variables as by the external stimulus. The research took off and even acquired a psychodynamic/clinical flavor. For over a decade, it seemed that unconscious processes might become central to academic psychological research. But it all came crashing down under the weight of methodological critiques and a hostile zeitgeist. There was a brief burst of research innovated by Spence on the restricting effects of consciousness/awareness, but it too died out. One stream we review remains. It is called subliminal psychodynamic activation and was innovated by Silverman to test dynamic psychoanalytic hypotheses via subliminal priming. It is still with us, but for the most part this avenue of research has closed down.

Nonetheless, the seeds had been sown. Work on what was termed the "cocktail party phenomenon" and on shadowing (consciously following one stream of information while not attending to a second parallel stream) resulted in the insight that what we are conscious of does not exhaust the information we process. Instead, we seem to be processing information that we are not attending to (i.e., unconsciously). This led to attention theories, which posited filters on incoming information that chose what to be conscious of and what to ignore. Attention theories led to the cognitive revolution, which, in turn, resulted in a new emphasis on internal processes.

Another barrier to accepting the existence and importance of unconscious processes was overcome by four related and roughly contemporaneous areas of study in psychology. These were implicit memory (Schacter, 1987), implicit learning (Seger, 1994), automaticity (Shiffrin & Schneider, 1977), and the study of brain-damaged individuals like those with so-called split brains (Gazzaniga, 1970) and blindsight (Weiskrantz, 1986). All of these areas embedded unconscious processes into their core theoretical structures, elevating them to normative status. The brain damage research explicitly did so by positing modules for explaining one's own behavior (Gazzaniga, 1999) and for the self (Kurzban & Aktipis, 2007), neither of which has any special access to the causes of the behavior they are tasked with explaining.

One paper, authored by Nisbett and Wilson (1977), deserves special mention. These authors reinterpreted classical social psychological phenomena like cognitive dissonance and bystander intervention as requiring the postulation of unconscious processes. They argued that people do not have privileged access to the determinants of their behavior and that unconsciousness should be the default assumption, with awareness having to be proved. This turned the zeitgeist on its head and radically changed the conversation in psychology.

The weight of theory and data finally forced the acceptance and investigation of unconscious processes. Kihlstrom (1987) published a paper in the journal *Science* on the cognitive unconscious, Uleman and Bargh (1989) edited a book on the relevant research, and Bornstein and Pittman (1992) edited a volume of papers from a conference they hosted that summarized research on unconscious processes from different areas. After centuries, the unconscious had been rediscovered and gone mainstream. The zeitgeist had shifted to one supportive of unconscious processes.

CHAPTER 5

The Beginnings of Experimental Work on Unconscious Processes

Experimental work on unconscious processes probably began with the word-association test invented by Galton (1907) in the mid- to late 19th century. Galton thought he could use this test to explore the hidden recesses of the mind (Ellenberger, 1970). The test was next picked up by Wilhelm Wundt, who employed it to investigate the laws of association of ideas. He improved upon it methodologically by standardizing presentation condition. The test next passed to psychiatry. Aschaffenburg and Kraeplin classified responses into what they termed "inner" (i.e., based on the meaning of the word) and "outer" (i.e., having to do with sound and speech—structural—properties of the word) associations. Ziehen found that negatively toned associations tended to cluster around common underlying themes, which he termed "complexes."

Bleuler, who believed that schizophrenia was characterized by a loosening of associations, thought that the word association test would be a good way to test this hypothesis. He assigned Carl Jung to the job. Jung (1906/1969) was particularly interested in further investigating the complexes discovered by Ziehen. Among the numerous findings reported by Jung and his collaborators were that complexes need not be negative, that members of the same family showed similar associations, and that the sexes demonstrated different patterns of complexes. Jung concluded that the mind was composed of unconscious, emotionally toned ideational complexes. This notion became a cornerstone of his later theory of the mind. Jung eventually (Jung, 1928) became disillusioned with experimental work and abandoned his investigations into the word association test. The rest of psychology followed suit. For reasons that are unclear to us, the use of the word-association test virtually disappeared from the armamentarium of experimental psychology.

One area of research that has faded in and out of favor but has never entirely disappeared from experimental psychology is the study of subliminal effects. The term "subliminal" derives from early classical psychophysics, which defined the limen as the stimulus threshold below which perception is impossible or the point at which differences between two stimuli are undetectable. Subliminal means below the limen (i.e., less than detectable). The first subliminal study was probably conducted by Peirce and Jastrow (1884), who were interested in finding out what would happen if differences between stimuli were reduced below the limen. They served as their own subjects and discovered that they could guess which stimulus was objectively heavier or brighter even when they subjectively reported that they seemed identical. Fullerton and Cattell (1892) replicated the findings. Other early work on subliminal perception focused on Freudian notions of unconscious processes. The earliest and best known such work was conducted by Poetzl (see Ionescu and Erdelyi, 1992). Poetzl was a Viennese professor of neurology and psychiatry who examined many gunshot wounds to the occipital cortex of World War I veterans. Some of his subjects could not see a stimulus presented centrally. Later, however, fragments of the apparently unseen stimuli entered consciousness in combination with ongoing peripheral perception. To Poetzl, this seemed like the condensation Freud said took place in dreams.

Poetzl's next step was to see whether he could obtain analogous effects in the dreams of individuals with undamaged brains. His subjects were unable to remember or reproduce a subliminally presented landscape scene. However, when Poetzl told them to have a dream that night, come back the next day, and draw elements of their dream, aspects of the landscape scene emerged in the postdream drawing. Subsequent experiments used different pictures but obtained similar results.[1] Poetzl's results were expanded upon by others, who obtained recovery in waking free associations (Allers & Teler, 1924/1960). Malamud and Linder (1931) reported that the recovered material often seemed related to subjects' conflicts. A later series of elegant studies by Erdelyi, to be reviewed later (see Ionescu & Erdelyi, 1992), shed further light on the Poetzl phenomenon and on memory recovery generally (Erdelyi calls it "hypermnesia").

Finally, there is the remarkable and prescient work of Bartlett (1932), who argued that memories and perception (phenomena abjured by behaviorists) were constructed affairs involving lawful cognitive processes (also prohibited by behaviorists). Bartlett had his subjects memorize narrative material. He then asked them to recall it on several occasions over extended periods of time. The memories of the stories changed in line with subjects' preexisting cognitive schemas. Bartlett thereby demonstrated that memories were not passive copies of events but active constructions of them.

THE NEW LOOK

The studies reviewed to this point were few and far between. The late 1940s and early 1950s, however, witnessed a sustained series of studies on unconscious processes (see Dixon, 1971). Many of these investigations employed subliminal presentations. Because this research directly challenged behaviorism, it had a revolutionary flavor. The work as a whole came to be called the New Look and became one of the most controversial areas of research in the history of experimental psychology. Studies burgeoned throughout the 1950s. The momentum could not be sustained in the face of constant resistance from the zeitgeist, however, and the research came to a virtual halt in the early 1960s. Nonetheless, New Look research is a watershed in the history of the study of unconscious processes.

It all began when Bruner and Postman (1947) wished to demonstrate that perception is not entirely controlled by stimulus parameters, as the received wisdom of the time averred, but is also affected by internal psychological variables as Bartlett had argued. This new way of conceptualizing perception led to the play on words "New Look"; coupled with a Parisian haute couture fashion influence at the time, the name took hold. To experimentally make their point, Bruner and Postman assessed the associative latency to a series of words (interestingly, they did not record the associations). They then chose words with short, middle, and long associative response times and presented them, via a tachistoscope, in a recognition threshold task. Recognition thresholds turned out to be uncorrelated with the previously determined associative response times. Instead, words that produced the longest associative latencies had either very high or very low recognition thresholds. This was presumed to be related to the emotional loading of those stimulus words. High threshold was termed perceptual defense; low threshold was labeled perceptual vigilance. Shortly thereafter, Postman and Bruner (1948) found that stressing subjects (by harassing them) during the recognition task led to even higher thresholds. This was seen as further support of the emotionality hypothesis. In a follow-up study, Postman, Bruner, and McGinnies (1948) demonstrated that the recognition threshold also depended upon the subject's hierarchy of values. Words related to subjects' values had lower thresholds (perceptual vigilance) than words unrelated to those values.[2]

Studies demonstrating perceptual defense, as this area of research was now called, began to appear with increasing regularity. Various studies demonstrated perceptual defense for red spade playing cards (Bruner & Postman, 1949) and for reversed letters (Postman, Bruner, & Walk, 1951). Postman and Solomon (1950) examined the classic Zeigarnik effect (people have better recall for uncompleted over completed tasks) and obtained both defense and vigilance for uncompleted tasks. Perceptual defense and vigilance seemed to be everywhere, but there was often no compelling theoretical reason for predicting one over the other. They simply appeared and were then said to have been found. This type of difficulty led Hochberg and Gleitman (1949) to aver that perceptual defense effects were ad hoc. If two comparison groups were unequal, one had to be higher, which was then adduced as proof of the phenomenon. Postman (1953), recognizing the cogency of this argument and the meaninglessness of studies that ignored it, proposed a sensible solution. Researchers were enjoined to make and justify predictions before conducting their experiments. For the most part, this advice was followed. Thus, Stein (1953) as well as Carpenter, Wiener, and Carpenter (1956) classified their subjects as sensitizers or defenders and obtained threshold effects in accord with those classifications.

It was a short step from studying values and using terms like defense to efforts to operationalize Freudian-type defenses. This step was soon taken by McGinnies (1949), and it set off an acrimonious debate in the literature. McGinnies presented taboo and nontaboo words to subjects in the usual recognition threshold task. He also assessed GSR (galvanic skin response, a measure of palmar sweating, usually thought to index affective arousal). He found that thresholds were higher for taboo than for nontaboo words and that the GSRs for prerecognition guesses of taboo words were higher than for nontaboo words. This set off a wave of studies and critiques because it seemed to imply an experimental demonstration of repression. That is, the taboo words were unconsciously recognized and arousing, as indexed by GSR, but not consciously available. In fact, they were harder to recognize than nontaboo words, even though people were obviously reacting to and being aroused by them.

Howes and Solomon (1950) argued that McGinnies's results were artifactual in two respects. First, they asserted that the taboo words appeared less frequently in language than the nontaboo words and were therefore more difficult to recognize. What no one pointed out until decades later (Erdelyi, 1974), however, was that the reference works Howes and Solomon used were created to help teachers determine what words to teach to children and when. That taboo words were rare in such venues is hardly surprising but says little about their scarcity in everyday speech. They may have been infrequent in the 1940s and 1950s. But that would mean that those times were radically different from our own.

In response, McGinnies (1950) more stringently controlled for frequency and still obtained defense effects. Other studies also obtained similar results when controlling for word frequency (Chapman & Feather, 1972; McGinnies & Sherman, 1952; Sales & Haber, 1968). On the other hand, McGinnies, Comer, and Lacey (1952) found that word length influenced recognition threshold. It appears, therefore, that although word frequency (and length) may not be irrelevant, they do not provide a complete account of perceptual defense effects. Such effects can still be obtained when appropriate controls are in place.

The second criticism Howes and Solomon leveled at the McGinnies study is more problematic. They suggested that subjects may have recognized taboo and neutral words equally well but that they were uncomfortable saying taboo words out loud in front of an authority figure like an experimenter. Before they utter a taboo word, they want to be absolutely certain that they have seen it. Thus, they require a longer exposure time.

With one exception, no one thought to ask the subjects in these studies if they had inhibited their responses. But it was the age of behaviorism, and subjective responses were suspect. In the one study we found where subjects were asked about suppression, Kissin, Gottesfeld, and Dikes (1957) found that inhibited subjects who displayed perceptual defense against sexual words reported consciously suppressing their responses. Moreover, Whittaker, Gilchrist, and Fischer (1952) obtained perceptual defense effects for the "N" word only when the experimenter was black. These studies favor the response suppression explanation of defense effects.

On the other side of the ledger, Zigler and Yospe (1960) presented a clearly visible word to their subjects followed by a recognition threshold task for a second word. When the first clearly visible word was taboo, subjects evinced a higher threshold for the second word even though it was neutral. The authors argued that there was no reason to suppress reports of the second word, yet it was defended against. Of course, it is simply possible that subjects were so distracted or made anxious by the first taboo word that they did not attend strongly to the second. Recall that Postman and Bruner (1948) found that stressing subjects raised recognition thresholds. If the results can be explained in this way, they have nothing to say about response suppression. However, in two other studies (Krauss & Ruiz, 1968; Zigler & Yospe, 1960), subjects still had higher thresholds for taboo words, even though they did not have to say them.

The results, in total, indicate that response suppression is a genuine phenomenon, but the data also show that it cannot fully account for perceptual defense effects. Other similar criticisms, involving subject expectations (Howie, 1952; Luchins, 1950) were also disputed and ultimately found insufficient to account for perceptual defense and vigilance.

Some critics resorted to logical argument to dispute the reality of perceptual defense effects. The argument went something like this: Perceptual defense as prevention of perception of a stimulus is a logical impossibility. A person cannot erect a defense against a particular stimulus unless he has first perceived it. Thus, the perceptual defense position involves what philosophers have termed a "category mistake"; it involves claiming that perception is both a process of knowing and a process of avoiding knowing (see e.g., Howie, 1952; Luchins, 1950). The flaw in this argument, as pointed out by Erdelyi (1974), is that it assumes that perception is a unitary, serial process. If we assume instead that multiple processes can occur simultaneously and at different rates, the problem evaporates. One process may be responsible for the defense, which then prevents the process charged with recognition from reaching fruition. Information-processing models, not available at the time these criticisms were made, assume exactly such processes. So do even more recent computational neuroscience models. We review these later. At the time, such arguments failed to check research because it seemed that perceptual defense was a real phenomenon and the various artifacts proposed to account for it could not explain it away. To say that it could not exist when there were data to the contrary could not stem the research effort.

The 1950s witnessed a veritable explosion of New Look studies. They filled the journals throughout this decade. Many were inspired by clinical lore and had clear implications for understanding psychopathology. Lazarus, Eriksen, and Fonda (1951) reported that patients judged by their therapists to employ the defenses of denial and repression evinced perceptual defense, whereas those said to employ intellectualization and counterphobic defenses showed perceptual vigilance. Eriksen (1951) reported that paranoid individuals showed perceptual vigilance for hostile words as compared to other words. He also obtained vigilance effects for aggressive pictures from subjects who wrote aggressive Thematic Apperception Test (TAT) stories. McGinnies and Adornetto (1952) obtained perceptual defense effects to sexual words in both schizophrenics and normals. Lindner (1953) reported that sexual offenders showed more perceptual vigilance to sexual pictures than to other pictures. Kurland (1954) reported perceptual vigilance for emotional words in hysterical and obsessive individuals when compared to normals. Greenbaum (1956) showed that highly anxious, as compared to low-anxiety individuals, evidenced perceptual vigilance for hostile faces. There were many other such demonstrations. Over 1,000 studies appeared in the literature during this period. For a review, see Brown (1961). Part of this mass of empirical work was a reaction to the constant criticism of positive findings. A search for viable artifacts continued unabated. If frequency, expectation, and response suppression could not account individually for the findings, perhaps in various combinations they could. Thus Davids (1956) argued that defense effects were a function of personal relevance rather than frequency per se. But since that was the point, this criticism did not get much mileage. Everything except unconscious defense was called upon to account for the phenomenon. Among other things, this had two effects. First, it sharpened the methodology. But, second, it kept attention focused on proving the authenticity of the phenomenon so that explaining it or moving on to test its implications rarely occurred. The former effect was salutary; the latter led to stagnation because experiments were endlessly repeated with new and more intricate methodological refinements.

However, not all of the work revolved around explaining away or demonstrating the existence of perceptual defense. There were also those who accepted the reality of the phenomenon and tried to explain how it could operate. The best of these efforts was probably that of Blum (1954). He proposed that threatening stimuli were quickly and unconsciously identified, triggering defensive processes before these stimuli were consciously recognized. That is, he proposed an early warning system that could trigger defense. This was closely akin to Freud's (1900, 1915) notion of a censor. Blum's model predicted that subjects ought to be more sensitive to threatening stimuli when they were very much below the conscious recognition threshold. The person would then be forewarned and on the alert (vigilant). Right around the recognition threshold, defense mechanisms would come into play, as the person was now in danger of becoming aware of the threat. This would then raise the recognition threshold (perceptual defense).

Blum empirically demonstrated that subliminally presented anxiety-inducing stimuli were reported to "stand out" more than neutral ones, even though subjects could not identify them. That is, accuracy was significantly below "stand-out" frequency (vigilance). Additionally, the recognition threshold for these anxiety-provoking stimuli was higher than it was for the neutral stimuli to which they were compared. Thus, as predicted, anxiety-provoking stimuli elicited a reaction (stand out) but were more difficult to recognize (higher recognition threshold) than neutral stimuli.

Several similar interpretations of perceptual defense (e.g., Byrne, 1959; Lazarus, 1956; Osgood, Suci, & Tannenbaum, 1957) appeared in the literature. These models all posited two interacting systems. One conducts some kind of unconscious analysis of stimulation. The models differ on the sophistication and outcome of this analysis. In some, the unconscious system analyzes meaning; in others, it only engages in gross discriminations of threat. In either case, it must somehow communicate the results of its analyses to a second, awareness-mediating, system.

There were now the beginnings of a coherent, if not yet fully formed, model of perceptual defense.[3] There were data that supported it and it fit in with clinical lore. It also could account, in a sensible and relatively parsimonious way, for all of the perceptual defense effects filling the literature. Attacks on the validity of perceptual defense, in contrast, seemed ad hoc. Variables such as frequency, suppression, expectation, and the like were important, but many studies obtained effects with them controlled for and there was no consistent unifying theme to them. For a while, there was significant support for the perceptual defense models. Even Eriksen (1954), who was to become a chief critic of perceptual defense and arguably the single person most responsible for putting an end to New Look research (see Eriksen, 1959, 1960), wrote that perceptual defense was a genuine phenomenon and subscribed to Blum's understanding of it. Alas, this was not to last.

The unifying theme for those opposed to the defense interpretation of New Look studies was provided by a major advance in psychophysics in the 1950s: signal detection theory (SDT). This struck at the heart of a sensory understanding of New Look effects. SDT declared that there was no such thing as a perceptual awareness threshold, no limen. As a result, all findings that depended upon stimuli presented below some awareness threshold or limen were now in question. These results were now said to be due to operant response variables; they were not sensory effects.

SIGNAL DETECTION THEORY

SDT was developed by Tanner and Swets (Swets, Tanner, & Birdsall, 1955; Swets, Tanner, & Birdsall, 1961; Tanner, 1955; Tanner & Swets, 1954) in response to problems presented by radar, telephone, and radio communication. Its tenets posed a major challenge to classical psychophysics and soon superseded it. In contrast to the classical view, SDT holds that there is no threshold or sensory cut-off point (limen). Instead, receipt of information is continuous, and no stimulus can be out of awareness in any absolute sense.

In the SDT model of perception, there is always some nervous system activity, regardless of the level of external stimulation. SDT calls this activity "noise" and argues that it forms a background to all nervous system responsivity to external stimulation, which is termed "signal." Since noise is always present, a signal adds a certain amount of neural activation to that noise. The charge in a threshold task is to determine whether a presentation belongs to the noise or to the signal-plus-noise distribution. The more energy in the signal, the more neural activation is increased and the easier it is for the receiver to differentiate the signal and noise from the noise-only distribution.

When the noise and signal-plus-noise activations are not that different, SDT assumes that the receiver sets some sort of neural activation cut-off point. This cut-off is a function of signal strength relative to noise (the only factor really considered by classical psychophysics), expectations, and the pay-offs for responding one way or another. Any stimulation exceeding that cut-off is responded to as if it contained the signal. Stimulation below that cut-off is treated as noise. If the receiver chooses a low cut-off, he will correctly identify more signals but also more often misidentify noise as a signal. If he chooses a high cut-off point, he will less frequently mistakenly guess signal present but will more often miss signals that are present. Since the cut-off that individuals choose depends upon many factors unrelated to stimulus energy, a stimulus-present or -absent response does not really mean that a person did or did not perceive the stimulus; it means that he prefers the decision that the stimulus was present or absent on the basis of several sources of information, only one of which is sensory energy.[4]

With this new understanding, all prior methodological criticisms of perceptual defense could be gathered under one roof. They all boil down to response bias. And no single one is critical. Word frequency, suppression, and expectation are all possible manifestations of response bias. Perceptual defense is no longer a sensory phenomenon but is a consequence of learned responses (see, e.g., Tanner, 1955). As this interpretation fit in with the behavioral paradigm of the time, it was generally welcomed and accepted. And indeed, there were some data that supported the SDT understanding of threshold and posed problems for perceptual defense (e.g., Tanner & Swets, 1954).

The oft-reported greater accuracy of forced-choice responses over assertions of phenomenal presence or absence were now adduced as supportive of SDT tenets. In fact, forced-choice seemed to have been granted some sort of privileged status as a true measure of awareness in SDT; it was seen as relatively immune to response bias (Birdsall, 1955). Thus forced-choice was deemed the preferred measure of awareness. The main thrust of SDT as far as the New Look was concerned was the claim that the effects obtained were *invariably* responsive. And it is on the truth or falsity of this assertion that SDT-based criticisms of the New Look rest. So the major question is: Are the obtained findings driven by preconscious psychological effects on the percept itself? Or are the findings always due to the way subjects choose to respond to their conscious perceptual experiences? If the former, defense interpretations make sense. If the latter, SDT would hold sway and the whole notion of perceptual defense could be jettisoned. Subliminal would then be redefined as simply not reported. Eriksen (1958) declared this to be the ultimate issue in the field. To truly test this question, the two possibilities must be present in the same experiment so that one could prevail at the expense of the other.

Several studies tried to make this comparison. Natsoulas (1965) provided a relatively comprehensive review of them. Dixon (1971) offered a less detailed summary. All of the studies reviewed involved comparing stimulus present with stimulus absent conditions, with the latter serving as an assessment of response bias (ß). If there proved to be no difference between the two groups, this was considered evidence for response and against sensory effects. If the two groups differed, sensory effects were considered likely. The results were mixed. It appears that both response and sensory effects may be operating. The most conservative conclusion that could be drawn on the basis of these studies is that the question of whether New Look effects are sensory or responsive in nature is moot.

SUBCEPTION

Another series of New Look studies was held to demonstrate subthreshold perception and so came to be termed "subception." They were related to perceptual defense in that they attempted to demonstrate the existence of emotional indicators of perception in the absence of verbal reports of awareness. They were inspired by McGinnies's (1949) finding that GSR could discriminate taboo words from neutral words when verbal report could not. Thus, both perceptual defense and subception had the same parent. Studies showed all sorts of conditioning of physiological responses to subliminal stimuli (e.g., pupillary responses and light: Baker, 1938; salivation and words: Razran, 1949; nonsense syllables and GSR: Lazarus & McCleary, 1951). The paradigm employed in these subception studies seemed robust with respect to the usual methodological critiques leveled at perceptual defense studies. As a result, they appeared to provide strong supportive evidence for the existence of unconscious processes.

It seemed therefore that perception without awareness had been clearly demonstrated. Alas, this was not to be, as a new set of potential methodological inadequacies were soon uncovered and debated. These revolved around response issues just like the SDT critiques of perceptual defense.

Howes (1954) pointed out that verbal reports were dichotomous whereas GSR was continuous. This means that there is no opportunity to signal uncertainty or partial information in verbal reports, whereas these could be communicated via GSRs.

The most telling critiques of the subception effect were expressed in a series of elegant experiments conducted by Eriksen. Eriksen (1956) picked up on Howes's idea that GSR can communicate more information than dichotomous verbal responses. He devised a control group that enabled subjects to communicate levels of uncertainty verbally and found that the subception effect was weaker in this second group, presumably because subjects had been presented with more options.

Eriksen went further and offered his own interpretation of the subception effect, which he termed the multiple concurrent response model. He found that GSR and verbal responses were imperfectly correlated with each other, as well as with stimulus discrimination. Therefore, he argued, verbal response and GSR are, at least partially, parallel systems. It is not that GSR is superior or more sensitive to stimulation or that affect is unconscious whereas verbal report is conscious. It is simply that the two are differentially related to correct discrimination. Any two response systems should therefore show subception because one could be correct when the other is wrong.

Eriksen (1957) tried to flesh out these implications by adding a third response system—a voluntary motor response. This paradigm was designed to show that neither an affective nor an involuntary response was necessary for obtaining the subception effect. The data supported his hypothesis. The three response modes were independently related to correct discrimination. That is, when Eriksen entered all three into a regression equation, significantly more variance was accounted for than any individual or pair of response modes could explain. Further, because the voluntary motor response was shown to be effective, the idea that affect and/or involuntary (unconscious) responding was somehow critical to subception was disproved. Finally, the idea that nonverbal judgment was superior to conscious verbal discrimination was also not supported. If anything, he found that the verbal response was superior. Moreover, he was able to replicate these results (Eriksen, 1959; Dulany & Eriksen, 1959). These studies and others, as well as Eriksen's meticulous reasoning, are contained in two review papers (Eriksen, 1959, 1960). They are deservedly classics and well worth reading by anyone interested in the New Look.

At the time, Eriksen seemed to have definitively debunked the unconscious perception interpretation of subception. If, however, we examine Eriksen's findings more closely, we see that this is not necessarily the case. Eriksen certainly demonstrated that different response systems are differentially and somewhat independently related to stimulus detection. But does this necessarily imply that all are imperfect indicators of a single perceptual process? And further, does it necessarily imply that they are all imperfect indicators of awareness? And if verbal responding is at least as sensitive to stimulation as any other response indicator, does this obviate the possibility of unconscious responding? These are all assumptions that Eriksen made.

At the time Eriksen wrote, psychologists believed in a single, serial perceptual process. Unconscious detection, if it existed, would have to occur early in this series and should therefore be more sensitive to subliminal stimulation than conscious detection, which should occur later in the same process. This was implied even in models proposed by such advocates of unconscious processing as Blum (1954). Eriksen clearly showed that so-called unconscious indicators (e.g., GSR, lever positioning) were no more sensitive and, for the most part, less sensitive than so-called conscious indicators (forced choice, phenomenal report of presence or absence). Eriksen therefore felt comfortable dismissing what he and other critics termed a "super-sensitive" unconscious.

Nowadays, no one believes in a single, serial perceptual process. Psychologists now hypothesize multiple parallel processes underlying perception (i.e., computational models; see, e.g., Sun, 2008). But even earlier than this, psychologists began to conceive of simultaneous parallel processes. The notion came into being with the rise of information-processing theories of perception (see Erdelyi, 1974, and Shevrin & Dickman, 1980). The assumption that unconscious processes have to be more sensitive than conscious processing is therefore no longer necessary. Nor is it necessary to assume that unconscious events must precede conscious events. This aspect of Eriksen's argument has therefore been overtaken by current developments and is outdated. Dixon (1971) and Erdelyi (1974) made these points decades ago.

Eriksen cannot be held accountable for his lack of prescience. He worked within the models available to him at the time. But there is another flaw in the arguments he and other critics of the New Look put forth that can be critiqued even from within their perspective. There is an apparent confusion throughout this literature between detection or discrimination and awareness.[5] Just because a person can detect a stimulus, it does not necessarily follow that she was aware of it. A thermostat can detect changes in temperature; few would attribute awareness to thermostats (but see Chalmers, 1996). Even forced choice, the sine qua non of consciousness for SDT advocates, does not have to be entirely due to awareness of stimulation. Recall that from early studies on (e.g.,

Pierce & Jastrow, 1884; Sidis, 1902), subjects insisted that they were only guessing when asked about how they made their choices. They routinely expressed zero confidence in their "guesses." Further, they frequently expressed surprise when informed of their accuracy. Adams (1957) said that this effect was so easy to get, it could function as a classroom demonstration. Anyone conducting such experiments today can see this for herself. Subjects are often astonished to learn that they had guessed correctly at a greater than chance level. They will insist that they saw nothing. How aware could they have been? What does awareness mean if this is an example of it? The issue of what is truly out of awareness and whether forced choice is the best measure of it has persisted to this day. For the most part, it is no longer considered the only way to demonstrate the veracity of unconscious processes (Merikle, 1992).

SUBLIMINAL STUDIES NOT RELATED TO DEFENSE

There was a relatively small body of data on subliminal responding that was not related to defense. These studies generally assessed the influence of subliminal stimulation on the interpretation of closely following supraliminal ambiguous stimuli. This work ranged from the study of illusions to the interpretation of social stimuli. Eventually, this kind of work came to be called subliminal priming. It is currently a major area of research and we review it later in this book. Briefly, the early studies in this area demonstrated that preceding cues, flashed subliminally, influenced subsequent perception of designs (Kolers, 1957; Smith & Henriksson, 1955), femininity/masculinity (e.g., Klein, Spence, Holt, & Gourevitch, 1958), positivity or negativity of a neutral image (Eagle, 1959), and of faces (Smith, Spence, & Klein, 1959). The meaning of these findings was debated. The argument was that the subjects had some kind of fleeting awareness of the so-called subliminal stimuli and that this controlled their responding. Guthrie and Wiener (1966) backed up a similar argument with some research. We review their study in the section on partial cues.

What no one talked about, however, was what it would mean if these results were genuine. They suggest that ordinary, real-life social interactions may be influenced by incidental, unconscious cues. This would imply that there are various and sundry influences all around us, of which we may be unaware. Our actions may therefore not be entirely due to the causes to which we attribute them. This possibility has enormous implications for psychological functioning. These possibilities lay unnoticed by research psychologists for decades. In a classic paper we review later, Nisbett and Wilson (1977) argued that people are often unaware of the causes of their behavior. They did not cite any of these studies, however. Decades later, researchers (see, e.g., Bargh, 1996; Niedenthal, 1992) picked up on these early studies and explored their implications in similarly constituted experiments. The idea that many of our social actions are controlled by stimuli out of our awareness is now flourishing in social psychology, and unconscious priming is seen by many to be ubiquitous (see, e.g., Bargh, 1997, 2006, 2017).

QUALITATIVE VERSUS QUANTITATIVE DIFFERENCES

The question of the existence of subliminal perception and, by extension, empirical verification of unconscious processes seemed to be at an impasse. And using the methods we have described, it was. But there is another approach to answering this question, one derived from what seemed to be a corollary of the SDT assertion that receipt of information and therefore the effects of stimulation are continuous. If this is the case, then so-called subliminal effects should be similar, albeit weaker, versions of supraliminal effects. If this proved to be true, it would support the SDT model. But if subliminal and supraliminal effects turned out to be qualitatively different from one another, it would strongly militate against the SDT model. Since the response mode would be identical in both conditions, the multiple concurrent response model could not account for such differences either.

This approach to testing for the existence of unconscious processes (qualitative vs. quantitative differences) assumed the status of a *via regia* to proof of unconscious processes to some (e.g., Brody, 1972; Shevrin & Dickman, 1980). The usual paradigm employed to examine this issue is what came to be called priming studies. In this early incarnation, they were usually termed "matching studies."

Murdock (1954) exposed his subjects to subliminally presented nonsense syllables. He then presented them with a series of supraliminal stimuli and asked them to guess which one they had seen earlier. They chose stimuli that bore a structural resemblance to the previously presented subliminal stimulus. Bricker and Chapanis (1953) reported similar results. These authors concluded that their findings indicated that their subjects must have been aware of part of the stimulus, which then governed their later guesses.

It seems clear that some information was imparted, but how can we tell if it was consciously or unconsciously processed? Results using nonsense syllables cannot unambiguously address the question of qualitative differences. After all, what else but structure is available from such stimuli? A better test would involve meaningful words, which is what

Postman et al. (1948) and Razran (1949) did. These studies suggested semantic processing of subliminal stimuli but did not directly compare subliminal and supraliminal stimuli. Zuckerman (1960) made such a comparison. He presented subliminal or supraliminal writing suggestions. The subliminal exhortation "Don't Write" led to shorter stories than either "Write More" or no subliminal stimulus. When the same suggestions were presented supraliminally, they had no effects. Dixon (1956) also reported results suggestive of qualitative differences between responses to subliminal and supraliminal stimuli. The subject's task was to write down the first word that came to mind after viewing a supraliminal flash of light. Each flash was preceded by a subliminal auditory presentation of an emotionally toned word. Dixon reported that the responses differed from those given to supraliminal presentations. In fact, responses to the subliminal presentations had a Freudian flavor (i.e., metaphorically and/or symbolically related—a response to subliminal "cow" might be "mother" whereas it might be "milk" to supraliminal cow.) A later study (Dixon, 1958) asked subjects to identify subliminal words. A week later, they viewed their guesses together with the correct stimuli and asked to match their guesses with the correct words based on common associations. Matching was better than chance and many of the mismatches were due to connecting a guess with a synonym of the correct word. Thus, subjects relied on meaning rather than structure.

A subsequent study cast doubt on Dixon's findings, however, and argued for partial cues underlying subliminal effects. Fuhrer and Eriksen (1960) presented their stimuli upside down and backward. Correct matching was greater than chance and not statistically different from that of the experimental group. Matching had to be structural for these subjects unless we are willing to assume that they could somehow unconsciously read a seriously distorted word as readily as they could a normal one. A second control group further supported the structural over the semantic hypothesis. In addition to the words presented to the experimental group, this group was offered words similar in structure but different in meaning to the subliminal words. There was no tendency for this group to match their associations with the "correct" words over the structurally similar control words. Another study (Guthrie & Wiener, 1966) also supported the structural hypothesis by demonstrating that subjects responded more negatively following an angular than a hostile picture, irrespective of content. This led them to conclude that subjects were responding to structure and not meaning. This conclusion does not flow from the study as clearly as the authors thought, however. Why should angularity be associated with hostility? Is this based on experience? Is it genetic? Would a person be conscious of this? That is, would the average person, when asked why one picture was deemed more hostile than another, declare that it was because of the greater angularity of one of them? Probably not. So, even if Guthrie and Weiner are correct about angularity, we are probably looking at an unconscious effect. The effect is that we unconsciously associate angularity with aggression and hostility. Other studies that showed semantic rather than structurally based responses to allegedly subliminal stimuli support unconscious effects that are qualitatively different from conscious effects (see, e.g., Arey, 1960; Pine, 1960, 1961, 1964). The work of Spence (1961) and his colleagues (Spence & Bressler, 1962; Spence & Ehrenberg, 1964; Spence & Gordon, 1967; Spence & Holland, 1962) is particularly interesting and relevant to the understanding of unconscious processing. We review it below.

The above review indicates that although some data argued for the importance of structural cues in subliminal perception, there were also plenty of data suggestive of qualitative differences between responding to sub- and suprathreshold stimuli. Moreover, even some of the results interpreted as supportive of conscious, structural effects can be seen as indicating unconscious effects. As a result, the notion of unconscious processes, although not proved, remained tenable. This parallels all of the other research areas we reviewed. These studies are particularly critical, however, because they not only argued for the existence of unconscious processes, they had something to say about their laws of operation. It seemed that at least some unconscious processes operated in a way that was closely akin to what Freud had termed primary process. And they differed in important ways from the laws of at least some conscious processes, which seemed to operate according to something like secondary process.

THE DEATH OF THE NEW LOOK

The New Look came to its end with the appearance of three papers (Eriksen, 1959, 1960; Goldiamond, 1958). None of them broke any new ground. Rather, they brought together the arguments that had been scattered throughout the vast literature in the area. The interested reader could now conveniently see all of the problems with the work in one place and evaluate them. The result was devastating for New Look research. Not only did work in the area come to a virtual halt, it fell into disrepute. The few investigators who continued this line of research were now seen as being on the fringes of the field, and their work was somehow tainted. The original work was rarely cited, except critically. Goldiamond (1958) repeated many of the artifactual interpretations of perceptual defense like word frequency, suppression, and expectation.

He also brought together and presented many of the SDT arguments leveled against New Look research.

Eriksen's (1959, 1960) reviews were even more devastating. He carefully went through each of the research areas constituting the New Look. He discussed possible methodological confounds in each. The implication, not always directly stated, was that the findings were either fortuitous or entirely due to these confounds (i.e., they were entirely artifactual). This reasoning was especially compelling for subception effects, where Eriksen could call upon his multiple concurrent response model as a viable alternative to unconscious processing.

Eriksen also argued that verbal forced choice trumped all other measures of awareness. According to Eriksen, even if a subject categorically denied awareness and had zero confidence in his guess, a correct verbal forced choice demonstrated that he was aware. But even forced choice could not always be trusted because it was not a perfect indicator. Eriksen seemed to be saying that any evidence of detection or discrimination should be construed as evidence of awareness. Thus, response to a stimulus, of any form, no matter the reaction of any and all other response systems, indicates awareness. He thereby made it impossible to demonstrate unconscious functioning (cf. Bowers, 1984). This essentially ruled unconscious processing out of psychology, a situation we have encountered before. The difference is that Eriksen's arguments seemed empirical, whereas the others we encountered were avowedly philosophical.

Although Eriksen was generally seen as having dismissed unconscious processing, his actual stated conclusion was that there did not yet exist any convincing evidence that people could discriminate or differentially respond to external stimuli presented at intensities too low to elicit forced-choice verbal report. Further, he stated that there is convincing evidence that behavior can be affected by *above-threshold* cues that the subject is unaware of: "The weight of experimental evidence indicates that not only is behavior without awareness a legitimate phenomenon but also that it has been amply demonstrated in the laboratory" (Eriksen, 1959, p. 211). Eriksen thereby was explicitly endorsing the concept of unconscious processes. He repeated this in his 1960 paper. He also showed sympathy for and belief in clinical demonstrations of unconscious processing. These conclusions were and are never referred to, however. (Perhaps an example of unconscious bias?)

Goldiamond's and, particularly, Eriksen's papers had enormous negative impact on New Look research, but the real reason the New Look passed from the scene is because it flew in the face of the prevailing zeitgeist. The 1950s were the heyday of radical behaviorism. Classical behaviorism had dominated from the 1930s on, and Skinner's even more extreme radical behaviorism was predominant during the 1950s (and on into the mid-1970s). His *Science and Human Behavior,* published in 1953, argued against positing any kind of internal variable or agent and had an enormous impact on the field. Internal processing was irrelevant at best. If responses could be predicted from stimuli, what need was there to understand what occurred in between these two variables? At worst, internal processing implied an internal agency that watched over and controlled behavior. Such a mystic, soul-like homunculus had no place in a science of psychology (or as radical behaviorists termed it more tellingly, a science of human behavior). Criticisms of the New Look were replete with pejorative terms such as "soul-like," "homunculus," "Judas eye," and the like. The whole New Look enterprise also had a Romantic flavor. The rejection of Romanticism preceded behaviorism; it was rooted in psychology from its inception as a discipline, as we have seen. The terms "Romantic" and "supersensitive" appear frequently in criticisms of this literature.

This is why, we believe, the field was so ready to dismiss the New Look. All it needed was to have all of the arguments presented cogently, and with the appearance of objectivity, in one place. The aforementioned three papers did that, while the zeitgeist provided the conditions in which the arguments grew and flourished. The sad part of all this is that, in many ways, it is as if the New Look literature had never existed. Dixon (1971, 1981) and Erdelyi (1974) tried to revive it but with little immediate success. Most modern-day psychologists are unfamiliar with this body of work and, to some extent, are reinventing the wheel. That is, now that the study of unconscious processes is part of mainstream psychological thinking, many areas investigated by New Look researchers are once again being examined. But it is as if no one has ever empirically addressed them before.

NOTES

1. Freud liked Poetzl's work, as he indicated in later editions of his master work *Interpretation of Dreams* (Gay, 1988), so he was not against experiments as has often been supposed.

2. These findings suggested that semantic processing of the stimuli was taking place. This is important to later debates over the contribution of partial (structural) cues to subliminal effects. At this point, however, its significance was not appreciated.

3. This model presages early information-processing models of perception like those of Broadbent (1958) and of Deutsch and Deutsch (1963). These will be reviewed in the next chapter.

4. SDT did not merely posit sensory and response effects; it also provided ways of measuring them. Sensory effects were operationalized as d'. This was defined as the difference between the means of the signal and the signal-plus-noise distributions, expressed in terms of their standard deviations. The value of d' could be approximated from data containing correct (hits) and incorrect (false negatives and false positives or false alarms) discriminations. These are converted into proportions and then into standard scores. The standard score for false alarms, conceptualized as an index of the person's response bias, is subtracted from hits, conceptualized as a combination of d' and bias. The resulting difference was seen to be a relatively pure assessment of d'. Different signal intensities had different d' values associated with them.

Response bias was labeled ß. It was the criterion the receiver adopted for deciding between observations he reported as signal present and those he reported as no signal. It represents his cut-off point. It is defined as the likelihood criterion that will maximize pay-offs or known values of the pay-off matrix (consequences) weighted by known or expected stimulus presentation probabilities (expectations). It is estimated from the standardized score for false alarms discussed above. After all, the person's claim to see something that is not there (false positive or false alarm) is compared to the claim that she did not see something that is there (false negative). This should reflect her bias.

5. I would like to thank Lou Primavera for pointing this out to me (J. Weinberger).

CHAPTER 6

Unconscious Processes Move from Outcast to Mainstream

After 1960, the New Look was rarely mentioned in the literature. And when it was, it was almost always as a failed enterprise. Its failure was seen to be so complete that some even suggested banning terminology connected to it. Trimble and Eriksen (1966) went so far as to suggest eliminating the term "subliminal" from the lexicon of psychology because of its association with the New Look. The perceived failure of the New Look had far-reaching effects on the study of unconscious processes generally. Many theorists argued that the dismal showing of the New Look demonstrated that there were no such things as unconscious processes (e.g., Bandura, 1969; Brody, 1972). As a consequence, systematic investigation of unconscious processes followed the New Look into virtual oblivion. For about the next 20 years, little sustained research or theoretical advance was made in the study of these phenomena. Recall that the same thing had happened to hypnosis a century earlier. History has a way of repeating itself. Even well-conducted research by prominent investigators tended to be ignored, often by the relevant investigators themselves. Thus, Broadbent and Gregory (1967) reported significant changes in d' (sensory effects), as opposed to ß (response bias), in a perceptual defense experiment employing auditory stimuli. Dorfman (1967) obtained similar results employing visual stimuli. Similarly, Hardy and Legge (1968) obtained changes in d' in two experiments that crossed sensory modalities. None of these studies caused a ripple. None were followed up, even by the investigators themselves, and none changed anyone's mind. As Broadbent was a major theorist and researcher of the time (and remained so until his death in 1993), this is particularly curious. Anyone who did try to make something of such findings and dissent from the prevailing zeitgeist (e.g., Dixon, 1971) was generally ignored or disparaged. This era did produce some valuable investigations, but they did not get the attention they probably deserved and died out.[1] Ironically, it was during this anti-unconscious period that the groundwork was laid for a change in the zeitgeist that would bring the study of unconscious processes back into the mainstream (see Erdelyi, 1974). This work made positing unconscious processes not just acceptable but necessary (see Shevrin & Dickman, 1980). The work we are referring to was the theorizing about attention and information processing begun by people like Broadbent (1958) and by Miller, Galanter, and Pribram (1960), which culminated in the cognitive revolution mainstreamed by Neisser (1967). The individuals who initially engaged in this enterprise did not at first realize that their work had these implications. Often, they drew exactly the opposite conclusions (e.g., Neisser, 1967). By the 1970s, however, some theorists had made the relevant connections (e.g., Dixon, 1971; Erdelyi, 1974; Shevrin & Dickman, 1980), and soon thereafter, so did the field. As a result of such theoretical innovations, work on unconscious processes began to burgeon in the 1980s and entered the mainstream once again.

SPENCE AND THE RESTRICTING EFFECTS OF AWARENESS

Spence conducted a series of investigations in the 1960s that are all but forgotten today. This is unfortunate because what he found has been repeatedly rediscovered in more recent work. Spence claimed to have uncovered one way in which unconscious processes differ qualitatively from conscious processes. Spence and Bressler (1962) presented one group of subjects with a subliminal presentation of the word "house." Another group saw "house" supraliminally. A third, control, group viewed a blank slide. All subjects then viewed a supraliminal but blurred array of nonsense words (strings of letters that looked like words but were not). All were then read a series of words and had to judge whether each had been part of the previously seen blurred set. The words read to subjects consisted of close or common, distant or rare, and nonassociates of "house." Their decisions as well as how quickly they made them were assessed. Both the subliminal and the supraliminal groups thought that close associates were present in the blurred array more often than distant associates or control words were. This effect was stronger in the supraliminal group. The subliminal group responded most quickly (shortest response latency) to the frequent associates and took longest to respond (greatest latency) to the infrequent associates. Clearly, the subliminal presentation was effective. Like the supraliminal presentation, but not as powerfully, it affected the decision variable. Uniquely, it affected the timing (latency) of the decision-making process. To Spence and Holland (1962), these results suggested that both subliminal and supraliminal stimuli activate a similar network of associates. The difference between the two kinds of activation is that a supraliminal stimulus narrows the band of these associates to the more popular ones. When the same stimulus is presented subliminally, this narrowing of associates does not occur. Instead, the entire network of associates is activated. This means that deciding whether a word is present or not requires matching that word to the entire (activated) associative network. The more distant the associate, the longer the process takes, as matching moves from central to peripheral associates. That is why distant associates had a longer latency in the subliminal than in the supraliminal condition of the Spence and Bressler study.

Based on this reasoning, Spence and Holland asked three groups of subjects to memorize a list of words, which included several associates of the word "cheese." One group was subliminally stimulated with the word "cheese." A second viewed "cheese" supraliminally. The third was not presented with any word (control group). As predicted, subliminally stimulated subjects recalled more "cheese" associates than either of the other two groups. The authors took this result as evidence that a larger network of associates had been activated in the subliminal than the supraliminal condition. That is, they found that more associates were available to the subliminal than the supraliminal group. The equivalence of the supraliminal and control groups was seen as evidence for the narrowing of associates, a phenomenon that Spence and Holland dubbed "the restricting effects of awareness."

Spence (1964) next conducted an experiment designed to demonstrate that these effects did not depend upon subliminality per se but on unawareness, however generated. He tested this hypothesis by embedding the relevant word (cheese) in a serial learning list that also contained associates of cheese. Spence argued that, until words from such a list are recalled, they are out of awareness. They are functionally equivalent to being subliminal. Once recalled, they enter awareness, which is equivalent to being supraliminal. If this conception is correct, more associates should be recalled before than after recall of the critical word. As a result, those subjects who take a long while to recall the critical word should generate more related associates than those who recall it quickly. In order to test these hypotheses, Spence had his subjects memorize a list of words consisting of cheese associates, noncheese associates, and filler words. The word "cheese" occupied the center of the list. As predicted, a larger number of cheese associates (relative to the other words) were recalled prior to recalling "cheese." After cheese was recalled, there were no differences. Late recallers produced more cheese associates than other kinds of words. Thus, Spence's hypotheses were completely supported. And so, by implication, was his model of the restricting effects of awareness.

Efforts were soon made to refute these findings. Researchers tried to dismiss Spence's findings as an example of associative clustering (Worrell & Worrell, 1966) or simple serial position effects (Jung, 1966). Unfortunately, none of these critics attempted an exact replication of Spence's (1964) study, and therefore their studies did not directly disprove Spence's results.

The results of this body of research are mixed. There are supportive, statistically significant effects, and effects in the right direction that were not statistically significant.[2] Clearly, more research needed to be conducted. Unfortunately, Spence's program of research was discontinued. The provocative suggestion that conscious and unconscious processes differ with regard to their activation of associative networks also lay fallow. This was really too bad because the idea appears to be correct. Studies on priming, particularly the classic experiments of Marcel (1983a, 1983b), reviewed later in this chapter, rediscovered this notion. Moreover, it fits in with subsequent conceptions of information processing like that of spreading activation (e.g., Collins & Loftus, 1975) and parallel distributed processing (to be discussed later; McClelland & Rummelhart, 1986). Spence's work suffered the same fate as did the New Look.

SHADOWING

Way back in the era of the New Look, Cherry (1953; Cherry & Taylor, 1954) investigated what he called the "cocktail party phenomenon." Basically, this refers to the common experience of being able to carry on a conversation with one or more people while other conversations are going on all around you. This happens all the time at restaurants, sporting events, and, of course, cocktail parties. We are not as completely tuned out of these other conversations as it appears, however. If someone mentions our name, for example, we often hear it and orient to the source of that sound. So somewhere, somehow, something of the other sounds is being processed. Cherry (1953; Cherry & Taylor, 1954) tried to investigate this phenomenon through a dichotic listening task. The test involves fitting a subject with earphones and sending a different stream of words and/or sounds to each ear. The subject's task is to attend to only one ear's information (one speaker or channel) and ignore what is being presented to the other ear (the other speaker or channel).

To ensure compliance and also to test for distractibility, the subject is asked to continuously repeat aloud what she is hearing in the designated, attended-to ear. This repetition is called "shadowing." Cherry found that people were pretty adept at shadowing (i.e., repeating without mistakes or hesitations), especially if the messages to the two ears differed on obvious physical characteristics.

The cocktail party phenomenon involves more than a capacity for tuning out, however. It also involves some processing of words and sounds the person had no conscious awareness of. Otherwise, how could she respond to a name? Moray (1959) was able to obtain this aspect of the cocktail party phenomenon in the dichotic listening paradigm. That is, his subjects responded to their names even though they showed no evidence of hearing the rest of the information played to them on the to-be-ignored ear. In other words, there seemed to be some unconscious processing going on.

Corteen and his colleagues took the next step and directly connected dichotic listening to unconscious processes. Corteen and Wood (1972) employed a traditional dichotic listening task but included words, presented to the unattended ear, that had been previously associated with or classically conditioned to electric shock. They demonstrated that the subjects were perfectly able to perform the shadowing task, claimed to have no awareness of the words being presented to the unattended ear, yet exhibited electrodermal responses to the shocked words and words associated to them. Attempts to replicate these results were mostly successful (see Corteen & Dunn, 1974, and Forster & Govier, 1978, for support, but also see Wardlaw & Kroll, 1976, for a failure to replicate).

Although it is not generally recognized (by most reviewers and even by the investigators themselves), the shadowing paradigm just reviewed represents a transposition of the New Look's subception effect from the visual to the auditory domain. In subception, previously shocked words are presented subliminally, via a tachistoscope, and elicit electrodermal responses, even though subjects claim not to have seen them. In shadowing tasks, previously shocked words are presented auditorially, via a dichotic listening task, and elicit electrodermal responses even though subjects claim not to have heard them. The criticisms of subception hinged on arguing that the stimuli were not truly unconscious (subliminal) or that different response systems were being confused with consciousness and unconsciousness.

ATTENTION MODELS

One effect of the dichotic listening paradigm, whatever its relevance to unconscious processes, was that it served as an inspiration for the attention and information-processing models that proliferated in the 1960s and 1970s. These models played a large role in ushering in the cognitive revolution in psychology. They also made the positing of unconscious processes not only a viable but a necessary part of psychological theorizing.

The first attention theory was formulated by Broadbent (1957, 1958, 1971). All subsequent models were offshoots of or responses to this seminal work. Broadbent (1957) noted that the dichotic listening data could only make sense if there were some kind of perceptual (auditory) selectivity operating on sensory input. He hypothesized a sort of bottleneck or buffer that held the information until the relevant selections could be made. What made it through this bottleneck was attended to; what did not was not. Broadbent placed this buffer and subsequent selection filter close to the level of the sense organ so that they operated on relatively unprocessed sensory input.

First, he said, all external information enters the perceptual system through a number of sensory channels (eyes, ears, skin, etc.). A great deal of information, from a large number of input sources, is therefore potentially and simultaneously available to the organism. All of these sensory inputs feed into memory stores, or buffers, where they are retained for a brief period of time (a couple of seconds). Broadbent referred to this buffer as echoic storage because virtually no processing has yet taken place and the information is in a raw form, a virtual echo of the external stimulus.[3] Beyond echoic storage exists a single storage space termed short-term memory, which has a limited capacity. Any information that is to be processed further must pass through this next storage area. A selection mechanism (filter) determines what reaches it and what does not. This filter is a rather primitive device, sensitive only to physical aspects of the input like location in space, frequency, and intensity. Dichotic listening is possible because the information from one channel (one ear) gets through the filter, whereas the information from the other channel (the other ear) does not.

Broadbent's model required some (albeit primitive) unconscious processing. That is, an initial sensory analysis of incoming information occurs prior to conscious awareness of that information. This processing is only of very elementary physical aspects of the information. Psychological meaning does not get analyzed preconsciously in this model, although Broadbent hinted that the selection filter might also be sensitive to some psychological aspects of incoming information. After all, the salience of one's own name is a function of its meaning and/or familiarity, not of its physical characteristics.

Treisman (1960, 1964, 1969) amended Broadbent's model by altering the selective nature of his filter and adding a second one. In her attenuation theory of selective attention, Broadbent's filter only attenuates those signals lacking the requisite physical characteristics. They then proceed to a second filter that has a permanently low threshold for stimuli with important psychological and survival characteristics. This means that if information, even if attenuated by the first filter, corresponds to meaningful psychological categories that the second filter is sensitive to, it may be passed on to short-term memory. The person will then become aware of it.

Broadbent (1971) was eventually persuaded by Treisman's work and adopted a version of her model. There is a logical problem with a Treisman-like model, however. If all information eventually reaches a second filter, why do we need the first one? What purpose does a first stage, concerned exclusively with physical characteristics, serve (see Dixon, 1981)? Why not simply posit a single primary site for all perceptual selection? This is exactly what Deutsch and Deutsch (1963) did. They suggested that selection into short-term memory and awareness follows a full analysis by something comparable to Treisman's second filter. In other words, all sensory signals reach higher-order analyzers where they undergo complex, meaningful analysis. Conscious perception is then a result or consequence of these higher-order (unconscious) analyses. Shiffrin and Geisler (1973) extended the Deutsch and Deutsch model from auditory to visual perception. Unconscious processing is quite sophisticated in the Deutsch and Deutsch model. In fact, virtually all processing is conducted unconsciously. Conscious perception is but the final output of these complex analyses.[4]

Posner (1973) held that encoding of stimulus information is the first stage of information processing and involves simultaneous registration and retention of multiple codes of the same event. For example, an event can be simultaneously encoded visually, auditorially, and symbolically. All of these different representations are encoded independently of one another. And all of it occurs unconsciously. After encoding is completed, the resulting representations are compared to and matched with the contents of long-term memory. This also occurs unconsciously. Only now does consciousness make its appearance. Its functions are to select one of the many available representations and respond to it. The other available representations must be suppressed. This means conscious functioning is code specific, sequential, and limiting.[5]

Neisser (1967) integrated these models to form a general theory of attention and perception that has become a classic in the field and helped to set the cognitive revolution firmly in place. In his general model, conscious attention mechanisms come into play only after unconscious global and holistic processes have completed their work. These unconscious processes function to organize the stimulus field into figure and ground. That is, they separate each figure or object from the rest of the stimulus field. Conscious attention then selects from this output and processes it further. In Neisser's model, much, if not most, processing (including complex and sophisticated processing) occurs unconsciously. Additionally, there is a qualitative difference between conscious and unconscious processes. Unconscious processes operate in parallel in a global and holistic manner. That is, several processing mechanisms are simultaneously active. The organism then chooses which of the various available representations to process further on the basis of the "pertinence" of the available information. This subsequent, conscious processing is sequential and analytic.

Neisser's model was quite prescient. By positing parallel rather than serial unconscious processing, it anticipated modern computational models, discussed later in this book (McClelland & Rummelhart, 1986; Sun, 2008). It is, parenthetically, ironic that Neisser helped to reestablish the importance of unconscious processes and contributed to an understanding of their nature. He was, after all, a severe critic of the New Look.

SHIFFRIN AND SCHNEIDER'S TWO-PROCESS MODEL OF AUTOMATIC AND CONTROLLED PROCESSING

Shiffrin and Schneider (1977) and Schneider and Shiffrin (1977) conducted an elegant series of perceptual accuracy and reaction-time studies. Their results led them to propose a two-process model of information processing. They then applied the model to apparently disparate findings from other information-processing investigations. Their model was able to account for these findings better than any available alternative. They termed their model "controlled and automatic information processing." This work was seminal, as the automatic and controlled processing distinction has become central to modern theory and empirical work on unconscious processes.

The model has several working parts. The most basic of these is the unit of information, termed a "node." Once any aspect or element of it is activated, the whole node becomes active. The constituent parts act together or not at all. This is the defining characteristic of a node and why it functions as the unit in this model. A node may activate another node or group of other nodes. The particular nodes that are activated, as well as the order of their activation, depend upon a host of conditions. These include the environmental context and the state of the organism. Thus, there are a myriad of possible connections between nodes.[6]

The repository of said nodes is memory. Memory is defined as a large and relatively permanent collection of nodes. As the person matures and learns, these nodes become interrelated in increasingly complex ways.

Nodes can be in one of two states in memory: long-term-store (LTS) or short-term-store (STS). LTS refers to currently inactive nodes. It is a sort of library of nodes waiting to be looked up and utilized. It holds an enormous amount of information. Most of memory is in this state most of the time. STS refers to whatever nodes are active at a particular point in time. Not many nodes can be in STS at any one time because its capacity is nowhere near that of LTS. Thus, STS and LTS are not different places; they are different states of nodal activity. When in LTS, the node is latent; when in STS, it is active. But it is the same node. The operation of the information-processing system consists of movement of nodes back and forth between STS and LTS.[7] Now that the components of the system are in place, it can be set into motion. And it turns out that it processes information in two qualitatively different ways. One of these is termed "automatic"; the other is termed "controlled."

Automatic processing involves activation of well-learned nodes (i.e., the movement of those nodes from LTS to STS). This activation is usually triggered or elicited by some internally or externally generated stimulus configuration associated with the nodes to be activated. Once activated, the sequence runs off mechanically, with no need for active attention, monitoring, or control. In fact, automatic processes are almost impossible to control. They proceed and run to completion in a predetermined, automatic manner. The more automatic a sequence, the more "fluent" it is. When an automatic process is running, the person can do other things without affecting that operation. More than one automatic process can run at once, in parallel, with no loss of efficiency. A control process (defined below) can also be active simultaneously with an automatic process and not affect it. Automatic processes are not constrained by the limited capacity of STS. In the lexicon of the model, automatic processing does not seem to have capacity limitations. The nodes just keep on coming.

There are costs associated with the apparently limitless capacity of automatic processing. Automatic processes are not easily created. They take a long time and repeated practice trials to develop. Shiffrin and Schneider and Schneider and Shiffrin reported that it required hundreds and hundreds of training trials to establish the automatic processes they investigated. Once automatic processes have been established, there is another cost: flexibility. Automatic processes are completely inflexible. Once begun, these processes are stereotyped, rigid, and very difficult to alter or stop. Although it is possible to alter and even reverse automatic responding, it takes much longer and requires many more trials than it did to create them in the first place. Additionally, the process of change or reversal is experienced as unpleasant.

As long as these processes are adaptive, their resistance to change poses no problem. But if circumstances change such that they become maladaptive, they can lead to serious, even dangerous, consequences. Think of an American-trained driver trying to drive on the left side of the road in England. Moving to the right is automatic for the American. Changing this behavior to driving on the left is extremely difficult, despite the life-threatening consequences of failing to do so. And trying to make this change would certainly not be fun. In fact, it is unpleasant. That is one reason we infrequently attempt to alter our automatic behaviors. We live with them instead.[8]

Control processes operate in a fundamentally different fashion from automatic processes. Like automatic processes, they involve the activation of node sequences. Unlike automatic processes, however, this activation does not involve well-learned node sequences. In fact, the sequences utilized in controlled processes are typically new. That is, they are put together from scratch to deal with a particular, just-encountered situation. As a result, controlled processing normally requires relatively sustained attention and monitoring. For the same reason, it is almost entirely dependent upon STS. It is therefore subject to the capacity limitations of STS. This means that controlled processes cannot operate in parallel with one another, as can automatic processes. Instead, they operate sequentially or serially. So controlled processes are very inefficient and use up resources; they are not "fluent."

The advantage of controlled processes is that they possess the flexibility that automatic processes lack. Controlled processes are quicker to establish and can be altered or even reversed much more easily than can automatic processes. They can be and are applied to situations for which automatic processes do not exist or would prove ineffective, thus allowing the person to adapt to novelty and change. Essentially, their lack of efficiency is compensated for by the ease with which they are created and altered. Further, controlled processes can and often are turned into automatic processes if the same situation recurs repeatedly.

Controlled and automatic processes complement one another. Automatic processing provides speed and efficiency. It enhances the person's adaptive resources by freeing up capacity (since it uses little or none). The person can then make use of these available resources for other endeavors. Control processes allow for the flexibility that automatic processes lack. This is advantageous whenever a situation not covered by an automatic process is encountered.

The two kinds of process can also be integrated. A control process can be carried out while an automatic process is operating. This combines efficiency and flexibility in the same operation. Together, they can make for smooth and highly adaptive information processing. If the same combination of controlled and automatic processes occurs frequently enough, the controlled process will itself become automatic and tied to the original automatic process. New control processes can then be built on top of this new, more complex, and more sophisticated automatic process. This process of building more and more sophisticated, capacity-free processing can go on indefinitely. In this way, extremely complicated behaviors may be developed and automatized.

What does all of this have to do with unconscious processes? As it turns out, quite a bit. Most of information processing takes place unconsciously. Information in LTS is, by definition, not in consciousness. Much of automatic processing is also unconscious. As Shiffrin and Schneider (1997) put it, "The subject may be quite unaware that the process took place" (p. 156). Even controlled processes are not necessarily available to consciousness. The authors divide such processes into two classes, one of which can be in awareness; the other is almost invariably not. The class that is potentially conscious is termed "accessible." In accord with the criteria listed above, *accessible* processes are both controlled and actively attended to. They can be instituted and modified by external instructions (e.g., rote rehearsal). *Veiled* control processes, on the other hand, usually take place outside of awareness. This class of controlled processes is not very open to instructional modification and usually takes place too quickly to be open to introspection (e.g., searching through a list of items for a previously designated target). Finally, the authors take it as a given that most sensory processes are out of awareness. They are particularly sympathetic to the Deutsch and Deutsch (1963) view in this regard.

So where is consciousness in this model? It is relegated to a subset of STS and is limited to what is both attended to and part of controlled processing. Again, as Shiffrin and Schneider (1977) put it: "The phenomenological feeling of consciousness may lie in a subset of STS, particularly in the subset that is attended to and given controlled processing" (p. 157). The controlled and automatic information-processing model does not just propose that most information processing takes place unconsciously. It explains why. Speed and lack of attention are the keys. The reader may recognize the tie this conception has to classical functionalism and the theories of William James.

Understanding of automatic and controlled processing has developed beyond the two-process model of Shiffrin and Schneider. Most of these changes have come from social psychology generally and John Bargh in particular (e.g., Bargh, 1989; Bargh & Ferguson, 2000). At first, modern social psychologists tended to be more like the functionalists and offered absolute conscious/unconscious splits, which they identified with controlled and automatic processing, respectively. The idea that automatic processes are all unitary and qualitatively different from controlled processes, which are also all unitary, has given way to more complex understanding, however (Bargh, 1989; Bargh & Ferguson, 2000). The field now recognizes that few processes are purely one or the other. We discuss this in more detail when we address current views of automaticity and control.[9]

SUMMARY OF INFORMATION-PROCESSING MODELS

In all of the models reviewed to this point, it is the job of consciousness to select one interpretation of the available information and to reject others. The various theories differ to some degree on where and when the selection takes place. They also vary as to what kinds of material get selected and what happens to rejected information. They all agree, however, that consciousness serves a restrictive function, whereas unconscious events involve broad and expansive processing. The reader may recall the restricting effects of awareness posited by Spence (1964). Spence seems to have been correct. Later data and theorizing further reinforce this conception, as we shall see.

The information-processing models reviewed above dominated psychology for about two decades (the 1960s through the 1970s) and were the beginning of a revolution whose effects are still being played out. It is clear that all of them posit unconscious processes in some form. Further, these points were made more and more explicitly as time went on. As a result, they brought unconscious processes back to respectability. As we stated earlier, however, this situation was rarely recognized by the authors of the theories themselves. And when it was, the implications were rarely explicated. It took others, more directly connected to the study of unconscious processes and New Look research, to make these connections (Dixon, 1971, 1981; Erdelyi, 1974; Marcel, 1983a, 1983b; Shevrin & Dickman, 1980; Silverman, 1976, 1983; Silverman & Weinberger, 1985; Weinberger & Silverman, 1987). In the next chapter, we review this work.

NOTES

1. This era also produced three separate research programs still active today: Perceptgenesis (e.g., Draguns, 2008), the work of the Shevrin group on brainwave responses to subliminal stimuli (e.g., Shevrin, Bond, Brakel, Hertel, & Williams, 1996), and subliminal psychodynamic activation (e.g., Silverman, 1976; Weinberger, 1992; Weinberger & Smith, 2011). All three shed light on unconscious processes but were not seen as mainstream and hence not much attended to.

2. Modern psychological researchers are more attentive to factors underlying statistical significance and effect size than were their progenitors in the 1960s. Two studies may yield the same effect size, but one may be statistically significant whereas the other is not. This could be because of greater power in one study than in the other. Sample size, for example, is directly related to power. Thus, an apparent failure to replicate may really be an exact replication (Weinberger, 1987).

3. Since Broadbent was trying to understand auditory processing, the name of his buffer reflected this sense. Neisser (1967) later termed this stage "iconic storage," thereby giving it a visual connotation.

4. These models are conceptually similar to Freud's topographical model. Recall that Freud posited a filter that determined what could and could not become conscious. In Freud's model, the critical variable was desire; in the attention models, various variables were offered. But the idea of a filter between the unconscious and the conscious mind is present in both types of model.

5. This sounds suspiciously like the restricting effects of awareness posited by Spence (1964), but this connection was never made. We will see this again when we review Marcel's (1983b) model, which also posits a constriction of associates due to conscious processing. Later, we will see a similar conception in parallel distributed processing (McClelland & Rummelhart (1986), as the brain/mind "settles" on a solution.

6. A node in this model is similar to what will be termed a unit (McClelland & Rummelhart, 1986) or a working (M. L. Anderson, 2010), in later computational neuroscience models, reviewed later in this book.

7. This is similar to Freud's topographical model's positing of the preconscious/conscious system.

8. This may partially explain why habits are so hard to break, why many maladaptive behaviors are so difficult to treat, and why relapse is so prevalent.

9. This seems to be an insight that psychology keeps having to learn over and over. Freud's (1900) topographical model posited an absolute difference between conscious and unconscious processes. His later structural model (Freud, 1923) argued, however, that there is no absolute differentiation. The functionalists never came to the realization that there is no absolute line between conscious and unconscious functioning. Automatic and controlled were originally seen as absolutely different (Shiffrin & Schneider, 1977) but are now seen as overlapping (Bargh & Ferguson, 2000). The same can be said for McClelland, Koestner, and Weinberger (1989) positing an absolute difference between implicit and self-attributed motives, Kahnemann's (2011) Type 1 and Type 2 systems, and dual-process theories generally (Strack & Deutsch, 2015). See Payne, Burkley, and Stokes (2008) for a demonstration that these two types of processes exist but are not absolutely separate from one another.

CHAPTER 7

Empirical Tests
of Unconscious Phenomena
The Effects of Subliminal Exposure

The next area of research we cover is termed "subliminal psychody-namic activation." It had two main sources of influence. One was a well-established phenomenon termed priming—the influence of a recent exposure (say of a word) on subsequent performance (like choosing a word from a list). Subliminal priming means that the initial exposure (the prime) is presented subliminally (i.e., outside of awareness). A simple example of subliminal priming was reported by Murch (1965, 1967, 1969). Subjects were supraliminally presented with ambiguously incomplete letters. They were then subliminally presented with one possible completion. Finally, they were asked to select a completed letter from a subsequent supraliminal display. Subjects tended to select the letter that matched the subliminal stimulation.

The second source of influence came from some of the findings of priming studies. Several of these studies (e.g., Dixon, 1956, 1958; Pine, 1960, 1961, 1964) reported results in keeping with psychoanalytic tenets. They showed that subliminal but not supraliminal presentations led to responses that were associatively related to the presentation in a way that seemed to reflect Freudian primary process. Also influencing this research were some New Look studies that reported that defense and vigilance could be predicted by diagnostic category in accord with psychoanalytic tenets (Eriksen, 1951; Greenbaum, 1956; Kurland, 1954; Lazarus et al., 1951).

SILVERMAN'S SUBLIMINAL PSYCHODYNAMIC ACTIVATION

In the late 1960s and early 1970s, Lloyd Silverman, himself a psychoanalyst, employed subliminal priming to test psychoanalytic propositions about unconscious processes. (The research was termed subliminal psychodynamic activation [SPA] for this reason.) The early studies focused on conflicts said by psychoanalysts to underlie particular behaviors/ symptoms. See Silverman (1983) and Weinberger and Silverman (1987) for listings and reviews of these studies. Several psychoanalytic theorists (e.g., Bak, 1954; Hartmann, 1939/1958) posited that some of the thought disorder and inappropriate nonverbal behaviors of schizophrenics was related to unconscious conflicts over aggression. An early set of SPA studies therefore examined the effects of priming schizophrenics with aggressive stimulation. The experiments involved presenting subliminal aggressive (e.g., a picture of a lion roaring) or neutral (e.g., a picture of a bird flying) stimulation to these individuals. Seventeen studies showed that aggressive stimulation increased the dependent variables whereas neutral stimulation did not (Mendelsohn & Silverman, 1982, review these studies).

Freud (1917) and Jacobson (1971) held that depression resulted from turning aggression against the self. Four studies (Cox, 1974; Miller, 1973; Rutstein & Goldberger, 1973; Varga, 1973) showed increased levels of depression on the Multiple Affect Adjective Check List following exposure to an aggressive stimulus (Destroy Mother) as compared to a neutral stimulus (People Walking). There were also failures to obtain this effect (Nissenfeld, 1979; Silverman, Bronstein, & Mendelsohn, 1976). Later studies indicated that this might have been due to there being more than one kind of depression. Blatt, Wein, Chevron, and Quinlan (1979) argued, and empirically supported the idea, that some depression was loss-based (anaclitic) and some was failure-based (introjective). Dauber (1984) presented the relevant primes subliminally and obtained supportive results. Psychoanalysts have also connected stuttering with anal conflicts (Fenichel, 1945; Glauber, 1958). To test this formulation, Silverman, Klinger, Lustbader, Farrell, and Martin (1972) presented anal primes to stutterers (a picture of a dog defecating). The subjects presented with this stimulus stuttered more than those presented with a neutral stimulus (a picture of a bird flying).

A more parsimonious explanation for these findings would be that priming with these stimuli raised anxiety levels, which then resulted in increases in the measured behaviors. No need to posit specific dynamic conflicts. Stress a stutterer and you get stuttering; stress a schizophrenic and increased thought disorder will result, etc. So Silverman et al. (1976) tested for specificity and found it. That is, they presented the stimulus predicted to be uniquely effective in a particular type of person (e.g., an anal stimulus for a stutterer, an aggressive stimulus for a schizophrenic), a stimulus that was not deemed to cause conflict in that type of person but was held to be conflictual in another (e.g., an aggressive stimulus for a stutterer vs. an anal stimulus for a schizophrenic), and a neutral stimulus. They found that only the relevant conflictual stimulus (e.g., aggressive stimulus for a schizophrenic but not for a stutterer; anal stimulus for a stutterer but not for a schizophrenic) had an effect in all of their groups but the depressives. Thus, the study supported psychoanalytic specificity. Geisler (1986), in one of the few studies to find effects analogous to repression, primed sexual guilt in college women (the phrase LOVING DAD IS WRONG, accompanied by a picture of a man and woman in a provocative pose) assessed to be high in this variable. Subjects showed more forgetting of verbal material presented subsequently than comparable women presented with a neutral stimulus. Finally, Silverman, Ross, Adler, and Lustig (1978) obtained support for Oedipal dynamics in men. They primed their male subjects with the subliminal stimulus BEATING DAD IS WRONG or BEATING DAD IS OK. The former resulted in worse dart-throwing performance than did the latter.

Silverman then moved from triggering negative reactions ("symptoms" in psychoanalytic parlance) to psychoanalytically based adaptation-enhancing priming. This work constitutes, by far, the largest literature in the area of subliminal SPA. See Silverman and Weinberger (1985) and Silverman, Lachmann, and Milich (1982) for reviews of the early investigations. One of us (JW) and his colleagues then expanded upon this work (see Siegel & Weinberger, 1998; Weinberger, 1992; and Weinberger and Smith, 2011, for reviews), as did Sohlberg and his colleagues (Sohlberg & Birgegard, 2003; Sohlberg, Birgegard, Czartoryski, Overfelt, & Strombom, 2000; Sohlberg, Claesson, & Birgegard, 2003).

The idea behind these investigations comes from the psychoanalytic clinical observation that most people harbor an unconscious wish to merge or become one with the good mother of early childhood. This was originally termed "symbiosis" (Mahler, Pine, & Bergman, 1975) and was conceived of as a return to an early developmental state wherein the infant could not differentiate herself from her surroundings. Triggering and symbolically gratifying this wish was deemed a positive experience that could lead to beneficial outcomes. This theory came under fire both because it was not based on actual observation and because later research (which was based on observing infants) seemed to have disconfirmed it (Stern, 1985). The phenomenon of unconsciously desiring a powerful connection with the early mother is still said to exist, however, and is not limited to psychoanalytic thinking. Silverman et al. (1982), Silverman and Weinberger (1985), and Weinberger and

Smith (2011) offer many examples, beginning with Plato and including the work of William James (1902/1929). Fitzsimons and Bargh (2003, 2004) presented data on the unconscious motivating effects of the good mother coming from a social psychological perspective. Weinberger and Smith referred to these desires as "oneness wishes" so as to lessen their theoretical baggage.

Silverman hypothesized that subliminally priming people with gratification of the wish to be connected with the good mother would lead to adaptation-enhancing effects. He therefore subliminally presented the message MOMMY AND I ARE ONE (MIO) or a control message (typically PEOPLE ARE WALKING) to subjects and then assessed their effects on various behaviors. Twelve studies with schizophrenics (e.g., Bronstein & Rodin, 1983; Fribourg, 1981; Jackson, 1983; Leiter, 1982; Silverman, Spiro, Weissberg, & Candell, 1969) found that MIO stimulation reduced thought disorder and inappropriate nonverbal behaviors relative to the control group. Weinberger, Kelner, and McClelland (1997) found that MIO stimulation led to improved implicit mood in college students, as indexed by spontaneously generated autobiographical memories, but did not affect explicit (self-report) mood. Sohlberg, Arvidsson, and Birgegard (1997) replicated these results. Moreover, alternative messages (MOMMY AND I ARE THE SAME, MOMMY AND I ARE ALIKE, MOMMY IS INSIDE ME) did not produce effects (Bronstein & Rodin, 1983), arguing that the specific message mattered and that it had to include oneness.

Silverman also examined the effects of MIO stimulation on treatment outcome, a direct test of their adaptation-enhancing properties. Specifically, researchers preceded intervention sessions with stimulation by MIO or a control stimulus. For example, Palmatier and Bornstein (1980) preceded a rapid smoking intervention with MIO or a control stimulus. At the end of treatment, both groups had stopped smoking. However, a month later, 67% of the MIO group but only 13% of the control group were still abstaining. Positive results were also obtained for adolescents receiving psychotherapy (Bryant–Tuckett & Silverman, 1984), college students in group therapy (Linehan & O'Toole, 1982), alcoholics in Alcoholics Anonymous (Schurtman, Palmatier, & Martin, 1982), insect phobics treated with exposure (Silverman, Frank, & Dachinger, 1974), and obese patients participating in a behavior modification program (Silverman, Martin, Ungaro, & Mendelsohn, 1978).

MIO intervention has also proven effective in other languages, using a different alphabet than the Latin of English. Thus, Ariam and Siller (1982) translated MIO into Hebrew and reported that their high school math students received a higher grade when each class was preceded by the Hebrew MIO than when each class was preceded by a Hebrew control stimulus. Sohlberg, working in Sweden, found that the positive effects of MIO stimulation seem to depend upon the relative differentiation from or identification with the mother (Sohlberg et al., 2000). His group also reported that MIO effects depend (in part) upon activating unconscious schemas relating to self with others (Sohlberg & Birgegard, 2003; Sohlberg et al., 2003). Finally, Sohlberg and Birgegard (2003) reported that the mood and relational effects triggered by MIO lasted for months. This parallels some of the implicit memory results reported later in this book. It seems that MIO effects are real and relate to internalized social representations.

As one would imagine, there was considerable criticism of this work (e.g., Balay & Shevrin, 1989; Fudin, 1986). These ranged from questioning the reliability of the phenomenon to wondering whether only Silverman-affiliated labs could obtain it to methodological critiques. Weinberger (1986, 1989) responded to these critiques. Further, Hardaway (1990) and Weinberger and Hardaway (1990) conducted meta-analyses of the MIO research. Their findings indicated that the results were reliable, of respectable strength (effect size of d = 0.41—a small to moderate effect), and were of comparable magnitude whether conducted by Silverman-associated or independent labs. Weinberger and Hardaway also conducted a file drawer analysis to determine whether the findings were attributable to selective reporting of positive results (where negative results get buried in file drawers and are never published). They found that it would require more than 1,500 null results to obviate the 70 positive results then reported. Thus, the findings are valid, reliable, and of decent effect size. Whether the results support a specifically psychoanalytic interpretation is less clear. Nonetheless, this work can be said to offer the strongest experimental support of psychoanalytic propositions in the empirical literature.

MARCEL'S PATTERN-MASKING STUDIES

A series of studies conducted by Marcel (Marcel, 1983a, 1983b; Marcel, Katz, & Smith, 1974; Marcel & Patterson, 1978) provides support for positing a qualitative difference between conscious and unconscious processes. They also support Spence's view of awareness as restrictive and unconscious activation as triggering a broad associative network. These studies utilized a technique termed "masking" to prevent stimulation from reaching awareness. (The following review of masking is necessarily limited. For a comprehensive review of masking and its intricacies, see Breitmeyer, 1984; Breitmeyer & Ögmen, 2006.) Masking involves the reduction or elimination of the phenomenal representation of one stimulus by another. The stimulus whose phenomenal representation is affected is called the "target." The stimulus that affects this representation is called the "mask."

The type of mask and its temporal relationship to the target critically affect its influence on the target. For our purposes, two types of masking are important. One is called energy masking or masking by light. A briefly flashed, uniformly illuminated field is used to obscure the target in this kind of masking. The other kind of masking is termed pattern masking. This refers to a mask consisting of forms and contours, which interfere with conscious perception of the target. The temporal relationship of target and mask is also very relevant. There are three possible temporal sequences of target and mask. The mask and target may be presented together (simultaneous masking); the mask may precede the target (forward masking); or the mask may follow the target (backward masking). These can also be combined (e.g., a mask may both precede and overlap with the target). The time between target and mask in backward and forward masking, termed stimulus onset asynchrony (SOA), is critical. Subliminality, especially for backward pattern masking, is achieved only within a certain window of time between the two (i.e., a certain SOA). We focus here on backward masking, as it was employed by Marcel and still is by most others who study unconscious processes. Marcel (1983b) conducted a classic study based on a series of earlier experiments conducted by Meyer, Schvaneveldt, and Ruddy (1972), Schvaneveldt and Meyer (1973), and Schvaneveldt, Meyer, and Becker (1976). Meyer et al. (1972) and Schvaneveldt and Meyer (1973) had shown that identification of a word, as a word (lexical decision), is quicker when it is preceded by an associated word. Schvaneveldt et al. (1976) went a step further. They presented three words to their subjects. The second word had two equally plausible meanings (e.g., *bank*, which can either be a place that holds money or the edge of a body of water). Words of this sort are called *polysemous*. The first of the three words presented to subjects was associatively related to one of the two meanings of the polysemous word (e.g., *money* or *water*). The third word was also associatively related to one of the two meanings of the polysemous word. The first and third words could therefore be matched or mismatched associates of the polysemous second word. Both conditions were run. The following examples should (we hope) clarify the structure of the two conditions:

1. *water, bank, river*
2. *money, bank, river*

It turned out that when the first word was associated to the same meaning of the polysemous second word as was the third word (like example 1 above), lexical identification of the third word was enhanced. If, however, the first word primed a meaning at variance with the third word (like example 2 above), reaction time to the third word was longer. Schvaneveldt et al. argued that their results were attributable to different patterns of associative linkage. That is, the word preceding *bank* set off one chain of associates when it was *water* and a completely different chain when it was *money*. The former was part of the associative network of *river* (*bank* as the edge of a body of water). It therefore sped up recognition of that word. The latter was not associatively linked to *river* but to a qualitatively different set of associates of *bank* (*bank* as a place that holds money). It therefore retarded word recognition time for *river*.

In the Schvaneveldt et al. study, all presentations were supraliminal and therefore in awareness. Marcel (1983b) brought this paradigm to bear on the study of unconscious processes by pattern masking the polysemous word in one condition and then comparing the results with those obtained in a supraliminal condition. We concretize the subliminal conditions for purposes of clarity.[1]

    1. *hand, palm* (pattern mask), *wrist*
    2. *tree, palm* (pattern mask), *wrist*

Marcel replicated the Schvaneveldt et al. results in the supraliminal condition. That is, the polysemous word facilitated reactions to the target word only when it was preceded by a word associatively connected to the target word. The findings were very different in the subliminal condition, however. When subjects could not detect the polysemous word (i.e., when it was pattern masked), it facilitated reaction to the target word regardless of what kind of word preceded it. That is, no matter how the first word was associatively connected to the polysemous word, reaction time to the third word was facilitated. Marcel explained these results by arguing that in a preconscious state, all possible meanings of a word are activated and capable of priming subsequent words. That is, the entire associative network of the word is active and available. This means that multiple meanings of the word can coexist, in parallel, unconsciously, which is why the influence of a masked polysemous word was not dependent upon the word that preceded it. On the other hand, said Marcel, conscious processing is a selective and restrictive process. Only one meaning of a word can exist in consciousness at any one time. Thus, in the supraliminal condition of Marcel's experiment, only the meaning of the polysemous word primed by the preceding word was available. If it was associatively related to the target word, it reduced reaction time; if it was not, it increased it. As the reader may recall, this is strongly reminiscent of Spence's (1964) ideas about the restricting effects of awareness (although Spence is not cited in Marcel's paper). It also accords with the various information-processing views that hold conscious processing to be serial and limited whereas unconscious processing is parallel and diffuse. A replication of Marcel's (1983b) findings by Fowler, Wolford, Slade, and Tassinary (1981) lent further credence to Marcel's model.

Marcel (1983b) tried structurally related words as well. A word structurally related to the polysemous word slowed reactivity in the subliminal condition. He also tried energy masking. An energy mask eliminated effects (i.e., there were no differences between conditions). These findings indicate that the effects obtained are unique to semantic relationships and to a particular kind of masking, namely, pattern masking. Marcel hypothesized that energy masking destroys information processing at its point of impact. Pattern masking, on the other hand, only interferes with phenomenal representation. All other information processing continues to completion. Additionally, it seems that semantic processing has priority over structural processing. These hypotheses were further tested and supported in another set of experiments (Marcel, 1983a).

Marcel (1983a) also showed that both graphical and semantic processing can exist in the absence of phenomenal awareness. In this study, subjects evidenced structural and semantic processing whether or not they consciously saw anything. They also processed meaning even when they could no longer discriminate structure. Contrary to the received wisdom of the time, phenomenal representation was the most fragile aspect of processing, whereas semantic representation was the most robust. This constituted powerful support for subliminal perception. This finding was also replicated by Fowler et al. (1981). A second experiment conducted by Marcel (1983a), however, showed that semantic processing may not be more robust than structural processing, as the previous experiment (and the Fowler et al. replication) suggested. As we shall see, this controversy concerning the primacy of structure versus meaning of stimulation evaporated in more recent research. The key was the notion that many kinds of processing go on at once, that is, in parallel. So the reason that the primacy of one or the other cannot be definitely established is not due to imperfect studies, but to the fact that neither occurs first; both occur simultaneously.

THE SUBLIMINAL MERE EXPOSURE EFFECT

In 1968, Robert Zajonc reported a phenomenon he termed the mere exposure effect. He found that repeated presentations of novel stimuli increased people's liking of them—a finding which has since been shown to be reliable and valid (Harrison, 1977; Bornstein, 1989). Curiously, this effect has since been obtained through repeated subliminal presentations of novel stimuli (Wilson, 1979; Kunst–Wilson & Zajonc, 1980). That is, people developed preferences for stimuli they had been exposed to but were unaware of having encountered. This was termed a subliminal mere exposure effect (SME). Even more curious, the SME is stronger than is supraliminal mere exposure (Bornstein, 1989; Bornstein & D'Agostino, 1992).

In what is now a classic and seminal study, Kunst–Wilson and Zajonc (1980) subliminally exposed subjects to what they described as Chinese ideographs. Most would probably call them irregularly shaped polygons. After these subliminal exposures, subjects viewed several pairs of shapes supraliminally. When subjects were asked which shape they recognized as having been presented to them earlier, they chose correctly 48% of the time, which was not significantly different from chance (50%). Furthermore, the confidence they felt in their judgments had no bearing on their accuracy. But when subjects were asked to choose the shape they *preferred,* they chose the previously experienced stimulus 60% of the time, which *was* significantly greater than chance. And now confidence did make a difference. The more certain subjects were about which stimulus they preferred, the more likely they were to have chosen the previously exposed shape. A similar effect for liking was also obtained for auditory stimuli by Wilson (1979).

This finding was quickly put to the test by other researchers and proved easy to replicate. Bornstein (1992) reported seven published studies and a total of 14 separate experiments that replicated, either directly or conceptually, Kunst–Wilson and Zajonc's (1980) findings. And there have been several since then (e.g., Bornstein & D'Agostino, 1992, 1994; Seamon, McKenna, & Binder, 1998). Moreover, the effect had been found for implicit as well as explicit emotional responses (Hicks & King, 2011). The effect has even been shown for individuals suffering from neurological impairment, prenatally, and across species (Zajonc, 2001).

The SME effect shows that subliminal exposures yield the same kinds of preference effects as do supraliminal exposures. But the strength of the effect differs systematically depending on whether the presentations are subliminal or supraliminal. Bornstein's (1989) meta-analyses showed that subliminal exposures yielded substantially *greater* effects—three to four times greater—than did supraliminal exposures. Interestingly, Bornstein found an inverse relationship between stimulus recognition accuracy and the magnitude of the affective preference effect. The more awareness, the weaker the effect. But Bornstein's meta-analyses compared studies utilizing exclusively subliminal presentations with studies employing exclusively supraliminal presentations. No study had both conditions present in a single experiment. Bornstein and D'Agostino (1992) filled this gap, comparing a subliminal and a supraliminal presentation condition in the same experiment. Preference was affected by frequency of exposure in both the subliminal and supraliminal conditions. The more frequently a stimulus was presented, the more it was liked, as expected. This was a main effect. There was also an interaction effect. Subjects in the subliminal condition showed a significantly more rapid rise in liking with increasing frequency than did subjects in the supraliminal condition. Thus, the mere exposure effect was stronger in the subliminal condition than it was in the supraliminal condition. The results of Bornstein's (1989) meta-analyses were thereby confirmed in a single experiment.

Explaining the SME Effect: Affective Primacy versus Perceptual Fluency

The counterintuitive finding that SME leads to stronger affective preference than supraliminal mere exposure has historically been explained in two ways (see Bornstein, 1992). Zajonc (Murphy & Zajonc, 1993; Zajonc, 1980, 1984, 2001) offered what he termed an "affective primacy" account. (Later in this book we critically evaluate this model and contrast it with a cognitive primacy model; see Lazarus [1984]; Storbeck, Robinson, and McCourt [2006]). We will conclude that what is important is not affect or cognition per se. Rather, the relevant variable is what is most salient and plausible to the person. Often, this is affect. But not always. The debate over what underlies the SME did not address this issue, however, so we present the arguments from that literature here and return to cognition versus affect later. We will allude to it in the discussion when warranted, however.) According to the affective primacy hypothesis, processing of affective information proceeds independently of and differently from processing of affectively neutral information. Affective information is processed on a rapidly conducting, preferred channel. Cognitive information, in contrast, is processed more slowly and on a different, secondary set of channels. The SME effect is a direct consequence of the primacy of affective processing. Subliminal presentations result in stronger effects because only affective processing can take place in so short a period of time. Given more processing time, cognitive processing can proceed and may override or at least interact with affective processing, resulting in weaker supraliminal exposure effects. Zajonc (1980, 1984) reviewed a great deal of evidence from various areas in psychology and neurophysiology to support his view, and LeDoux (1996), a decade later, offered neurophysiological evidence for two pathways carrying affective information. One is quick, bypassing cognition, whereas the other is slow and involves cognitive processing.

Bornstein (1992; Bornstein & D'Agostino, 1992, 1994) and Seamon (Seamon, Brody, & Kauff, 1983; Seamon, Marsh, & Brody, 1984; Seamon et al., 1995) offered an alternative account of the SME effect, which they termed the "perceptual fluency model." The term and the model come from work conducted by Jacoby (e.g., Jacoby & Dallas, 1981; Jacoby & Kelley, 1987; Jacoby, Lindsay, & Toth, 1992; Jacoby, Toth, Lindsay, & Debner, 1992; Jacoby & Whitehouse, 1989), which essentially holds that practice facilitates the encoding and processing of stimuli. That is, stimuli that have been experienced before are easier to encode and process than are novel stimuli. Jacoby has shown that perceptual fluency can be acquired automatically, without any conscious awareness. Jacoby and his colleagues have also demonstrated that perceptual fluency can be attributed (misattributed actually) to a variety of stimulus properties, thereby affecting a person's subjective experience of that stimulus. That is, because the person is unaware of the development of perceptual fluency, he may misattribute ease of processing to various and sundry stimulus properties (a kind of unconscious rationalization).

The perceptual fluency account of the SME effect is straightforward (cf. Bornstein, 1992; Klinger & Greenwald, 1994; Seamon et al., 1983; Seamon et al., 1984). It holds that when subjects are asked to choose between a previously seen and now fluent stimulus and a novel, nonfluent stimulus, they attribute the fluency or ease of processing to liking the stimulus. They therefore choose the previously presented stimulus. When asked to identify the stimulus previously seen, however (recognition task), a wholly different process, in which perceptual fluency is not a factor, is triggered. The subject sees recognition as a test of awareness and searches his conscious recollection for the stimulus. Since the relevant stimulus was presented subliminally, the person's search fails. Believing that there is a right and a wrong answer (which there is) but having no *explicit memory* for which stimulus was shown, the subject is prone to make random guesses. Performance is therefore at chance. As a result, affective choice is superior to recognition choice and we have the SME.

Essentially, the perceptual fluency hypothesis avers that the subject misattributes a vague sense of familiarity to liking because that was the adjective offered and there is no sense that an absolute right or wrong answer is required. If this is true, then offering other attributes for evaluation should work just as well, so long as the experimenter does not indicate that there is an objectively correct answer.[2]

Perceptual fluency is supported by Bornstein's (1989) meta-analyses. When affective ratings were collected immediately following supraliminal exposure, the affective preference effect size was $r = .184$; when affective ratings were delayed, the effect size was $r = .215$. Thus, delaying the affective evaluation in supraliminal mere exposure studies led to stronger effects (i.e., more preference for previously seen stimuli). Perceptual fluency accounts for these results quite nicely. When ratings immediately follow supraliminal exposure, the person is more likely to attribute a sense of familiarity (fluency) to actual familiarity. After all, the subject is quite aware that she just viewed the stimulus. Delay lessens the likelihood that subjects will attribute their ease of processing to stimulus familiarity because its familiarity is not so obvious or salient. They are therefore more likely to attribute fluency to other characteristics of the stimuli, like attractiveness or likability. Affective primacy would be hard put to account for Bornstein's findings. Why should delay have anything to do with the primacy of affect (or the lack thereof)? Fluency can also explain the SME effect. When something is subliminal, it is functionally equivalent to a delay in the supraliminal condition. It is hard to connect a sense of familiarity (perceptual fluency) with stimulus familiarity. After all, there is no conscious awareness of ever having seen the stimulus. The likelihood of misattribution to another attribute like affect is thereby enhanced.

There are also data that directly support the perceptual fluency hypothesis. Bonnano and Stillings (1986) asked their subjects to rate felt *familiarity* as well as affective preference in an SME study. They found that both a sense of familiarity and affective preference increased with repeated exposures. Recognition ratings, as usual, remained at chance. This constitutes powerful support for the perceptual fluency hypothesis for several reasons. First, a nonaffective quality was affected by SME. Second, familiarity is uniquely suited for testing perceptual fluency. It is exactly the variable that perceptual fluency predicts would be affected. Finally, although familiarity is conceptually similar to recognition, the latter was at chance. This supports the idea that consciously searching memory for right and wrong answers is fatal to the SME effect. A sense of familiarity is subjective and relative. Recognition is absolute and objective.

Other studies lend further support to the perceptual fluency hypothesis. Reingold (1990) and Merikle and Reingold (1991) reported the usual finding that recognition of nonshadowed words in a dichotic listening task was at chance, whereas recognition of the shadowed words was high. A wholly different result was obtained when subjects were asked to evaluate the extent to which the nonshadowed words or control, nonpresented words "stood out," however. Now, the previously presented words were chosen significantly more often. Since "standing out" is not an affective choice, these experiments support the perceptual fluency hypothesis. Further, it is intuitively reasonable that something that was easier to code and process (more fluent) would be more salient or noticeable than something that is more difficult to process. It stands out. Recall that Blum (1954) also reported that subliminal stimuli stood out even when they could not be consciously identified.

Bornstein and D'Agostino (1994) provided further support for the perceptual fluency hypothesis. They reasoned that if perceptual fluency resulted from transpositions of processing ease onto stimulus qualities, then offering a priori attributions ought to influence the SME effect. Their results demonstrated that providing individuals with information that enabled them to attribute their sense of fluency to familiarity resulted in a significant lowering of their affect ratings. Mandler, Nakamura, and Van Zandt (1987) took the perceptual fluency hypothesis to its limit. They argued that perceptual fluency could be attributed to *any* stimulus quality. It did not have to be related in any way to familiarity or affect. They termed this the "nonspecific effects of exposure." In order to test this extreme view of fluency, they conducted an SME experiment in which they asked for brightness, darkness, and disliking ratings, as well as the usual liking and recognition judgments. They found the typical liking and recognition effects. That is, affective ratings of previously seen stimuli exceeded those of control stimuli whereas recognition judgments did not. They also found that previously viewed stimuli were rated as both darker and brighter than matched but not-previously-seen stimuli, depending upon the question asked. There was no effect for ratings of disliking, however.

On the basis of these results, Mandler et al. argued that repeated exposures generated an unformed representation (i.e., a representation devoid of context or meaning). This representation could therefore be elaborated into or attached onto any available stimulus property. The property in question need not have any relationship to the actual stimulus presented. Even opposite qualities could serve this contextual, elaborative function. All that matters is that the property be made salient to the individual.

Seamon et al. (1998) presented data that argued against the Mandler et al. model. Seamon et al. were unable to replicate the bright and dark effects while successfully replicating the usual liking and recognition effects. The Mandler et al. nonspecific interpretation of the SME effect is therefore currently moot. There may be limits to the attributional flexibility of fluency. Further investigation is needed.

The value of the perceptual fluency hypothesis is not moot, however. It clearly can explain much about the SME effect. It also has ramifications for other findings in psychology (e.g., implicit memory, discussed in more detail later in this book). The perceptual fluency hypothesis may help explain a finding we have repeatedly come across in this book. Subliminal effects seem to be stronger when subjects adopt a passive (Dixon, 1971, 1981), nonstrategizing (Marcel, 1983a; Murch, 1965, 1967, 1969) approach to their tasks. Additionally, awareness apparently restricts the breadth of associations (Marcel, 1983a; Spence, 1964). This latter finding also turned up in the very early studies on word association. Aschaffenburg and Kraeplin (cited in Ellenberger, 1970) reported that subjects showed looser, more unconsciously tinged word associations (he termed them "outer" associations) when they were tired, feverish, or intoxicated. In other words, they had less restrictive associations when they were less alert and focused. These apparently inexplicable findings make sense in the context of perceptual fluency. When actively seeking right and wrong answers, when actively adopting a conscious strategy toward a task, the person sees her memories and thoughts as containing objective contents that must be searched actively and deliberately. Conscious awareness and restrictiveness are central to such an enterprise. The key is what can be explicitly recalled and/or thought about. When subjects do not behave in this proactive manner, memory and thought seem secondary. The person then relies upon a sometimes vague subjective sense of the familiar that requires no external justification. In short, the person relies upon more inclusive and broad unconscious processes. Specifically, he relies upon perceptual fluency.[3]

Although perceptual fluency is a very powerful concept that is relevant to a variety of unconscious phenomena, it may not be all there is to the SME effect. Murphy and Zajonc (1993) reported that their subjects were able to discriminate subliminal faces on the basis of affective expressions but not on the basis of the perceptually salient characteristic of gender. One might think that gender is a more obvious and salient characteristic than is affective expression but that proved not to be the case for subliminal exposures in this study. It seems that there is true equality of gender subliminally. Perceptual fluency cannot account for these findings. Gender should have been just as accessible, just as fluent, as affect, but it was not. There seems to be something special about emotional expression. Murphy and Zajonc interpreted their results (in conjunction with five other experiments they conducted showing subliminal effects for affective and supraliminal effects for cognitive stimuli) as support for the affective primacy hypothesis.

Other research also seems to be at odds with perceptual fluency. Blum (1954; see chapter 5) found that subjects reported that emotionally arousing stimuli (symbolic castration scenes) stood out more than neutral scenes, even when they reported no conscious recognition of them. Shevrin, Bond, Brakel, Hertel, and Williams (1996) reported that subliminally presented, personally meaningful stimuli affected brain-wave reactions in a way that neutral stimuli or the same stimuli presented supraliminally did not. Similarly, Silverman and his colleagues (Silverman, Lachman, & Milich, 1982; Silverman & Weinberger, 1985; Weinberger, 1992) showed that subliminally presented, psychodynamically meaningful stimuli affected all sorts of behaviors in ways that subliminal neutral stimuli or the same emotionally meaningful stimuli presented supraliminally did not.

None of the aforementioned research utilized stimuli that were familiar in any way. Blum's symbolic castration scenes are hardly the stuff of everyday experience. Shevrin et al. used phrases and words gleaned from intensive testing and interviewing of their subjects. And Silverman employed messages inspired by psychoanalytic theory (e.g., MOMMY AND I ARE ONE) that were unlikely to have been heard or uttered by subjects prior to the experiment. Perceptual fluency cannot account for such findings. There was no prior practice that could have led to ease of processing.

There are also neurophysiological data reviewed by LeDoux (1990, 1996) that argue against a simple perceptual fluency interpretation and seem to favor affective primacy. LeDoux (1996) concluded that the amygdala is an important part of an emotional memory system, whereas the hippocampus is a critical part of a cognitive or declarative memory system. LeDoux (1990) also reported that there is a point in the brain where only one synapse separates the thalamus from the amygdala. There are many more synapses between the thalamus and the hippocampus. This difference in access means that the amygdala can react more quickly to a stimulus event than can the hippocampus. LeDoux estimates this difference to be on the order of 40 msec. This provides the architecture for the affect before recognition posited by the affective primacy hypothesis.

There are also neurophysiological data that contradict affective primacy and support perceptual fluency, however. Johnson, Kim, and Risse (1985) conducted a mere exposure experiment with individuals suffering from Korsakoff's Syndrome—a form of brain damage usually attributable to alcoholism. Such individuals show both retrograde and anterograde amnesia. That is, they cannot recall recent events nor can they process new information. They also tend to be apathetic and unemotional. Johnson et al. found that despite demonstrating poor recognition for previously played melodies, these patients preferred them to never-before-heard melodies. In other words, they exhibited a typical mere exposure effect. This is damaging to the affective primacy hypothesis because Korsakoff patients have deficiencies in emotional responsivity. Perceptual fluency seems the only viable explanation for these results. Seamon et al. (1998) offer more such examples. Finally, LeDoux himself

(2015) has backtracked, acknowledging that the data cited in his 1996 book, which were largely collected on mice, may not apply to humans.

A Solution?

What can be made of all of this? Neither the affective primacy nor the perceptual fluency models can account for all of the data. We would like to suggest that some version of each may be correct. Thus, some version of affective primacy (or the salience model we discuss later) can be used to understand Silverman's subliminal psychodynamic activation, Blum's "stand-out" results, and the Shevrin et al. brain wave studies. All employ unfamiliar, emotionally tinged (and salient) stimuli, and all yield effects. Moreover, in all, subliminal stimulation results in more powerful effects than does supraliminal stimulation.

Fluency cannot explain such findings. Ease of processing does not seem to be relevant to any of them. On the other hand, perceptual fluency underlies the research program of Jacoby. It is also highly relevant to implicit memory findings. And it may explain why passive, non-focused responding seems conducive to obtaining subliminal effects and loose associations. Finally, some SME effects seem explicable in no other way (e.g., Bornstein & D'Agostino, 1992, 1994; Johnson et al. 1985).

Neither model seems to have a decided advantage over the other. In further support of this is Bornstein's (1992) report that the effect sizes for affective preference and other SME dependent variables were approximately equivalent. If all SME effects are due to affect, then other effects ought to be secondary, derivatives of the "true" affective response. Similarly, if fluency was primary, its most direct manifestation ought to be a sense of familiarity, with affect (and any other) effects representing a misattribution. If this were true, then affective (and any other) results would be weaker than familiarity effects. The equivalence of the two effects, in conjunction with all of the previously discussed findings, argues for the veracity of both views. This means that there may be (at least) two unconscious processes operating according to somewhat different principles. This should not be surprising.

There is no a priori reason to posit a single monolithic unconscious. Freud (1923) recognized this long ago. In the SME, the two systems happen to produce similar effects.

Both views also make evolutionary sense. An organism designed to quickly respond affectively or to whatever is personally salient in the environment is at an advantage in the struggle for survival. In a similar vein, it is in the organism's best interest to respond in ways that have worked before and to do so without effort. This saves having to constantly reinvent the wheel with every repetition of an experience.

It also frees up resources for other events and needs. The mechanisms underlying perceptual fluency make it easier for the organism to process such recurring events. This leads naturally to the efficient and adaption-enhancing process of automatization.

The relevant research questions ought not to be which process is more real. Instead, investigators might better spend their time determining how each functions, how they interact, and how they become integrated or conflict. Later in this book, we review evidence for both processes and discuss their relevance to psychotherapy. Perceptual fluency will be seen to partly underlie implicit memory, attribution, and automaticity, all of which have powerful implications for psychotherapy (and many other phenomena). We also review the data on affective versus cognitive salience, which has equally powerful implications for psychotherapy and many other phenomena. The integration we come up with favors neither fluency nor affect. Rather, we argue that what is important is what is most salient and plausible to the person. This can and often is affect, but it can be other things as well. The keys are *salience and plausibility,* not affect or any other quality.

In any case, the SME is a well-established, valid psychological phenomenon. Whatever underlies it, it provides powerful support for the existence of unconscious processes.

NOTES

1. We have not reproduced the exact design, nor all of the conditions for either the Schvaneveldt et al. (1976) or Marcel (1980b) studies. There were other sets of words and control conditions. Our purpose is to make the basic conditions clear so that the reader can follow the reasoning and understand the basic findings.

2. This parallels Eriksen's (1959) Multiple Concurrent Response Model understanding of the subception effect. Recall that he pointed out that recognition of the relevant stimulus in subception experiments was a two-alternative, right or wrong task. GSR, on the other hand, was continuous and therefore potentially more sensitive to relative degrees of certainty and doubt. In the SME effect, liking is neither right nor wrong. It can therefore reflect doubts and relative certainties better than can recognition. The 60% preference for the previously presented stimulus reflects this relative variable. The 50% recognition score reflects the absolute, right or wrong variable.

3. Another area where perceptual fluency may be operative is the "sleeper effect" of attitude change research. It has long been known that the more prestige and credibility a communicator has, the greater the likelihood that his message will influence an audience. However, Hovland and Weiss (1951) showed that this wore off after a few weeks. The message became influential

regardless of who had delivered it. The target had forgotten the source but was still influenced by the message. This was termed the *sleeper effect* because of the delayed change in message effectiveness. Although it has never been thought of in this way, the sleeper effect can be explained through perceptual fluency. The second time the message is delivered, sans source, it is somewhat familiar. It is therefore now easier to code and process (perceptually fluent). Since it is an effort at persuasion, the person misattributes fluency to force of argument or persuasiveness and agrees with the message. See also Kelman and Hovland (1953), as well as Bornstein and D'Agostino (1992).

CHAPTER 8

Attention Models Bring
the Unconscious to the Mainstream

The mainstreaming of attention models opened the door for theorizing about unconscious processes. In this chapter, we review some of the major early efforts in this area.

DIXON'S RETICULAR ACTIVATION MODEL

Dixon (1971, 1981) bridged attention theories and subliminal perception with unconscious processes. He pointed out that, whatever their differences, all attention models posit analysis and decision making outside of awareness. This is necessitated by the temporary storage and selection stages that are part and parcel of all the models. That is, all information is said to be stored in some temporary buffer. The information-processing system then chooses from among the stored inputs on some basis or another. In order for this selection to take place, the system must be able to differentiate among various properties of the inputs. And it must be able to do so prior to the emergence of phenomenal awareness. Selection therefore is also unconscious. What becomes conscious is only a subset of what is processed and selected. (Once again, we meet the restricting effects of awareness.)

Subliminal perception experiments demonstrated that when stimulus energy is reduced or masked, the subjective experience of the stimulus weakens and finally disappears. That is, the person can no longer report on, is no longer consciously aware of, the stimulus. Nevertheless, the stimulus still has measurable effects (i.e., the person still shows some response to it). Lack of awareness, coupled with measurable responsiveness, is the essence of subliminal perception. In order for this phenomenon to exist, the stimulation must have been processed to some degree; it must have made some impression on the nervous system, even if this impression did not rise to the level of awareness. This is in complete accord with attention theories. In the language of those theories, selective processing took place outside of awareness. Thus, unconscious processing and even subliminal perception can be logically deduced from attention theories.

Dixon described what a model that captured the aforementioned connections between subliminal perception and attention would have to include. Such a model would require a system in which all information could be temporarily collected and stored (like Broadbent's echoic storage [1958] or Neisser's icon [1967]). There would also have to be a monitoring system (or systems) that could compare the stored input to some sort of internal dictionary. Based on these comparisons, a regulatory channel would see to it that those signals meeting relevant criteria would be inhibited or enhanced. These outcomes would lessen or increase (respectively) their chances of achieving phenomenal awareness. Inhibited information would not be ineffective and disappear; it would affect behavior but not reach awareness. Noninhibited or enhanced information would both affect behavior and reach awareness.

Dixon's model sounds like a modified version of Treisman's (1969) or Deutsch and Deutsch's (1963) models. Dixon's model also resembles Freud's (1900, 1915) topographical model. Recall that Freud singled out attention as the variable that brought ideas into consciousness. His censors were selection devices, and information was processed by the preconscious–conscious system.[1] Dixon also made much of the enormous differences between the input (receptive and storage) and output (effector) channels of the information-processing system. Input channels are relatively economical in terms of the physical space they require and the energy they consume. Many such channels therefore evolved. This allowed for processing of vast amounts of input. Effector channels, on the other hand, take up a great deal of space and utilize large amounts of energy. They therefore did not proliferate in the nervous system and did not develop anywhere near the capacity of the input channels. This arrangement means that input channels can operate in parallel whereas output channels must operate sequentially.

To deal with this disparity in capacity and action, a decision mechanism evolved. Its function was to scan the vast amount of input and select the information most relevant to situational demands and the organism's needs. This more limited information was then passed onto the capacity-poor effector channels. Consciousness appears at the level of this limited, sequential output system and represents only a small subset of processed information. The higher sensory threshold required for conscious apprehension shows that it requires more energy for its activation. And, again, subliminal perception flows logically from this model.

ERDELYI'S MULTIPLE SELECTION MODEL

The next theorist to connect subliminal perception and the New Look with attention theories was Erdelyi (1974). Erdelyi was struck by the irony of the New Look being discredited by a model of perception that was itself in the process of being discredited by attention theories. What he added to Dixon's (1971) views was the notion that selectivity need not occur only once or in one place in the information-processing sequence. Instead, Erdelyi argued that selectivity took place at many levels of information processing. There are therefore many different selection processes operating throughout processing. Input progresses through a series of stores, processes, and transformations. Selectivity can therefore be found wherever one chooses to examine the information-processing system. The whole controversy over whether selection happens early (e.g., Broadbent, 1958) or late (e.g., Deutsch & Deutsch, 1963) was therefore a red herring, in Erdelyi's view. The real questions concern identifying the myriad points at which selection occurs and the nature of the selection at these various points. The effect of one set of selections and transformations on subsequent sets is also relevant.

Since much processing goes on in parallel, several selections may take place simultaneously. Moreover, such selections can be based on innumerable stimulus qualities including structural features, arbitrary stimulus characteristics, and meanings. Even Freudian qualities like drives, wishes, and defenses could, in principle, be bases of selection. Erdelyi (1985) offered a book-length monograph on how this could occur. Thus, Erdelyi's model can assimilate the Freudian unconscious into a multistage, parallel-processing information system.

SHEVRIN AND DICKMAN'S CRITICAL DURATION MODEL

A paper by Shevrin and Dickman (1980) was the next important step in bringing unconscious processes into the mainstream. These authors built upon the data and theoretical conceptions of attention and subliminal perception to assert that unconscious processes ought to become part and parcel of all psychological theorizing. They asserted that unconscious psychological phenomena parallel conscious psychological phenomena. That is, they include perception, judgment, cognition, affect, and so on. Further, unconscious processing is not rare, anomalous, or crude. Most processing takes place outside of awareness and much of it is complex. And, finally, unconscious psychological processes are not restricted to attention and subliminal perception. They pervade all of psychological functioning. About a decade later, Greenwald (1992) wrote an influential paper arguing for a simple and primitive unconscious, thereby disagreeing with Shevrin and Dickman. But years after that, Hassin (2013) and Dijksterhuis (e.g. 2004; Dijksterhuis & Nordgren, 2006) argued that the unconscious is broad and high level. They thereby supported a view similar to that of Shevrin and Dickman, without its psychodynamic overtones.

Models of unconscious psychological processes can take two forms, according to Shevrin and Dickman. A "weak" model of the unconscious simply asserts that unconscious processes exist and actively affect ongoing behavior and experience. A "strong" unconscious incorporates the weak unconscious but adds the belief that conscious and unconscious processes operate according to qualitatively different principles. Shevrin and Dickman reviewed the extant attention and subliminal models and concluded that virtually all of them were in accord with a strong model of unconscious processes. First, all posited a psychological, active unconscious (so far, the weak model). Additionally, processes outside of awareness were held to be qualitatively different from overtly conscious processes (strong model). For example, in virtually all of the models, unconscious processes operate on many channels and run in parallel, whereas conscious processes are restricted to a single channel and run off sequentially.[2]

Shevrin and Dickman also argued that unconscious processes do not all run off automatically and/or randomly. They proposed instead that there were psychodynamic aspects to unconscious functioning. (Shevrin was a psychoanalyst.) First, unconscious processes can be, and often are, motivated. That is, they are meaningfully related to the individual's needs, desires, and life situation. Second, Shevrin and Dickman suggested that events can be stored in long-term memory for extended periods of time, even years, before they affect ongoing behavior. Such memories may or may not have ever been conscious. These memories can be retrieved and affect behavior without ever reaching consciousness themselves. Attention and subliminal theories of that time did not explicitly call for such operations, although there was nothing in these theories that would militate against them. They simply were never considered. These kinds of phenomena were and are routinely discussed by psychoanalysts, however (albeit mostly without any supporting empirical data).

Later data and theory on implicit memory and on automaticity support both of these contentions. We review them in Chapters 12 and 15. So Shevrin and Dickman's work was prescient.

MARCEL'S MULTIPLE REPRESENTATION MODEL

The final model of unconscious processing of this era was proposed by Marcel (1983a, 1983b). It owes more to the theorizing of Posner (1973) than to any of the other models reviewed. We like to think of Marcel's model as a "shoot first and ask questions later" view of information processing. According to Marcel, all information impinging on the organism (i.e., all input) is processed every way the information-processing system is capable of processing it. There is no system, no overarching organizing principle. The strategy seems to be to make certain that nothing is missed. That more is processed than is needed is the cost of such an approach. Given the enormous number and low energy consumption of the input channels available, this is an evolutionarily acceptable price tag (cf. Dixon, 1981).

Although processing is characterized by overinclusiveness and comprehensiveness, it is not primitive or simply preliminary. Quite the opposite. Multiple complex and sophisticated processes are brought to bear on the data. It is just that there is no effort to classify and/or integrate the results. Later processes, culminating in consciousness, sift through the clutter. It is their job to pick and choose the most relevant and useful aspects of the processed information and make coherent sense of them. It is also their job to inhibit the information deemed less relevant and useful. This is necessary because, unlike input, output is biologically expensive. There are relatively few output channels, and they use up a lot of the organism's resources (cf. Dixon, 1981). All of this goes on outside of awareness. (A later and more sophisticated model with similar ideas of initial broad activation followed by restriction as the mind settles into a solution is offered by PDP [McClelland & Rummelhart, 1986], described in Chapter 21.)

If we had direct access to the processed (unconscious) information at this point, we could make little sense of it. Although it is highly processed and therefore transformed from the original stimulation that instigated it, it is not yet organized in such a way as to be related to the world as we are used to experiencing it (this is not dissimilar to the notion of unformulated experience put forth by psychoanalytic relationists described in Chapter 4). Numerous alternative representations of the information exist side by side. So what we have are multiple, alternative ways of looking at the same information. Some of these representations may be antithetical to others; some may be complementary; and some may be completely orthogonal. Figure is not separated from ground; there is no segmentation into events, objects, and episodes. There is no narrative structure. These representations are not even oriented to time and space. The information resembles what James (1890/1950) termed "a blooming buzzing confusion." Marcel was a bit less poetic and called it a nondisjointed flow. (Later in this book, we review embodied cognition and the neural reuse models that predict it [M. L. Anderson, 2014; Dehaene, 2005; Gallese, 2007]). These models predict that information is not transformed in some arbitrary disembodied fashion, as Marcel seems to believe, but by networks that also serve other purposes.)

The information-processing system must have some way of structuring and organizing these cacophonous representations into sensible, actionable forms. It must be able to sift through the various possibilities, pick the best, and organize or structure them properly. That it is not always successful is easily shown by all of the maladaptive behaviors people engage in. We say more about this when we cover heuristics, implicit memory, implicit learning, affective salience, attribution, and automaticity, as well as the clinical implications of each of these processes. But whether or not the end product is adaptation enhancing or not, some selection has to take place. This selection process must be able to inhibit other representations so that they do not interfere with the ones chosen. (Again, PDP offers a more modern model of a process like this one.) Consciousness is the end product of these selection and inhibition processes. Thus, the transformation of unconscious to conscious representations consists of imposing a definite structure, a particular interpretation, on what, to that point, consisted of multiple disconnected and disjointed (possibly even contradictory) interpretations. By performing these functions, consciousness makes coherent, adaptive sense of as much of the available information as possible.[3]

Consciousness appears late in this model. It is an end product of a great deal of prior processes. This means that the person becomes aware of higher-order, already organized percepts and meanings. The steps that went into the making of these percepts and meanings are not available to consciousness. Marcel's masking studies (Marcel, 1983a, 1983b) and other data (detailed below) support his (Marcel, 1983b) model. In Marcel's (1983a, 1983b) studies of polysemous words, the influence of a masked (unconscious) polysemous word was not dependent upon the word that preceded it. No matter what the preceding word was, the masked polysemous word enhanced the subject's ability to react to the target word. In the supraliminal (conscious) condition, on the other hand, only the meaning of the polysemous word primed by the preceding word was available. If it was associatively linked to the target word, it reduced reaction time; if it was not, it retarded it. Thus, more than one meaning of a word was simultaneously represented unconsciously, whereas only one meaning was represented consciously. This supports Marcel's (1983b) notion that there are multiple unconscious representations but only one achieves consciousness.

Other classic phenomena in psychology can also be explained through Marcel's (1983b) model. One such phenomenon is the reversible figure. Examination of this phenomenon goes all the way back to Rubin (1915). It also played a critical role in the development of Gestalt psychology (Köhler, 1947). Reversible figures can be seen in two ways but only one way at a time, sequentially. They had to have been processed both ways to be reversible, however. Consciousness inhibits one of the alternatives, which nonetheless continues to exist unconsciously. When this second interpretation of the figure emerges in consciousness, the previously conscious interpretation is inhibited.

Other evidence that supports Marcel's views is the work of Spence (1964) on the restricting effects of awareness. As long as a word on a list was out of consciousness, its associates were active. Once that critical word achieved phenomenal awareness, however, its associates were less available to recall. Thus, a wide range of representations was available unconsciously but was inhibited once a central representation was chosen.

New Look (discussed in Chapter 5) and shadowing research (Corteen & Dunn, 1974; Corteen & Wood, 1972; Dawson & Schell, 1982—discussed in Chapter 6) also support aspects of Marcel's model. Those studies showed that meaning and physiological reactivity could exist independently of awareness. Marcel's (1983b) model is therefore a compelling one. It can account for a great deal of data. Subsequent developments (to be reviewed later in this book) like massive modularity (Carruthers, 2006; Kurzban, 2010; Pinker, 1997), parallel distributed processing (McClelland & Rummelhart, 1986; Rogers & McClelland, 2014), and neural reuse (M. L. Anderson, 2010, 2014) may have superseded Marcel's views, but his model remains a landmark in the study of unconscious processes.

NISBETT AND WILSON BRING UNCONSCIOUS PROCESSES INTO SOCIAL PSYCHOLOGY

With the exception of psychoanalysis, the theoretical models and critiques reviewed up to this point derived their arguments from relatively low-level mental operations (i.e., simple perceptual and memory tasks). One influential paper of this era was different. Nisbett and Wilson

(1977) employed findings from classic social psychology studies to make their case. Their database, therefore, encompassed higher-order mental processes like motivation, inference, and complex judgments. This meant that unconscious processes were not limited to basic information processing; higher-order psychological processes also could be said to take place unconsciously.

The classical paradigms reinterpreted by Nisbett and Wilson (1977) were cognitive dissonance, attribution theory, and bystander intervention studies. None of these areas were originally designed to demonstrate unconscious processes, nor had they been thought of in those terms. Nisbett and Wilson ingeniously reinterpreted them and persuasively argued that their results only made sense if unconscious processes were at play. The two authors also offered data from some experiments they themselves conducted. We extend their analysis to the Milgram obedience studies and to experimenter expectancy effects so as to illustrate the breadth of their arguments.

Unconscious Processes in Cognitive Dissonance and Bystander Intervention Studies

Cognitive dissonance theory (Festinger, 1957; Zimbardo, 1969) holds that if a person knows things about herself (attitudes, behaviors, thoughts, feelings, or any combination of these) that are at variance with one another, a state of psychological discomfort or tension results. The person then acts so as to reduce that discomfort by changing or altering one of the discrepant bits of self-knowledge. If the conflict is between an attitude and some behavior that contradicts that attitude, the behavior cannot be altered. But a privately held attitude can be altered; it therefore is. The appeal of this model of human functioning is that it leads to predictions that run counter to common sense. For example, Festinger and Carlsmith (1959) paid subjects either $1 or $20 to tell the next potential subject (actually a confederate) that the task he had just completed (and the new person was about to begin) was enjoyable. In fact, it was horribly boring. Everyone complied with the experimenters' request. Those paid $1 rated the task as more enjoyable and were more likely to agree to do something similar again than those paid $20. Common sense might predict the opposite. Those receiving $20 should have a more benign view of the task and agree to do it again. But dissonance theory predicted the results that were, in fact, obtained. All participants experienced some dissonance in saying the task was enjoyable when it was actually boring. Those who received $20 could easily say, "I did it for the money." (Twenty dollars meant a lot more in 1959.) This would reduce the dissonance. But asking someone to tell a lie for a paltry dollar does not relieve dissonance. So something else has got to go and that something is the evaluation of the task. The person decides that the task was not so bad after all. This type of result has been reported many times. Dissonance findings are one of the more reliable results in the social psychology literature.[4]

Self-perception theory, also called insufficient justification, is dissonance theory's cognitive cousin. It is essentially dissonance theory without the motivation and discomfort. Instead, it hypothesizes that subjects perform a logical appraisal of their behavior and come to the same conclusions as are predicted by dissonance theory.

Nisbett and Wilson (1977) examined dissonance or insufficient justification studies in detail. They found that there was no evidence for the affect or the reasoning supposedly underlying dissonance reduction. Participants never stated that they had experienced discomfort, which they then needed to alleviate. Neither did they report that they had engaged in the type of cognitive strategy hypothesized by either dissonance or self-perception theory.

Nisbett and Wilson went so far as to contact some of the more prominent dissonance researchers and asked them if they had ever uncovered any conscious awareness of the processes underlying dissonance findings. They reported that they had not. Moreover, when the hypothesized dissonance or self-perception reasoning was presented to subjects, they denied having engaged in it. They were even unaware, for the most part, that their attitudes had changed at all.[5] Thus, whatever had occurred seems to have taken place outside of awareness.

Nisbett and Wilson (1977) did not only base their arguments on a lack of reported awareness. Many dissonance studies involved behaviors like eating grasshoppers (Zimbardo, Weisenberg, Firestone, & Levy, 1965) or agreeing to undergo electrical shocks (Zimbardo, Cohen, Weisenberg, Dworkin, & Firestone, 1966). This resulted in behavioral and psychophysiological findings to supplement the more cognitive attitudinal results. Nisbett and Wilson noted that these behavioral and psychophysiological results were usually stronger than were the verbal attitudinal results obtained. That is, the effect size for the amount of shock taken or for the originally counterattitudinal behavior engaged in was larger than the effect size of the subjectively experienced pain or the reported change in attitude. If the effects were mediated by attitudinal change, as both dissonance and attribution theory maintain, verbal reports should more directly reflect these attitudinal differences than should nonverbal behavior. The nonverbal behavior should have been mediated by said attitudinal changes and so should have been weaker.

But the opposite occurred. Moreover, the correlations between verbal and nonverbal results tended to hover around zero. If both came from the same source, they should have been positively correlated. But they were not. In toto, these results show that conscious, verbal cognitive processes cannot underlie the findings. Unconscious processes must be implicated instead.

Bystander intervention studies were inspired by news accounts of people not coming to the aid of others who were in dire straits. Sometimes, this inaction even resulted in death. Latane and Darley (1970) discovered that help becomes less likely as the number of witnesses or bystanders increases. That is, a victim is more likely to be helped if there are only a couple of people (or even just one person) around them than if a crowd is present. It is as if the bystanders assume that someone else will help so they do not have to. There is diffusion of responsibility to the detriment of the victim.

As in the dissonance experiments, participants in the bystander experiments showed no awareness or recognition of the relevant causal variables. They were unaware that the number of people around them affected their helping behavior. Further, they denied that this could be so when it was presented to them as a possibility. Even showing them the data could not get them to recognize the truth. Clearly, they were not aware of the reason for their actions or the lack thereof.

Extending Nisbett and Wilson's Analysis to Obedience and Expectancy Effects

In Milgram's (1974) obedience to authority studies, subjects believed that they were delivering electric shocks to another subject as part of a learning experiment. They began by administering mild shocks and were gradually asked to deliver more severe shocks. (A meter rated degree of shock from "Slight" to "Danger: Severe Shock 450 Volts.") In reality, the other subject was a confederate and the shocks were bogus. The purpose of the study was to see how powerful a shock subjects would be willing to administer at the behest of the experimenter. Milgram asked mental health professionals and laypeople to estimate the percentage of subjects who would administer an ostensibly deadly shock (450 volts). These consultants predicted that empathy, compassion, and a sense of justice would keep compliance below 2%.

In the actual experiments, about two-thirds of the subjects delivered the maximum, ostensibly deadly, shock. Moreover, they were willing to do so repeatedly. They did this despite protests from the "victim," which included banging and screaming. In some conditions, the victim stopped responding altogether so that he seemed unconscious or even dead. Subjects shocked him anyway. The subjects were often agitated and upset (there is a marvelous film of these studies that shows just how these subjects reacted: see *http://alexanderstreet.com/products/stanley-milgram-films-social-psychology*), but they continued to administer shock. Their only external justification for this brutal action was that the experimenter had asked it of them. Milgram could reduce compliance by bringing the victim physically closer to the subject. The lowest compliance was obtained when the subject had to physically place the victim's hand on the shock plate. Even in this condition, compliance was at 30%, well above any prediction.

Milgram debriefed his subjects and found that those who administered maximal shock showed remarkably little insight into the manipulations and conditions of the experiment. Many blamed the "victim." None recognized the importance of victim proximity, although this was the most powerful mediating factor uncovered by Milgram. Furthermore, no one, including experts, predicted anywhere near the level of compliance obtained. Milgram concluded: "The subject is controlled by many forces in the situation beyond his awareness, implicit structures that regulate his behavior without signaling this fact to him" (pp. 44–45). The Milgram studies represent another classic social psychology finding that fits Nisbett and Wilson's analysis.[6]

Another classic series of studies that appear to support Nisbett and Wilson (1977) are investigations on experimenter expectancy effects. Basically, when researchers, teachers, or supervisors expect something from their subjects, pupils, or supervisees, they seem to get it. Somehow, they treat these individuals in such a way as to induce the behavior. Alternatively, they somehow communicate their expectations, and the objects of these communications comply. This result has been found literally hundreds of times (Rosenthal, 1976; Rosenthal & Rubin, 1978). Most writings on the subject enjoin researchers to employ careful controls, like double-blind designs, so as to avoid having expectancy effects bias results (Rosenthal & Rosnow, 1991). There is very little about understanding what underlies the phenomenon, however (Adair, 1978). So little is known about it that some thinkers have even called on extrasensory perception (ESP) to account for the effects (Krippner, 1978; Rao, 1978).[7]

Experimenter expectancy effects would be uninteresting and easy to control if they were due to conscious events. They would then simply be a consequence of fraud, sloppy research, or overzealous, inexperienced researchers. Furthermore, any influence attempts or communications to subjects would be clearly detectable, probably even by the subjects themselves. There would be no need for difficult-to-implement double-blind controls if conscious processes were responsible for the effects. It is precisely because the causes of these effects are out of awareness and are difficult to detect that they are interesting and important. Experimenter expectancy effects are a ubiquitous unconscious part of all research focusing on humans. They are a higher-order phenomenon that must be attributable to unconscious events even though they have not been recognized as such.

Everyday Unconscious Higher Processes

Finally, Nisbett and Wilson described some studies they themselves conducted to demonstrate that higher-order unconscious mental processes occur in normal, mundane, daily events. In one experiment, the authors had subjects memorize word pairs that were associatively connected to one representative of a subsequently presented category. One such word pair was "ocean-moon." This was followed by a request to name a laundry detergent. A significant percentage of subjects named "Tide." When asked how they came up with their responses, subjects offered all sorts of explanations. But they did not offer the correct one (i.e., their responses were associatively related to the memorized word pairs). When the real reason was suggested, some accepted it as a possibility but denied any subjective awareness of its influence.

A second study took advantage of a commonly observed position preference. People seem to choose items on the right side of a display more often than they choose items on the left side of the display. Nisbett and Wilson displayed some clothing in a store and asked customers to pick out the ones they liked best. Subjects tended to choose the rightmost articles. They never identified position as relevant, however. Further, when the experimenter brought it up, they denied that it had any role in their deliberations.[8] Nisbett and Wilson described five other such studies. The point was the same in all of them. In every case, subjects responded in accord with some psychological principle but were completely unaware of doing so. They usually misattributed their behavior to a nonrelevant cause and (sometimes hotly) rejected the possibility that the relevant cause had any effect on them. These studies suggest that unconscious behaviors are common and can be found in virtually every aspect of our lives.

Nisbett and Wilson's Understanding of the Data

Nisbett and Wilson came to (what were then) some radical conclusions. They declared that individuals have no privileged access to the determinants of their own behaviors. That is, people are not aware of, have no introspective access to, the thought processes that actually determine their actions. These higher-order cognitive processes are almost entirely unconscious. What seems like introspective access to the aforementioned processes is actually an illusion. The subjectively felt causal links between stimuli and behaviors are really inferred by the person after the fact. Society, culture, previous experiences, and genetic proclivities combine to create implicit behavior and personality theories. These a priori theories represent "plausible" explanations of phenomena, which are then brought to bear on whatever the person is experiencing.[9]

Here is what Nisbett and Wilson think happens. If a stimulus implies a response or bears a family resemblance to the type of stimulus that ought to bring forth that response (i.e., is plausible), that stimulus is implicated as the cause of the response. Additionally, if the stimulus captures the person's attention, its probability of being judged a cause is that much greater. Thus, the major factors in causal judgments are plausibility and salience. If the actual causes are plausible and/or salient, the person will judge correctly. If they are not, she will be in error (cf. Wegner, 1989). Recall that Neisser (1967) said something similar when he suggested that the information-processing system chooses from all of the information available to it on the basis of its "pertinence." More recently, Bar-Anan, Wilson, and Hassin (2010) offered empirical proof for a similar argument. They implicated plausibility, accessibility, and self-promotion as underlying judgments and attributions.

If what Nisbett and Wilson aver is true, then a person ought to be no better at adducing a cause for his own behavior than would someone else who is merely observing the action. Both make causal judgments on the basis of implicit, a priori causal theories, not on the basis of privileged access to current information processing. Nisbett and Wilson make exactly this claim. Specifically, they argue that participant and observer causal judgments should be highly correlated. Further, their judgments should both accurately reflect causality when the actual causes are plausible and/or available (accessible). But both should be inaccurate when the actual causes do not plausibly flow from commonly held implicit theories and/or do not clearly stand out.

These predictions were supported in an experiment conducted by Nisbett and Bellows (1977). One group of subjects was asked to read a detailed description of a job applicant and make judgments about the suitability of that individual for employment. Another group of subjects was asked how certain personality characteristics would influence their judgments about hiring someone. Both groups arrived at exactly the same judgments. And in both cases, plausibility and salience predicted the judgments.

Finally, Nisbett and Wilson proposed a *new definition of awareness*. They rejected equating awareness with accurate verbal report. They said that this was insufficient. Instead, they argued that *participant verbal report must be shown to be more accurate than observer report before awareness can be safely inferred*. Note the radical change in assumptions and methods this definition entails. No longer is consciousness the default assumption with unconsciousness having to be rigorously demonstrated. Now there is a presumption that all processes are unconscious until rigorously proven otherwise. Related to this premise is the fact that stimuli need not be rendered subliminal or otherwise made to bypass conscious perception in order for a study to claim to be studying unconscious events. Stimuli can be fully conscious and so can the responses to them. Intervening events and processes are the focus of interest and these are presumed to be unconscious. This presumption of unconsciousness is a cornerstone of the influential work of Bargh (2011, 2016; Bargh & Morsella, 2008, 2010), some of whose work we review later in this book.

As one might expect, Nisbett and Wilson's views did not go unchallenged. These challenges generally took the form of defending the usefulness of self-report. Quattrone (1985) argued that a large body of dissonance and attribution studies revealed reliable changes in self-report. He also held that the superiority of behavioral outcomes over self-report had been exaggerated by Nisbett and Wilson. Mostly, they were not significantly different from one another. And when they were, it was due to the effects of the behavioral responses on self-report. This latter claim was a rehashing of an old argument against the New Look offered by Hochberg (1953). And, like Hochberg, Quattrone had no supportive data. Smith and Miller (1978) challenged Nisbett and Bellows's (1977) data analyses. Their reanalysis indicated a positive relationship between subject estimates of environmental effects and its actual effects, independent of "plausibility."

None of the critiques could account for the vehement denials often expressed by study participants when confronted with the true causes of their behaviors, however. And phenomena like experimenter expectancy effects cannot be explained without recourse to unconscious processes. At best, these critiques may have served to mitigate Nisbett and Wilson's absolute rejection of self-report. "We view their [Nisbett and Wilson's] argument for the inaccessibility of mental processes as sound in its application to some situations, but their claim that access is almost never possible is overstated" (Smith & Miller, 1978, p. 361). The Nisbett and Wilson paper was a watershed in the study of unconscious processes, especially for social psychology. It changed the nature of the debate and continues to be regularly cited. Its critics, on the other hand, seem to have fallen by the wayside.

NOTES

1. Freud (1900, 1915) may therefore have been an early (the first?) attention theorist. Erdelyi (1985) has so considered him.

2. The findings that subliminal effects can sometimes be stronger than supraliminal effects does not fit neatly into the Shevrin and Dickman scheme. The difference between subliminal and supraliminal effects in something like the SME effect (Bornstein, 1989) is a quantitative one so it seems to bespeak a weak unconscious. But subliminal effects are counterintuitively stronger, which seems to indicate a strong unconscious.

3. Marcel's model resembles the functioning of the id and ego of Freud's (1923) structural model. Of course, what is unconscious is not held by Marcel to be populated by inherently conflictual desires, object representations, self-esteem needs, and/or affect.

4. This seems to be a psychological operationalization of Nietzsche's (1906/2014) dictum, "I did this, says memory. I cannot do this, says pride and remains inexorable. In the end, memory yields" (p. 68).

5. This is really quite convenient. Say you are buying a new car and have to choose between two equally appealing options. As hard as the choice may be, as soon as you do choose, your unconscious will make sure that your conscious appraisals change. Whichever choice you make, you will almost always end up liking it better in the end.

6. The moral implications of these studies are far reaching. See Milgram, 1974, Appendix I, as well as Baumrind, 1964.

7. A similar problem exists for placebo effects. Researchers are more interested in eliminating them than in understanding them (Weinberger, 1995, 2014; Weinberger & Eig, 1999).

8. One of us (JW) decided to informally examine a famous advertising campaign termed "The Pepsi Challenge." The ads in this campaign presented what was claimed to be a blind taste test between Coca-Cola and Pepsi Cola. Since the campaign was launched by Pepsi, it should come as no surprise that Pepsi won. Various explanations have been offered for this result, ranging from Pepsi is really preferred, to one sip leads to a preference for the sweeter drink (Pepsi) but a full cup would show no differences or even a preference for Coke. What I did was simply see which side the Pepsi alternative was on. I was able to find 10 such choices from old ads available on the Internet. All, of course, showed Pepsi being preferred. In 9 of the 10 choices, however, Pepsi was on the right. This campaign, purposefully or not, may have capitalized on the position preference Nisbett and Wilson discussed.

9. Gazzaniga (2009) has posited a brain network he calls the "interpreter" that creates a plausible story to account for our behaviors. As with the Nisbett and Wilson (1977) model, the person infers causality from her behavior. Kurzban and Aktipis (2007) explicitly made a connection between a hypothesized module they term the social cognitive interface (SCI) and Nisbett and Wilson. The SCI has no access to the true causes of behavior, it just creates the best possible "spin" so as to enhance social interactions.

CHAPTER 9

Unconscious Processes

From Mainstream to Central Tenet

The final obstacle to full acceptance of unconscious processes was probably overcome by three related and roughly contemporaneous events in psychology. The first was the recognition of implicit memory as an important phenomenon requiring explanation (Schacter, 1987). The second was the related investigation of implicit learning as underlying much of our behavior (Seger, 1994). The third development was related to the first two in that it advanced their study as well. It was the systematic and integrated study of the functioning of brain-damaged individuals. All of these areas embedded unconscious processes into their core theoretical structures, elevating them to normative status. Further, previous findings relating to unconscious processes fit with and paralleled results reported by these three areas of investigation. We begin this chapter with brain damage research and then discuss how that work led to postulating unconscious processes as normative and central, even underlying consciousness and the self.

BRAIN DAMAGE STUDIES

Researchers have been studying individuals who had suffered serious brain damage, either as a result of surgery or through accident, for hundreds of years (Shelley, 2016). It has captured the popular imagination as well (Sacks, 1985). It seems that damage to different areas of the brain results in highly distinctive effects. What people can and cannot do subsequent to their injuries was said to reveal the functions of the damaged parts of their brains. That is, if one brain-damaged individual demonstrated one type of deficit whereas another showed a different kind of impairment, the logical inference is that the different insults to their brains damaged different, separable components of their information-processing system. By studying these individuals, investigators learned to identify and understand the functioning of some of these separable components. (Note the unquestioned assumption of isolable components—modules—having specific functions. We will return to that later in this book.)

The literature in the area of brain-damage is voluminous, so we focus on only a few examples here. These were chosen because some of the findings parallel unconscious phenomena in non-brain-damaged individuals, discussed earlier in this book. The reader interested in learning more about how the functioning of the brain can go awry is referred to eminently readable books by Restak (1994), Sacks (1985), and Ramachandran and Blakeslee (1999). Investigations of what has come to be called the split-brain (see Gazzaniga, 1998, for a review of the work in this area) probably did more to usher in the systematic study of brain damage and the modular view than did any other set of studies (Gazzaniga, 1999).[1] The split brain refers to the apparent independent functioning of the left and right hemispheres of the cerebral cortex. This independence of functioning is only apparent when the corpus callosum, a large fiber system that connects the two hemispheres, is severed. Although radical, this surgery is sometimes performed to manage epileptic seizures that begin in one hemisphere and are then communicated to the other. Once the cut has been made, there is virtually no way for the neurons in one hemisphere to send signals to the neurons in the other, thus limiting the spreading of seizures. This has effects that can be observed under controlled laboratory conditions. After the cut, each of the now separated hemispheres seemed to function independently, as though it were an autonomous, self-contained brain.

The original research on split-brain phenomena was conducted in the 1960s by Gazzaniga (e.g., 1970) and Sperry (e.g., 1968). In the 1970s, Gazzaniga, LeDoux, and Wilson (e.g., Gazzaniga & LeDoux, 1978; Gazzaniga, LeDoux, & Wilson, 1977) continued the work. This research capitalizes on the normal lateralized functioning of the human visual and tactile sensory systems. When a person fixates upon a point in space, all visual information to the right of that point is projected to the left half of the brain and all visual information to the left of the point is projected to the right side of the brain. Given enough time, a person will move his eyes and the stimulus will end up being projected to both sides of the brain. A visual stimulus must therefore be presented quickly enough to preclude eye movements if information is to be limited to one hemisphere. No speed requirements apply for touch, but an object must be kept out of view lest visual information concerning it be sent to both sides of the brain.

In an early experiment (Gazzaniga & Sperry, 1967), lights were flashed to either the left or right visual field. When the lights were flashed in the left part of the field (and therefore processed by the right half of the brain), subjects claimed to have seen nothing. But if they were asked to point to the lights as they appeared, they did so correctly. In another experiment in the same series, subjects were asked to identify objects, hidden behind a screen, by touch. They could do so when the object was placed in the right hand (the information went to the left hemisphere). They were unable to do so when the object was grasped by the left hand (and the right hemisphere received the information). They could identify it on a nonverbal test, however. Yet, even after this correct nonverbal response, they could not verbally name or describe it. In the final experiment of this series, the word "heart" was flashed on a screen. The "he" portion of the word was to the left of the fixation point; the "art" portion to the right. When asked what they saw, subjects replied "art." When asked to point to the word they had viewed, they chose "he."

These and other experiments led Gazzaniga and Sperry to conclude that the speech centers of the brain are located in the left hemisphere. Because of the commissurotomy, this hemisphere had no access to stimuli sent to the right hemisphere and could not speak of them. As nonverbal indices made clear, however, these stimuli were registered and processed. The radical nature of the separation of these functions is demonstrated by subjects' continued inability to verbally describe a stimulus even after it has been nonverbally identified. The left literally does not know what the right is doing.

Additional split-brain studies indicated that the left and right hemispheres serve several other distinctive functions (see Gazzaniga, 1998, for a review). This was explained by positing different modules housed in the two hemispheres. In general, the modules of the left hemisphere were said to operate analytically, focusing on details, whereas the modules of the right hemisphere were seen as operating more holistically, attempting to synthesize details into a unity.

Another type of brain damage is what Weiskrantz (1980, 1983, 1986; Weiskrantz, Warrington, Sanders, & Marshall, 1974) termed "blindsight." A patient (labeled DB) had a major part of his right striate cortex surgically removed in order to excise an arteriovenous malformation. One unfortunate result of this operation was that DB reported being blind in his left visual field. Nonetheless, he could correctly indicate the position of a point of light, reach for objects, discriminate between horizontal, vertical, and diagonal lines, distinguish between Xs and Os, and even between Ts and 4s. All the while, DB reported that he saw nothing and was simply guessing. More recent work has indicated that people suffering from blindsight can also recognize emotional facial expressions (de Gelder, Vroomen, Pourtois, & Weiskrantz, 1999) as well as display an emotional reaction to a face (Tamietto Castelli, Vighetti, Perozzo, Germiniani, Weiskrantz, et al., 2009) they claim not to have seen.

What makes these reports particularly important for our purposes is that they exactly parallel findings in the subliminal stimulation literature, going all the way back to Pierce and Jastrow (1894). In a myriad of such studies, subjects reported seeing nothing but could discriminate these "unseen" stimuli at greater than chance levels. If blindsight were a subliminal experiment, critics like Eriksen (1959) would probably have argued that DB really was aware of the stimuli he successfully discriminated. Holender (1986) in fact did doubt the veracity of blindsight. A signal-detection analysis would probably produce d's greater than zero, buttressing these arguments. But because this was a brain-damaged individual, most critics were willing to accept DB at his word. Later thinkers, arguing against the concept of massive modularity, did question these findings (Prinz, 2006). We discuss these critiques when we review massive modularity later in this book.

Prosopagnosia, another form of brain damage (Bauer, 1984; Tranel & Damasio, 1985), literally means loss of knowledge of faces and results from a bilateral lesion in the mesial portion of the occipital and temporal lobes of the cortex. Individuals who have sustained this form of brain damage cannot recognize others on the basis of their facial features. This includes highly familiar others like celebrities, friends, family members, and sometimes even their own faces in a mirror. Recognition occurs on the basis of nonfacial cues like hearing the person's voice or watching her walk. No other skill or ability seems to be affected, including correctly interpreting facial expression.

Some work on prosopagnosia has revealed subception-like effects. Individuals suffering from prosopagnosia show elevated GSRs to previously encountered faces. This occurs despite denials of recognizing or even finding said faces familiar. Recall that in subception (see Chapter 6), the (brain-intact) subject evinces chance-level verbal discrimination but above-chance GSR discrimination of a stimulus. Once again, although subception was controversial, because of the neurological insult known to exist in the person suffering from prosopagnosia, these subception-like effects were not questioned for decades (but see Holendar, 1986, and Prinz, 2006).

There are also modules that seem to correspond to the structure and meaning of words. Caramazza (1996) reported that the phonology (sound), orthography (spelling), and semantics (meaning) of words are represented independently in the brain. That is, they are controlled by different modules. Coslett (1986) and Shallice and Saffran (1986) reported that alexic individuals (severe difficulty reading even common words) were able to make lexical decisions and categorize words based on their meaning even when they could not consciously identify them. Blumstein, Milberg, and Shrier (1982) and Milberg and Blumstein (1981) reported that aphasic individuals with severe deficits in word comprehension nonetheless showed semantic priming for related words. This occurred despite their conscious inability to understand the semantic relationship that linked the words. Finally, Coltheart (1987) described a form of brain damage (deep dyslexia) characterized by substituting a semantically related word for the word the individual was asked to read (e.g., asked to read the word "peach," the person instead says "apricot").

These findings suggest that unconscious and conscious semantic understanding can be dissociated. More specifically, semantic understanding can exist unconsciously in the absence of conscious comprehension and can influence behavior (Blumstein, Milberg, & Shrier, 1982; Coltheart, 1987; Coslett, 1986; Milberg & Blumstein, 1981; Shallice & Saffran, 1986). Second and perhaps more importantly, it appears that structure and meaning may be processed by different modules (Caramazza, 1996). This means the understanding of a word can be independent of its structure. They are processed simultaneously and independently. It is therefore physiologically possible to have semantic processing in the absence of lexical or structural processing. Marcel (1983b), reviewed in Chapter 7, offered a model that anticipated this point of view. The whole structure-versus-content debate may therefore be based on a false premise. Structure was presumed to precede and be necessary to meaning. That is apparently not the case. When we review computational neuroscience models of brain functioning (in Part IV), we will see that this whole issue evaporates once we accept that the brain functions in parallel rather than serially.

ARE CONSCIOUSNESS AND THE SELF MODULES?

All of the work reviewed above suggests that most brain processing occurs unconsciously. Gazzaniga (1999) estimated that we may possess hundreds, if not thousands, of separate modules. We are certainly not aware of the operation of most (if any) of these modules. Nor do we have any awareness of the integration that must take place if their simultaneous operation is to result in the unified perception, thought, and feeling that we are aware of. Awareness of integration is not the only issue. Scientists and philosophers are generally at a loss to explain how said integration occurs at all. There is no master site in the brain to which all or most modules report which then integrates their output. Brain cells communicate with other brain cells, but there is no center where they all converge. William James's assertion from 1890 still stands: there does not seem to be a series of convergences culminating in some pontifical center. There is no apparent ghost in the machine, no seat of an overarching consciousness, no homunculus, no modern physiological substitute for Descartes' pineal gland. As Dennett (1991) poetically puts it, there is no Cartesian theater. Some have termed the problem of integration the "binding problem." Although some ingenious solutions have been offered (e.g., Crick & Koch, 1990), no one has yet solved the problem.

Consciousness seems to have no place in the modular view of the brain (or in any computational model of the brain/mind, as we will see). One interesting suggestion is that our conscious phenomenal experience actually reflects the operation of yet another module. Gazzaniga (1998, 1999, 2009; Gazzaniga & LeDoux, 1978) is the major proponent of this point of view. He calls this module the "Interpreter." According to Gazzaniga, our sense of subjective awareness arises out of a module, housed in the left (verbal) hemisphere, which serves to explain our actions. It notes the behaviors we have engaged in and constructs a consistent and orderly story to account for them. It sustains a running narrative of our actions, emotions, thoughts, and dreams. The interpreter is responsible for our sense that we are coherent, rational beings. But its narratives are constructions. It does not always have access to the true reasons for our actions, and when it does not, it makes up reasons that may or may not be true. They are, however, experienced as genuine. There is evidence that supports the existence of the interpreter, much of it gathered from split-brain patients, some of which has been summarized in Gazzaniga (1998). For instance, flashing the word "walk" to the right hemisphere induced a subject to stand up and leave the room. However, when asked why he was leaving, he replied "I'm going out to get a Coke." In a similar study, upon seeing the command "laugh," subjects duly laughed, offering various spurious explanations like finding it funny that the experimenter tested them every month. "What a way to make a living." In non-split-brain patients, evidence for the interpreter can be found in patients with anosognosia. These individuals have become hemiplegic and blind on their left sides, due to parietal damage, but often deny having any problems. More bizarrely, they often respond to someone pointing out their impairments by claiming that all or part of the left side of their bodies does not belong to them. For example, Bisiach, Vallar, Perani, Papagno, and Berti (1986) described a 65-year-old woman who insisted that her left hand actually belonged to someone else (see Peskine & Azouvi, 2007, for a review).

Gazzaniga's understanding of findings like these is that whenever the right hemisphere cannot communicate with the left, the interpreter cannot "know" why a behavior occurred or failed to occur. Since its job is to interpret our responses to what we encounter in the environment, it fabricates reasons. In the case of the split-brain studies, cited above, these were plausible (getting a Coke; finding the occupation of the researchers amusing). In the cases of severe right hemisphere damage, the explanations were absurd and fantastic (the hand is not mine). It appears that the interpreter is neither self-critical nor self-conscious. Any explanation will do in a pinch, and it has no capacity to critically evaluate that explanation. If this is true, our sense of consciousness, our subjective awareness, is illusory, and its mode of operation occurs outside of awareness.

If the interpreter exists, it should not only reveal its foibles under conditions of serious brain damage. It should also be possible to observe its erratic operation in individuals with intact brains, in the everyday course of their lives. Psychoanalysis is filled with examples of people offering spurious and sometimes even fantastic explanations for their behaviors. In fact, this is at the core of psychoanalytic thinking. The true sources of our behaviors are unconscious; we then invent spurious explanations that fit in with our sense of safety and decorum to account for these behaviors. In the extreme, we can end up with delusional thinking.

The findings of Nisbett and Wilson (1977) can also be understood through the operation of the interpreter. Recall that they concluded that people have no privileged access to the actual causes of their behaviors. They observe their behaviors and then offer "plausible" explanations to account for them. Whatever captures their attention (is salient) is likely to figure prominently in such explanations. If actual causes are plausible and salient, explanations will be correct; if they are not, explanations are likely to be wrong. Later in this book, we review Bar-Anan et al. (2010) who come to essentially the same conclusion.

The interpreter fits both the psychoanalytic and the Nisbett and Wilson model. If the causes of behavior do not reach the interpreter, it will have no way of knowing why something is happening. It will then invent a reason. In psychoanalytic thinking, access to the interpreter is blocked by inhibitory processes (defenses). The phenomena discussed by Nisbett and Wilson (unconscious thought processes and affective reactions) are not available to the interpreter because of the architecture of the information-processing system (i.e., the modules or neuronal networks are simply not strongly connected to the interpreter). In the case of brain-damage, normally connected networks are physically severed from the interpreter.

To the interpreter, all of the above three scenarios lead to the same outcome: Make something up. Since the brain-damage situation is the most information-deprived and "unnatural" of the three (in the brain intact individual, the interpreter usually does have access to the relevant information), the explanations offered by the interpreter are the least satisfactory and the most far-fetched. In all three cases, however, what we experience as conscious understanding may be illusory.

Kurzban and Aktipis (2007) offer a different modular explanation of these types of phenomena. They argue that a module instantiates what we usually refer to as the "self." This module developed as a way to present oneself to others in the best possible light so as to enhance social relationships. Like the interpreter, it does not have access to all information and much of its functioning is unconscious. It has a more obviously adaptive function than does the interpreter, as it is designed to grease social interaction in the service of survival and procreation. Presumably it developed during the course of evolution because it did these things successfully. We return to this when we discuss massive modularity in our section on computational models of the mind.

UNCONSCIOUS PROCESSES FINALLY BECOME MAINSTREAM

Virtually all operations described in this chapter take place, in fact must take place, unconsciously. We could not be aware of the operation and output of the hundreds and possibly thousands of systems operating and performing different functions within us. And we certainly could not possibly be aware of them all operating simultaneously. Moreover, if Gazzaniga's (1998, 1999, 2009) interpreter or Kurzban and Aktipis's (2007) modular self exist, phenomenal awareness is just the operation of a module/network providing a running narrative or spinning reality in order to advance social relations. In either case, it generally operates outside of awareness so that we have no privileged access to our internal states. Even consciousness may not exist but just be an illusory outcome of the operation of some modular unconscious processes.

It was in the context of these developments that the existence of the unconscious became widely accepted. In 1987, John Kihlstrom (1987a) published a short paper in *Science,* which summarized the extant data relating to the operation of unconscious processes. It was a landmark publication because it represented scientific recognition of the reality and importance of unconscious processes. In 1989, Uleman and Bargh, published an edited book on unconscious processes. In 1992, Bornstein and Pittman edited a book entitled *Perception without Awareness.* Leading researchers presented their latest work in the area. In the same year, the *American Psychologist,* flagship publication of the American Psychological Association, published a special section on unconscious processes. None of these events elicited any negative response. After almost a century of denial and resistance, unconscious processes became a mainstream position in scientific psychology.

DIFFERENTIATING CONSCIOUS AND UNCONSCIOUS PROCESSES

It should now be clear that no strategy for differentiating conscious from unconscious processes is ideal. It may also be clear that, although discussion of these strategies may be couched in methodological terms, the issue is really conceptual (cf. Erdelyi, 1992) or even philosophical. If I strongly believe in unconscious processes, any behavior exhibited to stimuli below a subjective threshold is proof positive of their existence. If I adopt the even more liberal Nisbett and Wilson (1977) position (see Chapter 8), unconscious processes would be even easier to demonstrate. Everything is unconscious until proven otherwise. On the other end of the spectrum, if I doubt the existence of unconscious processes, I will demand incontrovertible proof, or I will conclude that consciousness is operating. This would take the form of a forced choice task consisting of many trials wherein the subject is asked to discriminate between two stimuli or between a stimulus and its absence. Nothing short of unequivocal responding to stimuli below this objective threshold will convince me. And respondents' denials of awareness will be meaningless to me.

The problem of choosing between these alternatives can be likened to a problem that bedevils statistics and methods in all areas of psychology (and all science for that matter). There are two kinds of errors one can make when using significance testing to judge the veracity of a hypothesis. One can conclude that a relationship exists when, in fact, it does not. This is termed a Type I error, and its probability is termed alpha. The other kind of error is to conclude that no relationship exists when one really does. This is called a Type II error, and its probability is called beta (Rosenthal & Rosnow, 1991). One type of error is not inherently more dangerous or worse than the other; it depends on what we are measuring and what the costs of being wrong are. What is worse: to mistakenly claim a cure for cancer (Type I error) or to miss noticing one (Type II error)?

As far as unconscious processes are concerned, those who favor a subjective threshold or the Nisbett and Wilson (1977) position are risking Type I errors; those who favor an objective threshold risk Type II errors. It is a preference. And preference in science is usually a function of prevailing theory and Zeitgeist. For most of the history of psychology, theory and Zeitgeist opposed unconscious processes. As a result, an impossible standard of objective threshold was demanded. Nowadays, unconscious processes are in favor, and so studies using subjective thresholds now routinely get published. Our theories not only allow, they require, unconscious processes. They have become obviously true. Bornstein and Masling (1998) reported that, from 1990 through 1998, not a single paper challenging the concept of unconscious processes appeared in a mainstream psychology journal. That has changed somewhat (see, e.g., Lahteenmaki, Hyona, Koivisto, & Nummenmaa, 2015) but is still largely the case. Old rejected studies showing the same kind of findings that are accepted today have been forgotten because they were conducted in a different, hostile culture. It is as if there was an absolute break at the changing of the Zeitgeist.

NOTES

1. Actually, the lineage of modules probably goes back to the work of Mount-castle (e.g., 1958; Mountcastle & Hennemann, 1952) who discovered that neurons within small, circumscribed regions of the cortex were related to the same part of the body. If an electrode penetrated straight down (90° vertically), all the neurons it encountered responded to the same stimulation. When the electrode deviated from the vertical, the neurons it encountered responded to different stimuli. The neurons that all functioned similarly were called "columns" because of their vertical setup. Eventually, the operative word became "module." Modules can also be likened to phrenology, which posited localized functions of the brain. If we accept that lineage (cf. Fodor, 1983; Simpson, 2005), then the idea of modularity can be traced back to Gall's (e.g., 1822–1825/1835) introduction of phrenology in the 19th century. We discuss this in more detail later in this book when we review modularity and massive modularity.

PART III

THE UNCONSCIOUS REDISCOVERED

It took psychology about a century to come to grips with the existence of unconscious processes. Except for psychoanalysis, no movement in psychology evinced any sustained interest in examining unconscious processes. In fact, such efforts were discouraged and even met with hostility. We reviewed this history in an effort to explain how and why this happened.

Despite this negative environment, studies of unconscious processes kept cropping up in every school, knowingly or unknowingly. All such efforts were ultimately suppressed. The New Look represented the longest and most productive such effort, but it too was finally stamped out. Even the efforts of psychoanalytic theory eventually stagnated because most theorists and practitioners eschewed empirical research. Only with the development of modern theories of attention did the study of unconscious processes begin to appear and develop in a systematic way. Only recently has the field really begun to focus on these processes in any kind of sustained fashion. Even so, there is no consensus on what model fits the data best or on the best methods for studying these phenomena.

In the chapters that follow, we review current systematic research to see what it has to teach us about unconscious processes, as well as to examine its implications for psychotherapeutic work. Now that we acknowledge that these processes exist, what do we know of their operation and influence? What is the nature of their effects on human functioning?

WHERE DID MORE THAN A CENTURY GET US?

Throughout the first century of psychology, unconscious processes were identified, forgotten, and then rediscovered. This discontinuity and inefficiency led to slower progress than would otherwise have been the case. We detailed this history in Parts I and II of this book. Nowhere is this ignorance of prior work more apparent than in the identification of the general characteristics of unconscious processes, described in Parts I and II. In the early 1960s, Spence (1964) asserted that unconscious processes are broad and expansive whereas consciousness is narrow and restrictive. The attention models of the late 1960s and early 1970s made this model central to their theorizing. It was also a core tenet of Marcel's (1983b) model. Yet, neither the attention theorists nor Marcel seemed to have been aware of Spence's work. The idea that unconscious processes are more likely to appear under conditions of weakened critical faculties goes all the way back to the 19th-century work of Aschaffenburg and Kraeplin (cited in Ellenberger, 1970) who catalogued the likelihood of inner and outer associations, depending upon the alertness and physical health of the respondent. Dixon (1981) later referred to the advantages of being relaxed and uncritical. Marcel (1983a, 1983b) made a similar observation. None of these authors referenced their predecessors. There are also more specific examples of this kind of reinventing the wheel. These include automaticity and subception. Automatic versus controlled processing was a sophisticated, empirical rediscovery of the functionalist view of unconscious processing. The idea in both cases is that conscious or controlled processes are brought to bear when the person faces a novel or problematic situation. When such episodes are mastered and then repeat themselves, responding to them becomes unconscious or automatic.

In a similar way, shadowing and some brain-damage studies rediscovered subception without realizing it. Subception involved a dissociation between electrodermal (unconscious) responding and (conscious) visual recognition. Shadowing studies demonstrated a dissociation between electrodermal responding and auditory awareness. And prosopagnosics show elevated electrodermal responding to faces they are unable to recognize. Here, the gap is only 15 to 25 years, but this is still a major loss of time. Furthermore, the connection between these phenomena has still not been recognized.

Accomplishments

Most of the work on unconscious processes conducted over the last century involved the question of their existence. That issue has finally been answered affirmatively. In fact, it is hardly possible to describe psychological functioning without resort to unconscious processes (see Hassin, 2013). The data seem unequivocal and the theories require them. (But see Searle, 1991, for a philosophical alternative, which denies unconscious thought. Also see Lahteenmake et al., 2015, for an empirical argument of this nature.) Now that we know that unconscious processes exist, what do we know of their operation? Not nearly enough. We do know that rather than being aberrant or unusual, *unconscious processes are normal and ubiquitous.* Rather than being peripheral and unimportant, *they are central and critical to psychological functioning,* which will remain a central theme in the rest of this book.

The field has also identified some differences between conscious and unconscious processes that support what Shevrin and Dickman (1980) termed a "strong" unconscious and what we termed qualitative differences between conscious and unconscious processing. Unconscious processes are frequently broad, expansive, and uncritical. They are often global and holistic. Several unconscious processes can operate simultaneously. They can be stereotyped, rigid, and difficult to change. Conscious processes, on the other hand, are selective and restrictive. They occur sequentially, one at a time, and are easy to disrupt. They are flexible and open to change.

Many models have identified such differences. Psychoanalysis differentiated between primary and secondary processes. Modern cognitive psychology and neuropsychology have described implicit and explicit learning and memory and have differentiated between automatic and controlled processing. There are differences in all of these conceptions. But what they all have in common can be summed up in Spence's (1964) felicitous phrase "the restricting effects of awareness." Unconscious processes are more likely to hold sway when a person is relaxed and not actively strategizing. Intuitive, spontaneous responding tends to rely on unconscious processes. Unconscious processes are also more likely to be relied upon when critical faculties are weakened, as is the case in brain damage, fever, extreme fatigue, sleep, or stress/heightened cognitive load. They can be artificially induced through degrading stimuli (e.g., subliminal stimulation), especially if participants adopt a passive, receptive attitude. Finally, a careful review of the work seems to indicate that these differences are not absolute. There are no "pure" unconscious or conscious processes. Everything is a mix of the two to varying degrees. This represents a rediscovery of Freud's (1923) realization, although this too is never acknowledged.

There is, as yet, no overarching theory of unconscious processes that can tie all of these phenomena together. That is not surprising for two reasons. First, systematic, sustained acceptance and study of these processes is only about 25 years old. Second, given the centrality we now attribute to unconscious processes, we would need a pretty comprehensive theory of mind to understand them. And we are nowhere near such a theory. Psychoanalysis, which professed to offer such models the longest, had a very productive beginning and then languished. Computational neuroscience offers promise, and we devote space to it later in this book.

Psychology has gone down a lot of blind alleys, suppressed a good deal of quality work, and discouraged thinking about unconscious processes for a long time. It seems now to finally be on the right track. In Part III, we see how systematic, ongoing efforts in cognitive and psychological science have shed further light on unconscious processes. We then sketch a model of unconscious processes that takes into account recent work while respecting the contributions of the first century of effort in this area. In Part IV, we tie it all together using recent models of computational neuroscience, specifically massive modularity, parallel distributed processing (or connectionism), and neural reuse. Finally, we summarize how our knowledge about unconscious processes applies to psychotherapy.

CHAPTER 10

The Normative Unconscious

In the last three decades, significant advancements in cognitive and social psychology, as well as in cognitive neuroscience, have systematically advanced the study of unconscious processes. Several such processes, considered to operate to various degrees in all individuals, have considerable empirical support. We regard these processes as *normative,* because they are not conflictual or motivated as is the dynamic unconscious posited by psychoanalytic theories; rather, they are universal and operate independently of repressed material, defenses, or deprivation experiences. Eight processes that seem to have garnered empirical support are cognitive heuristics, implicit memory, implicit learning, implicit motivation, automaticity, attribution, affective primacy and salience (or salience generally), and embodied cognition. In the next few chapters, we present advances in the study of these processes and their effects (e.g., how they impact decision making, problem solving, and interpersonal behaviors). We also describe important clinical implications of each. Before we enter the realm of present-day *normative unconscious processes,* we provide a brief overview of the contributions of cognitive science and its role in making unconscious processes mainstream.

COGNITIVE SCIENCE

Cognitive science developed in order to understand internal processes, specifically encoding, processing, storing, and retrieving information (cf. Gardner, 1985; Thagard, 2005). When research demonstrated and theory required that many of these processes take place outside of

awareness, the cognitive unconscious was born (Kihlstrom, 1987). Theories of attention provided a sensible context for previously disparaged
subliminal perception (now seen as an aspect of priming) as well as an
organizing theme for apparently disparate phenomena now subsumed
under implicit memory and learning. The study of automaticity also
developed as a result of an information-processing approach (Schneider
& Shiffrin, 1977; Shiffrin & Schneider, 1977). Modularity (e.g., Carruthers, 2006; Fodor, 1983; Kurzban, 2010; Pinker, 2005), connectionism (e.g., PDP [McClelland & Rummelhart, 1986]), and neural reuse
(M. L. Anderson, 2010, 2014) came into being to account for the manner
in which information was processed under ordinary and extraordinary
(brain-damaged) circumstances. It is largely because of these developments in cognitive science and cognitive neuroscience that unconscious
processes became mainstream in the research literature.

The actual term "cognitive unconscious" was coined by Rozin
(1976), although, as we have seen, the work subsumed by this term
began far earlier. Kihlstrom (1987) brought much of this work to the
attention of the scientific world in a seminal paper published in the
prestigious journal *Science*. He (Kihlstrom, 1987, 1999) populated the
cognitive unconscious with implicit perception, implicit learning, and
implicit memory. It could also have been said to include automatic processes. We add what has been termed cognitive "heuristics" (Kahneman,
Slovic, & Tversky, 1982; Kahneman, 2011) to this framework as well.
Conspicuously absent in early work in cognitive science were affective
and motivational processes, even though they had long been a topic of
exploration in social and clinical psychology (e.g., Kihlstrom, Mulvaney,
Tobias, & Tobis, 2000; McClelland, 1987; Stoycheva, Weinberger, &
Singer, 2014; Weinberger, Siefert, & Haggerty, 2010). (See Weinberger,
Siegel, & DeCamello, 2000, for a discussion of the absence of motiva-
tion and affect from cognitive science at that time.)[1]

HEURISTICS

A heuristic is a strategic shortcut for solving a problem or reaching a
conclusion that bypasses effortful, logical reasoning. It functions as a
cognitive rule of thumb, allowing for quick and effortless judgments and
decision making. Tversky and Kahneman (1973, 1974, 1981; Kahneman
& Tversky, 1979) determined that people employ such nonrational strategies to solve problems, make decisions, and come to conclusions, even
when they are patently wrong. They do so with no understanding of the
assumptions inherent in these heuristics and with no awareness of using

them at all. This can lead to specifiable, systematic, and unconscious biases. These heuristics and the unconscious biases that accompany them are not motivated; rather, it seems that we humans are simply built to process information in these ways, presumably as a result of natural selection (A. Reber, 1992). That is, these heuristics were generally beneficial in our environment of evolutionary adaptiveness (see Bowlby, 1969). (For a high-level popular discussion of heuristics and the theory behind them, see Kahneman, 2011.)

Tversky and Kahneman identified three major heuristics, which they termed the representative heuristic, the availability heuristic, and the adjustment from an anchor heuristic. The availability heuristic employs ease of recollection to judge the likelihood of an event. Whatever is familiar or comes easily to mind is assumed to be common or typical. For example, Tversky and Kahneman (1973) presented people with lists equally divided between names of men and women. In one condition, the women on the list were more famous; in another, the men were. When asked whether the list contained more male or female names, respondents overestimated the frequency of the gender with the more famous names. They made this mistake because the famous names came to mind more readily, and this was confused with frequency. This result is closely akin to, if not identical with, the perceptual fluency phenomena discussed earlier. It is also related to the organization of associative networks, as described by connectionist models like PDP (reviewed later in this book).

In the representative heuristic, people base their categorizations on similarity to a prototype and ignore information relating to probability. For example, Tversky and Kahneman (1973) told one group of participants that they had collected personality descriptions of 70 lawyers and 30 engineers. Another group was told that the sample consisted of 30 lawyers and 70 engineers. Participants were then presented with a few of the descriptions and asked to determine the profession of the person described. Judgments were unaffected by the numbers (i.e., by the base rate of lawyers or engineers in the sample). Instead, the judgments were controlled by the perceived fit of the descriptions to profession, regardless of the objective odds. This too seems in line with how associative networks operate in connectionist models. It also has great relevance to bias and prejudice.

The adjustment from an anchor heuristic refers to the fact that people's opinions and estimates are influenced by their immediate past experience. Tversky and Kahneman (1974) had their participants spin a wheel of numbers and then guess whether the number that came up was greater or less than the percentage of African countries in the United

Nations. They were then asked to guess the actual percentage. The number that happened to come up influenced their guesses—the lower the number, the lower their estimate and vice versa. Thus, just having something in mind influences subsequent judgments. And this is not only true for numbers. Factual knowledge and social judgments are also affected in this way (Russo & Shoemaker, 1989; Zuckerman, Koestner, Colella, & Alton, 1984). Wilson, Houston, Etling, and Brekke (1996) offer a nuanced analysis and demonstration of this phenomenon.

We would like to offer an alternative explanation of these heuristics that places them more firmly into the model of unconscious processes we present in this book. This explanation retains their unconscious nature but integrates them into a single, associative network framework without the need to posit three independent, evolutionarily based problem-solving strategies. Our argument is that heuristics can be subsumed under either chronic, long-established associative networks or under acute, short-term associative networks. We begin with the availability heuristic. The idea here is that whatever comes most easily to mind is judged as typical or more frequent. The example given was looking at a list of famous names of men and women. When more famous names were female, the respondent thought that more names on the list were female as well, even though the number of male and female names was equal. When more famous names were male, the results were the opposite.

What is triggered by a famous female name? More famous female names. Associative networks related to frequency are not triggered by this intervention. So the associative network activated by this intervention did, in fact, have more female names. As a result, the person relied on her associative network rather than on the actual numbers presented. Clinically, a depressed person has chronically activated negative networks. She will then tell the therapist that most things in her life have been negative and that she feels hopeless, regardless of the actual frequency of negativity in her life. Anyone who has dealt with a depressed person has experienced this phenomenon. Similarly, when a personality description is presented, it activates associations to that description. If the personality described is more closely aligned with that of a lawyer than that of an engineer, the person will guess lawyer and vice versa. The numbers representing the percentages of 30 to 70 are not part of this chronic and strong associative network. As a result, the associations related to the description will trump those related to the math. This can explain the representative heuristic.[2] In the real world, a white person might be more likely to perceive an object as a weapon in the hands of a young black male than in the hands of an older white woman because, unfortunately, this is the associative network many white people have. Thus, this heuristic, explained as a result of associative networks, can help us to understand stereotyping and prejudice. We all carry around associative networks that relate to different groups of people (Devine, 1989) (e.g., men, women, African Americans, Jews, gay people, immigrants, Muslims, liberals, and conservatives). When we are asked to evaluate such groups, our evaluations tend to be in line with these stereotypes, regardless of our conscious beliefs concerning them (Greenwald, McGhee, & Schwartz, 1998). And so are our actions. When we are talking about lawyers, engineers, and artists, this can be harmless. When we are talking about minority groups or outgroups, this can represent some of the most serious problems our society faces. And it seems as though part of the problem comes from normative unconscious associative processes.

Finally, the adjustment and anchoring heuristic demonstrates that people's judgments are influenced by immediate past experience. This is not a new finding. Harry Helson's (1964) adaptation-level theory demonstrated this phenomenon and developed an entire model of psychological functioning based on it decades ago. These results can be understood associatively as well. The "anchor" triggers an associative network for that situation. A number or a fact (or an experienced weight for that matter) sets up a temporary associative network with that number or fact as central. Subsequent judgments will then be related to that newly activated network. As a result, judgments will be made in the context of that newly activated network. Thus, the view of human nature of a homicide detective will be much grimmer than that of a social worker. The detective may see the social worker as naive, whereas the social worker will see the detective as cynical. Both are operating out of a context of their anchoring associative networks.

This model has the advantage of positing one mechanism, activated associative networks, rather than three separately evolved heuristic strategies. But no matter how one conceptualizes heuristics, be it as unconscious strategies or as unconscious associative networks, the data show that a great deal of our thinking is unconscious and nonreflective. Thinking and judgments are often automatic, unconscious, and arational. If one accepts the Tversky and Kahneman formulation, these judgments follow rules (heuristics) that were adaptive probabilistically and historically in our evolutionary past. The biases and flaws of these heuristics can be made apparent under special circumstances. If one accepts our associationist interpretation, these judgments are strongly influenced by normatively activated associative networks that do not require a particular evolutionary past beyond the adaptive value of associative networks. The connectionist model of PDP, reviewed later in this book, can account for such findings, as well as many others, relatively easily. That is why we prefer this interpretation. It handles the data with one principle rather than three separate processing mechanisms. In either case, these types of erroneous conclusions can be overridden by conscious processes if they are noticed, but even then only with difficulty. They remain the default. If the reader doubts this, he has merely to read the experimental examples of Kahneman and Tversky or try JW's classroom demonstration to see how these operate in himself and how difficult it is to get past them.

NOTES

1. As an example of this purposeful early neglect, consider the following quote from Gardner's (1985) otherwise excellent book on the emerging discipline: "The third feature of cognitive science is the deliberate decision to de-emphasize certain factors which may be important for cognitive functioning but whose inclusion at this point would unnecessarily complicate the cognitive-scientific enterprise. These factors include the influence of affective factors or emotions" (p. 6).

2. One of us (JW) tested this in an even more extreme way than did Tversky and Kahneman. He told his audience that the odds were 90/10 and substituted artist for lawyer (so the differentiation was between artist and engineer) and obtained the same results. Participants ignored the probabilities and chose the profession that more closely matched the associative network connected to it. These results are so reliable that this test can be used as a classroom demonstration.

CHAPTER 11

Implicit Memory

Implicit memory cannot be defined without contrasting it with explicit memory. Explicit memory refers to a person's conscious, verbalizable recollection of some event. In contrast, implicit memory is inferred when a person does something that indicates she was influenced by a previous event, even though she denies having experienced or recalling that event. That is, there is a measurable effect of past events that the person does not consciously recall experiencing. Implicit memory is therefore indexed by changed behavior in the absence of conscious recollection. Memory of the experience is implicit in the behavior (see Schacter, 1987).

Explicit memory is measured through recall or recognition tasks. The person is asked to deliberately recall or identify (recognize) some past experience and then to use that knowledge. Measurement is straightforward and direct: "Do you remember your previous experience? Prove it through this test of recall or recognition." Implicit memory is measured by performance changes on tasks that are known to be responsive to prior experience, even if the person does not recall having had those experiences. These include completing sentences or graphemic fragments of a letter, indicating a preference for one of several stimuli, performing a skilled task, and the like. In all such cases, the person must profess to have never had the relevant experience. Some would add that the person must also perform poorly on tests of explicit memory. This is termed dissociation (Kihlstrom, Dorfman, & Park, 2007).

Research on implicit memory represents a major contribution to the belief in and understanding of unconscious processes. It also relates to, supplements, and supports earlier studies of unconscious processes. Graf and Masson (1993) and special editions of *Consciousness and Cognition*

(1995, 4[4]; 1996, 5[1]) offer extensive reviews of the early research and theory in this area.

Although Schacter (1987) and Squire (1987) are correctly credited with bringing implicit memory to the attention of modern psychologists, it actually has a long and venerable history (much of which Schacter reviewed in his paper, as did Squire in his book). There are two branches to this history. One relied upon the study of brain-damaged individuals suffering from what has come to be called the "amnesic syndrome." The second branch of this history relied upon studying people with intact brains. Priming, subliminal perception, and skills learning were the methods of choice here.

THE AMNESIC SYNDROME

The amnesic syndrome is caused by damage to the medial temporal and diencephalic regions of the brain (Kuhn & Bauer, 2013; Moscovitch, 1982; Parkin & Leng, 2014; Squire, 1986). The sufferer is said to be unable to transfer information from short- to long-term memory. This is manifested by an inability to explicitly remember recent events and newly acquired information. New information is lost within minutes. A momentary distraction is enough to trigger forgetting of what has just transpired. The phenomenal experience is probably like constantly waking from a dream, when the contents of the dream fade, apparently forever. Other cognitive functions like perception, language, and general intelligence are held to be spared in the amnesic syndrome.

One of the earliest accounts of implicit memory in the amnesic tradition was supplied by Claparède (1911/1995). He reported the case of a woman suffering from Korsakoff's syndrome. Korsakoff's syndrome is a disorder usually resulting from alcoholism in which the diencephalon has been damaged (Paller et al., 1997). The woman studied by Claparède did not recognize the doctors or nurses she saw daily and had to be constantly reintroduced to them. She would forget things told to her and events that had transpired within minutes.

Claparède hid a pin between his fingers, which pricked the patient when he took her hand. She quickly forgot the incident. Yet, when he subsequently reached for her hand, she precipitously withdrew it. She could not explain why. When pressed, she first insisted on her right to refuse a handshake; she then evinced suspicion of a hidden pin. She denied any memory of the pin itself, however.

Decades later, Milner (1958, 2005; Milner, Corkin, & Teuber, 1968) studied an individual she labeled HM. HM had undergone surgery to put an end to intractable seizures emanating from his temporal lobe. Among the parts removed were the medial temporal lobe, the amygdaloid complex, and most of the hippocampus (Augustinack et al., 2014). The result was amelioration of the seizures and amnesic syndrome (a tragic case of "good news and bad news"). Milner studied HM for years. Each time they interacted, they had to be reintroduced. HM would forget a list of words he was asked to memorize moments after they were removed from his presence. He did not even remember having engaged in the task. Thus, he had virtually no explicit memory. But he did show evidence of an intact implicit memory. He learned the words more quickly when given the list again. He also showed a tendency to use the words in sentence completion tasks. Finally, he could acquire some rather complex motor skills like pursuit rotor (which involves tracking a moving target) and mirror tracing. Moreover, his performance on these tasks was hardly different from that of individuals with intact brains.[1]

Many more such cases, with similar explicit–implicit dissociations, were reported. Thus, amnesiacs completed word stems using previously exposed words, with about the same level of success as nonamnesiacs (Warrington & Weiskrantz, 1968, 1970, 1978). Amnesiacs acquired motor skills as quickly as did intact individuals (Eslinger & Damasio, 1986; Starr & Phillips, 1970). They picked up complex cognitive skills like reading mirror-inverted script (Cohen & Squire, 1981; Moscovitch, 1982), puzzle solving (Brooks & Baddeley, 1976), and recall of spatial location (Postma, Antonides, Wester, & Kessels, 2008). There was even a case of an amnesiac learning to program a microcomputer (Glisky, Schacter, & Tulving, 1986). Earlier, we described a study reporting that amnesiacs demonstrated the mere exposure effect (Johnson et al., 1985). That is, amnesiacs preferred a previously observed but nonremembered stimulus to a novel one, even though both were subjectively unfamiliar. Schacter (1987, 1992, 1996, 2001) reviewed much of the classic work. (See Kuhn and Bauer, 2013, and Parkin and Leng, 2014, for more recent reviews.) In all of these cases, subjects did not even recall having worked on the tasks, let alone seeing the stimuli or learning the skills. And, in most cases, the speed with which they improved or the judgments they made paralleled that of intact individuals.

One set of interesting findings showed how trying to rely upon explicit memory can impair performance on implicit memory tasks. Graf, Squire, and Mandler (1984) found that correct completion of word stems deteriorated when amnesic subjects were told to use previously studied words to fill in the missing letters. Similarly, Schacter (1985) reported deterioration in performance in a sentence completion task when subjects were told to use the words they had just studied to fill in a missing word. In both cases, performance was comparable to that of nonamnesiacs when amnesiacs were asked to just respond with whatever came to mind. Priming effects were only adversely affected by instructions to rely upon recall (explicit memory).

What makes this particularly relevant is that it parallels an effect we have found repeatedly with nonamnesiacs. Recall that unconscious effects seem to be weaker when subjects actively search for right and wrong answers and/or actively adopt a conscious strategy. Conversely, effects are stronger when subjects rely upon some vague subjective sense (Berry & Broadbent, 1988; Dixon, 1981; Marcel, 1983a; A. Reber, 1993). This difference may reflect the differential operation of implicit and explicit memory. Searching for "correct" answers is an explicit memory strategy. If stimuli are presented so as to be out of awareness, they cannot be explicitly remembered. Attempting to rely upon explicit memory will therefore result in poor performance. Guessing or just going with what comes to mind, on the other hand, relies upon implicit memory. Since the material was processed implicitly, performance benefits. (This parallels the reasoning behind the transfer–appropriate processing approach [TAPA], reviewed below; see Roediger, 1990.)

Amnesiacs are said to have no explicit memory because of neurological insult. In subliminal experiments with non-brain-damaged individuals, stimuli are held to bypass explicit memory. In both cases, stimuli make it into implicit memory. And, in both cases, reliance upon explicit memory is a maladaptive strategy. Use of implicit memory, subjectively experienced as a guess or feeling, is the adaptive strategy. Performance in both amnesiacs and subliminal studies reflects this. Dijksterhuis, Bos, Nordgren, and van Barren (2006) presented data indicating that this is true for everyday decisions as well.[2]

The data on brain damage are not as definitive as they appear, however. First, some investigators have reported poor implicit memory functioning in amnesiacs (Chun & Phelps, 1999; Jernigan & Ostergaard, 1993; Ostergaard, 1999; Ryan, Althoff, Whitlow, & Cohen, 2000). Prinz (2006) also critically reviews brain damage findings. Perhaps more compelling than the existence of contradictory findings is an old argument going back to Eriksen's (1956) multiple concurrent response model critique of New Look findings on subception (a dissociation between physiological findings [GSR] and verbal report in forced choice discrimination; see Chapter 5). Recall that Eriksen pointed out that GSR and verbal report are separate response systems that are not highly correlated with one another and that therefore have uncorrelated error terms. Further, GSR is not nearly as precise and reliable as is verbal report. A similar argument can be made concerning the relationship between priming and recall/recognition. Like GSR, priming is less reliable than recognition or recall (Buchner & Brandt, 2003; Buchner & Wippich, 2000; Meier & Perrig, 2000). As a result, priming is less likely to yield an effect than is recognition on purely statistical grounds (see Berry, Shanks, & Henson, 2012) but can also evidence effects when recall/recognition does not. Another problem with studies based on brain damage, like the amnesic syndrome, is that conclusions tend to be based on very few cases. Often, an investigator only has one case to work with. At most, she has a few. The results are then generalized to the human race. It is dangerous to draw universal conclusions from such a small and unique database. The damage is often not perfectly known, compensatory mechanisms cannot be determined or accounted for, etc. That this may matter is evidenced by studies that show general rather than specific deficits (Prinze, 2006) and others that do not show the dissociations expected from a model positing localized brain functions (cf. Berry et al.; Reder, Heekyeong, & Kieffaber, 2009). On the other hand, we cannot simply dismiss so much work on brain damage and its assertion that there is some localization of function. We address this issue below and look at it again when we review neuroscience computational models.

IMPLICIT MEMORY IN INDIVIDUALS WITH INTACT BRAINS

Study of implicit memory in people with intact brains also has a long and distinguished history. The first to experimentally assess implicit memory in this population was probably Ebbinghaus (1913/1964). He noted that the savings method for measuring retention demonstrated memory in cases when recall did not. In the savings method, the researcher records the number of trials or amount of time it takes to reach a certain criterion of performance (e.g., perfect recall of a list of words). At some later time, the subject is again asked to perform the task and reach the criterion. Savings refers to the decreased time or lower number of trials it takes to reach the criterion on this (or any subsequent) occasion. McDougall (1923) was the first to employ the terms "implicit" and "explicit," in the sense that they are used today, to refer to different ways of demonstrating memory.

We have already covered the remainder of the relevant history. Subliminal and priming studies, reviewed in previous chapters, can all be considered examples of implicit memory in people with intact brains (see Squire, 2009). After all, behavior was affected by stimuli people could not recall having seen. Graf and Schacter (1985) first recognized the commonalities between the memory phenomena displayed by amnesiacs and certain kinds of memory performance displayed by persons with intact brains under special conditions. It was they who labeled these phenomena implicit memory.

HOW IS IMPLICIT MEMORY TO BE UNDERSTOOD?

Although few dispute the phenomenon of implicit memory, there was and is disagreement concerning what underlies it and how it should be understood. This disagreement reflects the two branches of its study. Those who came from the amnesic tradition (e.g., Benoit & Schacter, 2015; Schacter, 1987, 1992, 1996, 2001; Schacter, Gallo, & Kensinger, 2007; Squire, 2009; Tulving & Schacter, 1990) tend to understand the phenomenon in terms of separate networks in the brain. Those who came from a tradition of studying nonamnesiacs (e.g., Berry, Shanks, & Henson, 2012; Roediger, 1990; Roediger, Gallo, & Geraci, 2002) preferred explanations that rely on aspects of normal processing with one system underlying all. And then there is Reder (Reder, Park, & Kieffaber, 2009) who used drugs (midazilam) to emulate the amnesic syndrome in nonamnesiacs. She is also in the one-system camp. We begin with the normal processing approach.

Normal Processing Views of Implicit Memory

Fluency

We already encountered an example of the normal processing approach when we covered the subliminal mere exposure effect (SME). There, it went under the title of "perceptual fluency" (see Chapter 7). Recall that the argument was that experience with a stimulus facilitates its subsequent encoding and processing (it becomes more "fluent"). Further, this is an unconscious process. When asked which stimulus is liked more (or seems more familiar, or brighter, etc.), the person chooses the more easily processed (fluent) stimulus. When asked to identify the stimulus previously presented, however, fluency is not a factor. There is now a "correct" answer and conscious recollection is examined. This search fails because the stimulus was never in awareness, having been presented subliminally.

Perceptual fluency was called upon, in SME studies, to account for affective preference (or a vague sense of familiarity, or a misattribution of a quality to a stimulus) in combination with a failure of recognition and/or recall. Something like it can also be applied to implicit memory performance tasks (see Berry, Shanks, Speekenbrink, & Henson, 2012). The person fills in missing letters or words with whatever is fluent at the moment. Several theorists offered this kind of interpretation of implicit memory (e.g., Graf & Mandler, 1984; Mandler, 1980; Morton, 1979; Rozin, 1976). Basically, a recently activated and now "fluent" representation "pops into" the person's mind on implicit memory tasks. On an extrinsic memory task, the person searches awareness for the "correct" answer and fails because that answer never was in awareness. A study by Conroy, Hopkins, and Squire (2005) illustrates the fluency position well. A stimulus, that was initially unrecognizable, was gradually made clearer until it was identifiable. The task was to press a button as soon as an accurate identification could be made. The participant was then asked to determine whether the stimulus had been viewed earlier in the study. The judgment of whether the stimulus had been seen before is the explicit, recognition measure, whereas the time until identifying the stimulus is the priming/implicit measure. Amnesiacs showed the same level of fluency as nonamnesiacs did. The authors saw this study as evidence for independence between recognition and priming because the amnesiacs showed very little recognition but good priming effects. Berry et al. (2008) came to a different conclusion, however. They reanalyzed the data using signal detection methods and concluded that the data better support a single-system model. We review a more detailed example of their model (Berry, Shanks, Speekenbrink, & Henson, 2012) below.

One problem for the fluency argument is the duration of implicit memory effects. They are quite persistent. Priming effects can be demonstrated over a period of hours, days, weeks, and even months (e.g., Cave, 1997; Jacoby, 1983a; Jacoby & Dallas, 1981; Komatsu & Ohta, 1984; Tulving, Schacter, & Stark, 1982). At least one study reported effects that lasted many years. Mitchell (2006) asked individuals to identify fragments from black-and-white line drawings, some of which they had seen for 1 to 3 seconds, in a lab, 17 years earlier and some of which were new. Mitchell found that rates of identification were significantly higher for previously seen fragments than for novel fragments. This effect was present even in individuals who reported that they were unable to recall anything about their experience in the lab 17 years earlier. Mitchell concluded that implicit memory is "an invulnerable memory system functioning below conscious awareness" (p. 1). So, unconscious—or implicit—memory may be "timeless." We do not know what to make of such a remarkable finding. But it would be difficult to explain it in terms of fluency. According to a fluency argument, this finding would mean that a representation remains active or fluent indefinitely. This does not make sense. There should be a severe dropoff with time. Other representations should become fluent in the interim. Otherwise, all experiences would be fluent forever. This clearly cannot be the case (see P. Reber, 2013). A finding like this presents a real difficulty for a fluency interpretation of implicit memory.

It also does not take much time or many repetitions to obtain a long-term implicit memory effect. The drawings in the Mitchell study were presented for just a couple of seconds, yet showed effects almost two decades later. Thomson, Milliken, and Smilek (2010) mentioned a less referenced United States state during a classroom lecture. Four to 8 weeks later, students were asked to recall as many state names as they could in 10 minutes. As anticipated, they were significantly more likely to list a state name when it had been verbally presented weeks earlier than when it had not. This study not only demonstrates the aforementioned long-term (weeks) effects of conceptually based priming. It also suggests, as did Mitchell, that one-time "incidental exposure" to a stimulus may be sufficient for a long-term implicit memory to form. This aspect of the Mitchell and of the Thomson et al. findings also poses a problem for a fluency-based understanding of implicit memory. It would be difficult to argue that a single exposure could lead to weeks-long (let alone years-long) fluency. Both the Mitchell and the Thomson et al. findings argue for separate memory systems (or processes) and against a single fluency-based system.

These findings have not gone unchallenged. McBride and Dosher (1997) reported equivalent explicit and implicit recall of word stems for up to a 1.5-hour delay. Moreover, the rate of forgetting was the same for both. These findings have been replicated (McBride & Dosher, 1999; McBride, Dosher, & Gage, 2001). The authors interpreted the findings as indicating that there is only one memory system but could offer no explanation for the many reports of dissociation and long-term implicit memory effects. Perhaps explicit memory would have deteriorated beyond implicit memory effects had a longer time frame been used. We know of no study that compares the two over long stretches of time. What we have are several studies showing long-term and dissociated effects and a few showing no dissociation. On a strictly numerical basis, there are more studies showing the effects than not. Schacter, Chiu, and Ochsner (1993) interpreted these different findings as indicating that dissociation depends on what materials are used to assess explicit and implicit memory. But until the critical variables are identified and the effects can be reliably obtained or not, based on differences in these variables, the argument is moot.

Transfer–Appropriate Processing Approach

Roediger (1990; Roediger & Blaxton, 1987; Roediger et al., 2002) offered another normal processing model. The key to this approach is the degree of similarity between learning and performance conditions. In this model, performance on any memory task is enhanced to the degree to which conditions mirror those of learning. To the extent that learning and performance vary, performance will suffer. It therefore emphasizes context as critical to memory performance. Roediger et al. called their model the "transfer–appropriate processing approach" (TAPA). In TAPA, explicit memory tests draw on the elaborative coding of meaning. If performance on such a task is to be successful, learning must entail meaning or conceptual elaboration. Roediger et al. called such tasks "conceptually driven." Conceptually driven processes require active, controlled, participation by the person because elaboration, organization, and/or reconstruction are part and parcel of such processing. It is deep processing. Implicit tasks, on the other hand, rely on more surface features of stimuli. A perceptual sort of processing is involved. Learning that focuses most on perceptual factors will therefore result in the best performance. Roediger et al. refer to this as "data-driven" or perceptual processing. Data-driven processes are more passive and automatic than are conceptually driven processes. They are controlled by stimulus properties and not by the person's intentions or efforts.

When someone is asked to recall or recognize stimuli, conceptually driven processes are being called upon. Learning that stressed such processes will result in the best performance. When someone is asked to fill in blanks with whatever comes to mind, data-driven processes are implicated. Performance will be optimal when learning calls upon this same kind of processing. Performance in either case will deteriorate when learning and performance processes differ. Memorization is not enhanced by a strategy of responding with whatever comes to mind; filling in blank words is not enhanced by trying to recall subliminally presented stimuli. So this model can explain the finding (e.g., Schacter, 1985) that trying to get it right results in poorer performance on implicit tasks.

There are problems with the TAPA model, however. One involves the functioning of individuals suffering from the amnesic syndrome. Proponents would have to assume that the damage in amnesiacs is somehow related to conceptual processing but that perceptual processing is spared. But how can a process be damaged or intact? Only the structures underlying processes can be affected by physical damage. And if different structures underlying the two kinds of processes can be differentially affected, how does this position differ from a modular or network understanding of implicit memory? One module or distributed network underlies data-driven processes. This is spared in amnesia. Another module or distributed network underlies conceptually driven processes. This is damaged in amnesiacs. Another problem is Glisky et al.'s (1986) finding that an amnesiac could learn to program a computer. This seems to require more than perceptual/surface learning. It seems to require deep processing.

Source of Activation Confusion

Reder et al. (2009) offered what they termed a source of activation confusion (SAC) model to account for both explicit and implicit memory. The basic idea is that all memory is attributable to activation of a concept but that the presumed cause of that activation may be in error. Instead of modules, the SAC model posits experience-based connections between nodes. In addition to the concept node, there are context as well as feature nodes that comprise a concept's meaning and physical properties (semantic, perceptual, lexical, phonemic, etc.). (This model sounds very much like James's 1890 model of the stream of consciousness with its fringe of relations.) The rule of operation is that the strength of a concept is a function of the frequency of its activation. The strength of its connection to a particular context and/or feature is also a function of frequency of experience. (This part sounds like James's 1890 conception of habits [see Chapter 3] or of fluency, just reviewed above. It is also a main tenet of PDP. See McClelland and Rummelhart, 1986, reviewed later in this book.)

What is usually termed episodic memory actually consists of connections between concepts and contexts. Recognition or recollection is based on the strength of the episode node (the connection between the concept and the context). If the activation is weak or the episode node was never formed to begin with, recognition is only based on the activation of the concept node, which is indexed by familiarity (fluency). Reder et al. argue that a concept node has a higher base level of activation than an episode node because it has been experienced more often. Explicit memory tasks are held to be dependent upon the activation levels of both the episode and the concept nodes. Implicit memory tasks only involve the activation level of the concept node. In this conception, the connection of the concept to its context (episode node) is necessary for recollection (explicit task) but irrelevant for implicit tasks that tend to depend upon familiarity (activation of the concept node alone). What makes this a one-system model is that the representation that underlies explicit memory tasks (like recognition) and the representation that underlies implicit memory tasks (like fragment completion) are one and the same. And both depend upon activation of that representation (the concept). The difference is in the connection to other nodes. Recognition depends upon an additional connection to a context (episode node). People suffering from the amnesic syndrome have difficulty connecting to context and therefore to forming episode nodes. The reason is said to be damage to working memory and to the hippocampus, both of which are impaired in the amnesic syndrome. What is not affected in the amnesic syndrome is activation of the concept node itself. Hence familiarity-based outcomes are not affected. In cases of subliminal priming, the relevant episode nodes are not created because the structures necessary to their creation are bypassed. The superiority of implicit outcomes with delay is due to the greater base activation of the concept node over the episode node (which consists of the concept node in combination with the episode node). After all, the concept node is strengthened with every experience, whereas the episode node is only strengthened when the experience includes a connection between the concept and the context.

Reder et al. support this model in two ways. First, they review studies that did not show dissociations between implicit and explicit memory tasks behaviorally, in brain damage, in neuroimaging, and across development. The problem here is that there are also studies that do show such dissociations. So the reader must accept the authors' assertions that the studies they cite are superior and more valid than those that do not support their conception. But there is no a priori reason to do so. Their other support concerns their use of the drug midazolam, which mimics the effects of the amnesic syndrome. After administering midazolam, Reder et al. obtained results in line with their model—specifically, implicit performance on their task was not spared relative to explicit performance. Both implicit and explicit outcomes deteriorated. There are problems here as well. Equating drug-induced performance with brain damage is a risky enterprise. There could be differences between the two. Additionally, Reder et al. did find effects on procedural memory. That is, performance improved over trials in the drug group as much as in the control group. The SAC model must be considered tentative at this point, pending further investigation. But even if it is correct, the strongest conclusion one can draw from it is that there are no separate modules for the two types of memory. But the SAC model does posit differences in nodal connections. These differences are due to connection strength based on frequency of experience. So there is still a neurophysiological difference; it is simply more fine-grained. Further, Reder et al. see the operation of the hypothalamus as critical to its conceptions. This is surely a structure in the brain, and its presence/activation or absence/nonactivation is predictive of implicit versus explicit memory.

Berry, Shanks, and Henson's Single-System Model

The final normal processing view we review was offered by Berry et al. (2012). These authors did not set out to defend a specific single-system model, which they regarded as superior to multiple-system models. Rather, they tested both types of models in a general way using signal detection theory. They then fit each model to data that they generated experimentally and to already existing amnesiac data (Conroy et al., 2005) that they reanalyzed using their signal-detection, curve-fitting, model. The experimental task in each case was to decide whether a stimulus was old or new (recognition as explicit measure) and to measure reaction time to identifying the stimulus (priming as implicit measure). They tested four possible models. One was a straight single-system model, that is, the same memory system controls recognition, priming, and fluency. This model predicts that recognition and priming effects are not independent. More specifically, when recognition is high so is priming, and when recognition is low, priming effects are weaker if not nonexistent. The second model was a strict dissociation model. That is, there are at least two memory systems underlying recognition, priming, and fluency, and they are completely orthogonal. This model would predict that priming performance would be completely independent of recognition performance.

The third model was a modified dissociation model. This posits separate memory systems, but they need not be completely orthogonal. If this model is correct, there can be some independence of recognition and priming, but it does not have to be absolute. That is, the two systems (explicit and implicit) exist, but performance on the two can be correlated. The magnitude of the correlation would be expected to vary based on such factors as type of task or level of sustained attention. The fourth model was termed the dual-process signal-detection model. This is a single-system model except that there is another process, indexed by signal detection, which can affect recognition.

First, Berry et al. conducted three experiments. The results were consistent in rejecting the strict dissociation model. The experiments were not consistent concerning the other models, however. In the first, the single system provided the best fit. In the second, all but the strict dissociation model fit, with the dual-process signal-detection model providing the best fit. In the third experiment, the single-system and the modified multiple-system models provided good fits, whereas the strict dissociation and dual process, signal detection model did not.

Next Berry et al. reanalyzed the Conroy et al. (2005) data using their signal-detection models. Again, the strict dissociation model did least well, just as in their experiments. The single-system model did better for some of the brain-damaged patients, whereas the modified multiple-system model did better for others. Berry et al. combined the results and concluded that the strict dissociation model had been disconfirmed. They also concluded that the single-system model fit the overall data best. They argued that it was more parsimonious than the modified multiple-system model, even though it did equally well. They justified this conclusion by pointing out that the correlation between recognition and priming in the studies varied. The modified multiple-system model was therefore less precise since any correlation was acceptable.

We understand these data a bit differently. First, if these findings are to be taken at face value, we cannot conclude definitively whether there is a single system or multiple systems. The results were not consistent across experiments or among brain-damaged patients. Second, this is one set of studies, based on one kind of measure, and one set cannot definitively prove things one way or another. There could be facets to the study that uniquely result in the findings. After all, the same measures of explicit and implicit memory were used throughout, including in the amnesic data. The model would have to be applied to other tasks as well. We believe that what we can conclude is that we need to be open to several possibilities. There may be two systems despite these findings. After all, many studies seem to confirm this theory, and it is still the modal position in the field. There may be only one system, and previous studies have simply not analyzed their data comprehensively enough (this is the Berry et al. position). And, finally, there may be two systems, but they are not as completely independent of one another as has been heretofore thought. This would be the Berry et al. modified multiple system. We have found again and again that there are no "pure" conscious or unconscious processes. Everything seems to be a mix of the two in varying proportions. Consciousness seems to be a quality of a process not a structure or set of structures in the mind/brain. That is, consciousness and unconscious processes do not have separate loci in the brain. All brain processes have aspects of both. Some processes are more unconscious or conscious than others, but there is no place in the brain where consciousness resides and no place where it is prohibited from having an effect.

Multiple-Memory Systems: A Modular View of Implicit Memory

Schacter (Benoit & Schacter, 2015; Schacter, 1987, 1992, 1996, 2001) and Squire (2004, 2009; Squire & Dede, 2015; Squire & Wixted, 2016) have been major proponents of a modular point of view. They have attributed the differences in implicit and explicit memories to the functioning of different memory systems, or modules. This can be and has been called the "multiple-memory systems" view. In this model, explicit memory systems or modules have been damaged, whereas implicit memory modules have been spared, in those suffering from the amnesic syndrome. Memory studies of non-brain-damaged persons that show dissociation over time indicate that implicit and explicit memory decay at different rates. Studies that show dissociations at the time of test obtain their results by bypassing the explicit systems and thereby reflect the functioning of the implicit systems.

As with perceptual fluency, there is a parallel for the multiple-memory systems model in subliminal mere exposure (SME). Recall that Zajonc (1980, 1984; Murphy & Zajonc, 1993) argued that the affective preferences he obtained were due to separate affective and cognitive systems. Affective systems were said to function more quickly and unconsciously than do cognitive systems. Brain sites and processing were invoked to support this position (see Chapter 7). Also, see the work of LeDoux (1996) on the high and low roads of affective functioning that indicate the same thing. Essentially, Zajonc was arguing for affective modules operating somewhat independently of and differently from cognitive modules. These affective modules operate quickly and outside of awareness. Cognitive modules, in contrast, process information more slowly and effortfully. Their functioning is more related to conscious awareness. The affective preferences manifested in the SME, like implicit memory, are due to separate and independently operating brain structures. Although memory researchers do not generally speak of affect versus cognition when they discuss multiple-memory systems (but see Cahill, Uncapher, Kilpatrick, Alkire, & Turner, 2004; Kensinger & Schacter, 2008; Squire, 2009), the form of reasoning and appeal to proof is similar.

Graf and Schacter (1985) theorized that explicit memory is a function of what they termed a "declarative" memory system, whereas implicit memory relies upon a "procedural" memory system. Declarative memory refers to verbalizable knowledge. It is involved in the formation of new representations or data structures. Procedural memory is motor memory. It involves knowing how to do something and is involved in the development of skilled behavior. The procedural versus declarative memory view provides a straightforward account of the finding that amnesiacs show normal acquisition of skills they have no recollection of having learned. Skills are housed in procedural memory, which is spared in amnesiacs. Memory of participating in the learning task is normally housed in declarative memory. This is impaired in such individuals so they have no verbally conscious recollection of having learned the task. They have the skill but not the recollection of developing the skill. Normative examples would include riding a bicycle, tying shoelaces, and so on. We know how to do these things but, once learned, consciousness plays no role, and we seem to forget the learning but not the skill. We know what to do but cannot verbalize what that is.

Schacter (1983) provided an example of these systems in action. He ingeniously examined the differential operation of an amnesiac's explicit and implicit memory in a naturalistic setting. He took a man suffering from Alzheimer's disease golfing. The man had golfed regularly before the onset of the disease. This individual could not remember the location of his shots and even forgot that he had hit them in the first place. He had no idea of what his or Schacter's score was. And, finally, he denied that he had ever played golf with Schacter as they were about to begin their second round. Thus, his declarative memory was severely deficient. Despite this, he knew the rules, terminology, and etiquette of the game. He hit the ball properly and was able to execute specialized shots. His overall score, which he was unaware of, was commensurate with his premorbid functioning. Thus he displayed a fully intact procedural memory for golf.

Schacter's study seems to identify procedural memory with implicit memory. But it is not that simple and straightforward. The problem with differentiating explicit and implicit memory into declarative and procedural memory, respectively, is that amnesiacs show implicit but not explicit memory for events that should be stored in declarative memory. Priming of words in sentence completion tasks is an example. Filling in the missing word should fall to declarative memory. Yet, amnesiacs show implicit memory for such words even though they cannot recall or recognize them. The declarative-procedural distinction cannot account for such effects (see Kihlstrom et al., 2007).

Tulving (Habib, 2009; Tulving, 1972) differentiated between episodic and semantic memory. Some viewed this as a critical distinction between implicit and explicit memory (e.g., Cermak, Talbot, Chander, & Wolbarst, 1985; O'Reilly, Bhattacharyya, Howard, & Katz, 2014; Parkin, 1982; Schacter & Tulving, 1982). Semantic memory refers to the complex network of knowledge, concepts, and associations that make up a person's general understanding of the world. It is part of implicit memory. Episodic memory refers to memory of autobiographically recent events, just completed episodes in a person's life. The episodic memory system underlies explicit memory. This distinction can account for the sentence and word fragment completion data so problematic for the declarative–procedural distinction. Implicit memory exhibited on these priming tests is attributed to the semantic memory system, which is spared in amnesiacs. Explicit recall and recognition depends upon episodic memory, which is damaged in amnesiacs. As research on implicit memory progressed, it became necessary to postulate even more systems. For example, Schacter (1992, 1994; Schacter, Israel, & Racine, 1999) soon posited what he termed the perceptual representation system (PRS). This consisted of at least three separate implicit memory systems (word–form—both visual and auditory—structural–descriptive) in addition to the explicit (conceptual–semantic) system.

The two views (procedural–declarative and semantic–episodic) can be combined into one meta-view to account for more of the findings. Procedural memory remains as is. Declarative memory is divided into the various semantic and episodic distinctions. This would create at least three memory systems. Only episodic memory is damaged in the amnesic syndrome. This leads to poor explicit memory. Procedural and semantic memory remain intact; this is why skill learning and priming are normal. Squire offered something along these lines. He posited declarative and "nondeclarative" memory systems (Squire, 2004, 2009; Squire & Dede, 2015; Squire & Wixted, 2016). Nondeclarative memory systems consist of everything that is not episodic, which is identified with declarative memory. Nondeclarative memory is made up of semantic memory, procedural memory, and possibly others that we have not identified yet. Nondeclarative memory systems underlie implicit memory, whereas declarative memory, which boils down to episodic memory and which is identified as located in the medial temporal lobe and consisting of the hippocampus and the adjacent anatomically related cortex, underlies explicit memory (Squire & Zola-Morgan, 1991). So what we seem to have is a very specific explicit memory system, instantiated as the medial temporal lobe (MTL) memory system and a vaguely identified implicit memory system defined as anything related to memory that is not part of the MTL system (cf. P. Reber, 2013).

Roediger (1990) estimated that up to 25 independently functioning modules may be required to account for the various dissociations in implicit and explicit memory discovered as of 1990. And it has only gotten more complex since then. This can be a serious problem for this approach. If modules begin to multiply exponentially, they will come to explain everything and nothing. In philosophy, this kind of problem doomed Aristotelian properties. In psychology, the seemingly endless number of instincts postulated by McDougall (1908) brought about the demise of his system. The fact that humans have billions of brain cells organized in a modular fashion (tightly connected to one another) and that numerous modules have already been identified lessens the danger for the multiple-memory systems model. Nonetheless, the relevant memory modules will have to be located and their relationship to memory functioning empirically demonstrated if the problem is to be averted. We therefore take a cursory look at some neurologically relevant research in order to see whether the idea of such a plentitude of specialized memory modules has empirical support. Later in this book, we review massive modularity and neural reuse, both of which can account for such multiple housings, the former by literally positing thousands of modules (Carruthers, 2006), the latter by positing overlapping neuronal networks (M. L. Anderson, 2010, 2014). Heisz, Vakorin, Ross, Levine, and McIntosh (2014) offer a model of this sort to explain episodic and semantic memory.

There are also data that dispute the existence of multiple-memory systems. We cited some when we discussed brain damage data (see Chapter 9).[3] Some researchers (Dew & Cabeza, 2011; Reder, Park, & Kieffaber, 2009; Roediger & McDermott, 1993; Shanks & St. John, 1994) argue against the idea that there is a qualitative difference in memory based on consciousness. Schacter et al. (1993) suggested that underlying the debates over whether there is a single or multiple-memory systems may be subtle differences in the materials used to measure implicit and explicit memory. But when Schacter, Wig, and Stevens (2007) found that similar regions in the brain support both repetition priming and recognition, they suggested that there might be some overlap between the systems. In essence, Schacter and his co-workers entertained the possibility of a modified multiple-memory system (see Berry et al., 2012). Heisz et al. (2014) report overlapping neural circuits for episodic and semantic memory, evidence that would support our view that there are no pure conscious or unconscious structures in the brain. This is an area that requires further work. Below we review P. Reber (2013) who offers a way out for implicit memory and learning. Later in this book, we discuss neural reuse models (M. L. Anderson, 2010, 2014) that may be able to account for such a hybrid system and that offer comprehensive views of the brain/mind.

Are There Separate Implicit and Explicit Memory Systems?

Indirect proof for the modular point of view comes from work on the development of memory over the life cycle. Children's performance on explicit memory tasks improves with age (Kail, 1990; Naito & Komatsu, 1993). Performance on priming and other kinds of implicit memory tasks, on the other hand, is virtually constant through development (Naito & Komatsu, 1993; Schacter, 1996). We know that cortical structures continue to develop up to adolescence, whereas subcortical structures mature much earlier (Casey, Tottenham, Liston, & Durston, 2005). If cortical structures underlie explicit memory, we would expect positive change in explicit memory over this period. If subcortical structures underlie implicit memory, we would expect little change in performance on implicit tasks as the person develops. And that seems to be what happens. A normal processing view would be hard put to explain these developmental dissociations. Similarly, there is a general decline in explicit memory performance as we age (Craik & Jennings, 1992; Einstein & McDaniel, 1990; Fleischman, Wilson, Gabrieli, Bienias, & Bennett, 2004). There is far less, if any, decline in performance on implicit memory tasks late in life (Fleischman et al., 2004; Graf, 1990; Light, 1991; Russo & Parkin, 1993; Schacter, Kaszniak, Kihlstrom, &

Valdiserri, 1991). We know that cortical structures slowly deteriorate in old age, whereas subcortical structures are more likely to remain intact (Prull, Gabrieli, & Bunge, 2000). Once again, a multiple-system understanding can account for the data, whereas a normal processing account would be hard put to explain such findings. But, again, there are also some contrary data. For example, Pilotti, Meade, and Gallo (2002) reported that although cross-modality priming was equivalent in older and younger adults, modality-specific priming was worse in older subjects. The preponderance of the data seem to favor the implicit/explicit distinction, but the case is not closed. And an overlap model could fit more of the data than could a single system or a completely orthogonal multiple-system model.

There is also more direct evidence for the existence of relevant memory modules/networks. Animal research, involving selective lesioning of different sections of the medial temporal lobe, has implicated the hippocampus in explicit but not implicit memory (Squire & Zola-Morgan, 1988). This has also been supported in humans in studies using neural-imaging techniques (Gabrieli, 1998; Gluck & Myers, 1997; Squire, 1992, 2009). Thus, a modular locus or at least support for some localization of explicit memory (possibly in the hippocampus) seems supported. Further research has focused on more specialized loci for different kinds of explicit and implicit memory. Brain-damage data support the distinction between procedural and episodic memory. Individuals with Alzheimer's disease invariably demonstrate impaired episodic memory but usually show intact procedural memory (see Schacter, 1983). For patients with Alzheimer's disease, the damage is in the medial temporal lobes. The medial temporal lobes have been repeatedly implicated in declarative and episodic memory, as we discussed above. In contrast, people suffering from Huntington's disease show intact declarative and episodic memory but have impaired procedural memory. Huntington's disease is characterized by degeneration of the subcortical basal ganglia but intact medial temporal lobes (Butters, Heindel, & Salmon, 1990). Procedural memory has been related to the basal ganglia (particularly the striatum; see Packard & Knowlton, 2002), which are usually spared in Alzheimer's sufferers.

The episodic–semantic distinction was also supported in studies of brain functioning. Wheeler, Stuss, and Tulving (1995) and Shimamura (1995) reported that individuals exhibiting damage to the dorsolateral prefrontal cortex have severe deficits in episodic memory but no measurable deficits in semantic memory. Neuroimaging studies also supported this connection. PET scans of intact subjects demonstrate greater activation of prefrontal regions when engaged in an episodic memory task than when trying to retrieve semantic information (Nyberg, 1998). Other neuroimaging studies, using event-related potentials (ERPs), have supported the existence of separate activations for implicit and explicit tasks (Paller, Hutson, Miller, & Boehm, 2003; Rugg, Schloerscheidt, & Mark, 1998; Schott, Richardson-Klavehn, Heinze, & Duzel, 2002; Woollams, Taylor, Karayanidis, & Henson, 2008). Some investigators have used fMRIs and reported different brain areas activated in the two types of tasks (Donaldson, Petersen, & Buckner, 2001; Henson, 2003; Schott et al., 2006). More recent studies, however, indicate shared activation between implicit and explicit priming (e.g., Turke-Browne, Yi, & Chun, 2006). Heisz et al. (2014), as cited above, also reported overlap in a study employing magnetoencephalography (MEG). Schacter et al. (2007) hypothesized two types of priming in the brain to account for this. We would suggest that there is probably some overlap between the two types of task. As has been reported many times in this book, there does not seem to be any "pure" unconscious process. It is a quality of the various processes with some more unconscious than others. Overlap between somewhat separate implicit and explicit systems can account for this as well.

An even more fine-grained analysis reveals separate modules for different aspects of episodic memory. Baddeley (1995; Baddeley & Hitch, 1974) identified three separate episodic memory systems (and there could be more; see Baddeley & Hitch, 2000). One memory storage system was for temporary visual storage; another was for temporary storage of verbal information. A third system seemed to function in an executive fashion, overseeing processes like rehearsal and conscious decision making. Neuroimaging studies have indicated that verbal and visual episodic memory tasks activate different regions located in the left and right hemispheres, respectively. Thus, Smith, Jonides, and Koeppe (1996) reported that recalling letters (verbal episodic memory) activated areas of the left prefrontal cortex along with left temporal and frontal regions. D'Esposito et al. (1995) found that remembering the location of three dots on a screen (visual episodic memory) activated areas in the right prefrontal cortex along with regions of the right visual cortex.

Combining the Multiple-System and Normal Processing Views

Some evidence seems to suggest that implicit and explicit memory may be separate systems. But Berry et al. (2012), Berry, Shanks, Li, Rains, and Henson (2010), Reder et al. (2009), and Roediger et al. (2002), reviewed above, dispute this view and offer a single-system view. And, even within the modular view, there is dispute. Thus, one modular understanding is that explicit memory involves higher, cortical networks whereas implicit memory is more related to lower, subcortical networks like the basal ganglia (Hasan et al., 2013). But it is not quite this neat. For example, the cortex—specifically the anterior prefrontal cortex—is implicated in associative processes that are implicit in nature (Dutta, Shah, Silvanto, & Soto, 2014; also see Schacter, 1992; Schacter et al., 2007). Eichenbaum and Cohen (2001) as well as P. Reber and Squire (1999) also report implicit memory phenomena that are independent of the basal ganglia. But that does not mean that these views are a hopeless muddle and/or are mutually exclusive. As we proposed for the subliminal mere exposure effect, each of these views can be partially true. Recently activated networks may be more likely to influence subsequent information processing than are quiescent networks. In this way, perceptual fluency can be incorporated into a network model. Additionally, networks or modules must operate according to certain principles. Different networks may follow different sets of rules. The liver and the kidneys are systems in the body that operate differently. Certainly, brain systems can process information differently (cf. Carruthers, 2006). Some networks may be conceptually driven whereas others may be data driven. In this way, TAPA can be incorporated into a multiple-memory system account. Tulving and Schacter (1990), Hayman and Tulving (1989), and Schacter (1990) proposed this sort of solution early on. Subsequently, Schacter, Wig, and Stevens (2007) proposed a less localized, more distributed neural underpinning to memory. Restivo, Veter, Bontempi, and Ammassari-Teule (2009) also proposed this sort of distributed model of memory. Berry et al. refer to nodes rather than networks. This makes the relevant structures more basic and smaller than modules or what are usually referred to as systems but does not rule out some localization of function.

P. Reber (2013) offers an innovative model that focuses on a nonlocalized view of implicit memory in contrast to a localized, specific locus for explicit memory. His model can account for many of the apparently contradictory findings described above. It also offers a way of understanding both implicit memory and implicit learning (reviewed in the next chapter) as two sides of the same coin and thereby has more explanatory power than a model that accounts for only one or the other. As P. Reber (2013) conceptualizes it (O'Reilly et al., 2014, offer a similar model), explicit memory depends upon specifiable and localizable neural circuitry, located in the medial temporal lobe (MTL). This is supported by the data that show that damage to the MTL results in explicit memory problems, commonly referred to as the amnesic syndrome. As a consequence, explicit memory is correctly described as a memory system that is coordinate with what Squire (2004, 2009; Squire & Dede,

2015; Squire & Wixted, 2016) refers to as declarative memory. Reber terms it the "MTL memory system." The purpose of the MTL memory system is to rapidly acquire (largely episodic) information. It has a relatively low storage capacity, which necessitates a gradual consolidation process by which the information is stored long term into a separate long-term episodic memory system (cf. O'Reilly et al., 2014). If the system is damaged this consolidation cannot take place, and we have the amnesic syndrome. In contrast to the MTL memory system for explicit memory, there is no identifiable system for implicit memory. What the data show is that there are memory processes that are independent of the MTL memory system. These processes become evident when the MTL memory system is compromised either through damage or through being bypassed. But they occur normatively as well. These processes go under the summary term implicit memory. What the research has not shown is where in the brain this takes place or how it works. Some investigators have assumed that there exists a coherent, localized, and specialized non-MTL memory system, which they term the implicit memory system. The basal ganglia have been implicated as a possible location for this system. However, implicit memory processes do not always depend upon the basal ganglia (e.g., P. Reber & Squire, 1999). Additionally, these structures are implicated in nonmemory activities so that they cannot be solely dedicated to memory processes. This provides one explanation for why neuroimaging data and brain damage studies have not been able to locate a locus for implicit memory.

What can we say about implicit memory? Perhaps we simply have not found the system yet. Alternatively, there may be only one memory system, investigated in different ways. P. Reber (2013) offers a third alternative, in effect, a mixed model. There is a system underlying explicit memory (the MTL memory system). There is, however, no single system underlying all of memory. And there is no underlying specifiable system or systems underlying implicit memory. Thus, both single-system and multiple-system models have it wrong. What is actually going on, according to Reber, is that one type of memory (i.e., explicit) is dependent upon the operation of a specifiable system (the MTL memory system), whereas implicit memory has no underlying neuronal system. Instead, it is attributable to how neuronal circuits behave in general and cannot be limited to any specific location or system. In this conception, implicit memory is distributed throughout the brain. Reber argues that the neural circuits of the brain are inherently plastic and change with experience (see Eichenbaum & Cohen, 2001). As a result, implicit memory is not a neural system parallel to the MTL memory system but a principle of change that is part and parcel of how neural circuits in the brain function (i.e., experiences change the actual connections between neural units). These ubiquitous changes result from plasticity within all of the neural circuitry in the brain, not just in the MTL memory system.

Because these changes are not unique to any single brain system, there is no specific location for implicit memory, no unique localized center controlling implicit memory. Because plasticity in brain functioning is part and parcel of virtually every circuit and connection in the brain and because the nature of this plasticity is to reflect experience, Reber argues that implicit memory phenomena should be present whenever a perception or action is repeated. In effect, neural circuits reflect experience. The more often the person has the experience, the stronger the changes in the neural circuits and the more powerful the implicit memory. In addition to reflecting memory, this mode of operation represents a form of learning termed "implicit learning." We will come back to this topic in the implicit learning chapter. Since this kind of memory and learning is instantiated by physical changes in the connections of various parts of the brain, it follows logically that much if not the vast majority of this is unconscious.

The P. Reber (2013) model sounds a lot like James's (1890/1950) view of habit except that the memory/learning does not have to have ever been conscious. Additionally, there is a computational neuroscience model that details exactly how such a system would operate and from which one could derive implicit memory and learning (as well as other cognitive phenomena). It is called PDP, and we review it in detail later in this book. When we do that, we also review other computational neuroscience models like massive modularity and neural reuse that we believe, in combination with PDP, can comfortably handle Reber's model and offer viable general models of unconscious processing be it implicit learning, implicit memory, or other kinds of unconscious processes we have reviewed.

CLINICAL IMPLICATIONS OF IMPLICIT MEMORY

Whatever their neuroanatomical underpinnings and regardless of whether one is completely conscious and the other completely unconscious, or anything in between, implicit and explicit memory do seem to operate somewhat independently of one another at the functional level. This has significant clinical implications for reframing our understanding of processes that analytically inclined therapists may conceptualize as resistance or dynamically motivated defenses. To explicate, implicit memory reaches maturity earlier (Naito & Komatsu, 1993; Schacter, 1996), shows less variability across individuals, and deteriorates with age far less than does explicit memory (Kail, 1990; Naito & Komatsu,

1993). In short, implicit memory is pretty much the same across individuals and across most ages within those individuals. This also means that most of a person's earliest memories (before age 3) are implicit, as explicit memory systems have not yet developed sufficiently to process experiences for long-term retention. This explains the so called "amnesia" of early childhood. People also develop implicit memories relatively easily and retain them for lengthy periods of time (Thomson et al., 2010; Mitchell, 2006). As a result, they can behave in accord with these memories for long periods of time but often have no explicit recollection of them. The lack of explicit memory can arise for a variety of reasons. Perhaps a great deal of time has passed since the event (decay). Perhaps the person's explicit memory was not well developed when the event occurred (early childhood experiences). Perhaps the person was explicitly focused on a distracting experience so that his explicit memory failed to encode the event or important aspects of it. In any case, these patients cannot recount the origins of many of their behaviors and reactions. It is not because they have defended against such memories; it is because they were not coded explicitly or because the explicit memories have decayed. This dissociation between implicit and explicit memories is not motivated. There may not have been an original integrated memory that was later broken up or repressed because it was unacceptable. The behavior is pathological or maladaptive because the patient continues to respond as though a now nonexistent situation is still operating. The patient does not understand why he keeps doing this because the explicit memory associated with the pathology decayed or never existed. Instead, the patient keeps remembering the experience through his actions (implicitly). It may seem at times that the patient does remember some of it explicitly, but this could be due to the imperfect correlation between implicit and explicit memory processes rather than a break in defense. (This is not to deny the presence of dynamically motivated defenses, but we caution the clinician to be aware of and to consider implicit memory processes before making a determination.)

The long-lasting (invulnerable) nature of implicit memories is particularly important. Simple and unimportant phenomena like recall of pictures survive for weeks, even months, and years, without intervening practice or reminders (Mitchell, 2006). This means that implicit memories from early childhood may exert influence well into adulthood. As a result, implicit memory, originating in early childhood, may be implicated in some adult pathological behavior (e.g., phobias, fetishes, negative relational patterns, difficulty with affect regulation). Thanks to childhood amnesia (lack of explicit memory), the person does not explicitly remember the event but still implicitly "remembers" it through his actions and behaviors. Implicit memory subsequent to childhood amnesia may also be important clinically. After a while, a person may evidence behaviors, thoughts, and emotions based on implicit memory and yet remain totally unaware of the source of these psychologically important phenomena. The explicit memory has decayed; the implicit memory is in full vigor. Again, this is not motivated but normative.

NOTES

1. HM's real name was Henry Gustav Molaison. At age 9, he struck his head after being hit by a bicycle. His seizures began shortly afterward. He had his surgery in 1953, at age 27. He died in 2008. He was 82 years old (Carey, 2008). Dittrich (2016), the grandson of the surgeon who operated on HM, has written a wonderful book that humanizes the people involved.

2. Gut feelings, intuitions, and déjà vu have a powerful reputation among the lay public. They are often attributed to ESP or some mystical source. This kind of thinking was central to the Romantics and to the philosophers of nature. Scientists then and now tend to doubt the veracity of such events and attribute confirmatory anecdotes to selective memory. It may be, however, that anecdotal tales of the prescience of gut feelings and intuitions reflect implicit processes. After all, a person with no conscious recollection, who consistently guesses correctly, may also appear to be demonstrating ESP or a mystical communion with the ultimate. It probably feels that way to subjects in subliminal experiments and would to amnesiacs if they could reflect upon their own performances. We know, however, that scientifically respectable and measurable processes are involved. The same may be true for gut feelings, intuitions, and déjà vu. Djiksterhuis (2013; Djiksterhuis et al., 2006) makes a similar point and provides supportive data.

3. Berry et al. (2012), Reder et al. (2009), and Prinze (2006) cite others. Also see Benjamin (2010), Buchner and Wippich (2000), Dunn and Kirsner (2003), Kinder and Shanks (2001, 2003), and Newell and Dunn (2008) for arguments against multiple-memory systems.

CHAPTER 12

Implicit Learning

Implicit learning involves acquiring knowledge of relations between experiences without intention, without realizing that one is doing so, and without being able to verbalize what one has learned (Berry & Dienes, 1993; Seger, 1994). Implicit learning is closely related to implicit memory: A person cannot demonstrate implicit learning if she has no memory of what was learned; likewise, a person cannot implicitly remember what she has not learned (P. Reber, 2008, 2013). The two areas are separated because they emerged from different research traditions (Kihlstrom et al., 2007; Weinberger & Levy, 2005). As reviewed above, the study of implicit memory developed largely through examination of brain-damaged individuals, only later to transition to examining people with intact brains. Research into implicit learning, in contrast, focused on unimpaired children and adults (Berry & Dienes, 1993; Seger, 1994) and, even earlier in the history of psychology, animals (Tolman, 1949).

Implicit learning is not a motivated process. It is not purposeful but rather occurs automatically, as a by-product of moment-to-moment interactions with the environment (i.e., incidentally). Information acquired in this way can be quite complex and even abstract (cf. Howard & Ballas, 1982; A. Reber, 1989; P. Reber, 2013; Seger, 1994). Correct use and recognition of the underlying structure and grammar of language, for instance, can be attributed to implicit learning. Indeed, this is one of the earliest areas of implicit learning studied by researchers. Children learn grammatical rules yet cannot communicate what they are. Most adults cannot either. People just "know" when something is correct and when it is not.

165

Implicit learning can probably be traced back to Tolman's classic studies of latent learning in rats (e.g., Tolman, 1949). Chomsky's groundbreaking work on the underlying structure of language (Chomsky, 1957) was also seminal. The subject matter of implicit learning has traditionally been and continues to be more complex than that of implicit memory. For early comprehensive reviews of implicit learning, see Berry and Dienes (1993), Seger (1994), and Stadler and Frensch (1998). Frensch and Runger (2003) offer a short, more user-friendly, review.

ARTIFICIAL GRAMMAR AND PROBABILITY LEARNING

The earliest areas of investigation, relevant to systematically understanding implicit learning processes, were artificial grammar and probability learning. In fact, the term "implicit learning" was originally an attempt to describe the subjective experience of people in artificial grammar studies (P. Reber, 2013). Study of artificial grammar was innovated by Arthur Reber (1967). (See A. Reber, 1989, for a review of much of the early work.) The basic methodology involves presenting participants with strings of letters that follow a set of (often complex) rules specifying the sequences that the letters may take. These rules constitute the artificial grammar. In some studies, participants are asked to memorize the strings (e.g., A. Reber, 1967); in others, they are just asked to observe them (e.g., A. Reber & Allen, 1978). In neither case are they asked to figure out what the underlying rules are. After viewing 15 to 25 such strings, participants are asked to memorize a second set of strings and/ or to judge whether the individual members of a second set are consistent with the first set. It turns out that the ability to memorize the strings improves with practice. Additionally, participants are able to determine which strings are or are not grammatical with 60 to 80% accuracy, which is well above chance. The only explanation for such findings seems to be that the underlying rules have been learned unconsciously.

Training and testing need not be conducted in the same sense modality. Manza and Reber (1997) used auditory presentations to train and visual strings to test their participants. They also employed the opposite sequence (i.e., visual training and auditory testing). The "grammar" of the visual stimuli was based on spatial location, whereas that of the auditory stimuli was based on pitch. Despite these differences, there was transfer between the two sense modalities. That is, the usual artificial grammar effects were obtained when both had the same underlying properties. Scott and Dienes (2010) told their subjects that the training strings they had been asked to learn (which, e.g., might be letter-based) followed a complex set of rules. They were then asked to categorize test strings, half of which would follow the same rules but which might be in a different form (e.g., number-based). Switching modalities did not impair learning. These studies showed that transfer of learning was the same whether it occurred between different sense modalities or the same modality using different vocabularies. So artificial grammar learning is central, not sense- or modality-specific.

Smith, Siegert, and McDowall (2001) reported that patients with Parkinson's disease were capable of demonstrating implicit learning not only on an artificial grammar task but, surprisingly, also on a verbal version of a serial reaction time (SRT) task. This is curious because an SRT task involves motor sequence learning, thought to be located in brain areas that are significantly impacted by the disease. These data also point strongly to a central role of unconscious processes in implicit learning. They also suggest, as we found in implicit memory (see P. Reber, 2013), that there may be no specific location for implicit learning as there seems to be for explicit learning (and for explicit memory). Cleeremans and McClelland (1991) reported that individuals were able to successfully acquire artificial grammar even when some of the elements in the strings were occasionally incorrect. Such inconsistencies are usually fatal to an explicit learning task. This study testifies to the robustness of artificial grammar. Participants can pick up the underlying regularities of strings despite varied and difficult transformations. This holds for complex and even flawed strings.

An even more critical finding of these studies was that, despite undeniable evidence of understanding the rules, participants are usually unable to describe them. They typically claim to be guessing or to be guided by a feeling or by intuition. They are even unaware that they have learned anything at all. So this sophisticated, complex learning is apparently unconscious (A. Reber, 1967, 1976, 1989; P. Reber, 2013; A. Reber & Allen, 1978; A. Reber & Lewis, 1977). Further, participants in artificial grammar studies are not simply unable to articulate the rules underlying their performance. Efforts to determine what the rules are may actually worsen performance. Scott and Dienes (2010) asked their participants whether their decision strategy was based on random selection, intuition, familiarity, rules, or recollection. Only the "random selection" judgments were significantly more accurate than chance. A. Reber (1976), A. Reber, Kassin, Lewis, and Cantor (1980), and A. Reber and Lewis (1977) compared individuals who were asked to determine the nature of the rules (conscious hypothesis testing) with individuals who received the usual passive attention instructions (unconscious or implicit hypothesis testing). Those who were trying to determine what was going on tended to be worse at identifying which strings were grammatical than those who simply attended passively. A. Reber and Lewis (1977) reported that people in the conscious condition even reported incorrect rules on occasion. Fallshore and Schooler (1993) also found that asking participants to describe what they knew before they tried to differentiate grammatical from nongrammatical strings resulted in worse performance than just allowing them to make their decisions in the usual, nonreflective way.

The idea that not only are these processes unconscious but that conscious processes can interfere with them was further supported in an innovative study by Whitmarsh, Udden, Barendregt, and Petersson (2013). These investigators experimentally demonstrated that enhanced consciousness adversely affects implicit learning. Whitmarsh et al. reported that the personality trait of mindfulness (defined as being aware in the moment) disrupted implicit learning of artificial grammatical structures. More specifically, they concluded that the nonreactive, observant stance that mindfulness presupposes, calling on one to be more present (conscious) in the moment, reduced the tendency to automatically and unconsciously acquire knowledge and develop habitual responses to this knowledge. This finding held even after participants were debriefed about the existence of grammatical rules in the stimuli they had been presented with. Thus, a tendency to process experiences consciously adversely affected unconscious processing. This result strongly suggests that the oft-repeated finding that consciousness can be detrimental to implicit processes is genuine. This, in turn, seems to confirm that explicit and implicit processes follow different rules.

Dulany, Carlson, and Dewey (1984), as well as Dienes, Broadbent, and Berry (1991), were unable to replicate this differential performance, however. They therefore concluded that explicit, conscious processes could not be ruled out as affecting implicit learning tasks. (Also see Dulany, 1997.) In support of this conclusion, Frensch and Runger (2003) reported that subjects asked to indicate which letters in the letter strings enabled them to differentiate grammatical from nongrammatical strings could do so to some degree. They also found that forced-choice paradigms often revealed some awareness of what was learned in various implicit learning tasks. So there are data both for and against dissociation between implicit and explicit learning processes.

Matthews et al. (1989) conducted a more fine-grained study on the differential roles that conscious and unconscious phenomena play in learning artificial grammar. They had participants in one group provide detailed statements about what they knew and what criteria they were using to determine whether novel strings were "grammatical." These statements were then given to another group of individuals, who did not undergo a practice phase, to help them to decide whether or not strings presented to them were grammatical. The protocols were helpful to the nontrained individuals. By the fourth day of this procedure, the nontrained participants performed almost as well as the trained participants. However, the trained participants plateaued on the second day and always performed somewhat better than their nontrained counterparts.

These findings suggest two things. First, some knowledge about the nature of the artificial grammar was conscious. Otherwise, it could not have been communicated. This supports Dulany et al. (1984), Dienes et al. (1991), and Frensch and Runger (2003). However, some of the knowledge was also apparently unconscious since the trained group learned more quickly and always performed better than did the untrained group. So both conscious and unconscious processes seem to be involved. Batterink, Reber, Neville, and Paller (2015) showed this to be the case neurophysiologically. They looked at brain potentials during learning. The brain potentials they examined revealed statistical learning on both an explicit (recognition) and an implicit (reaction time) measure of learning. Accurate responses on the recognition test (explicit measure) were associated with a subjective sense of better recollection and with late positive potential. Reaction time (implicit measure) and P300 amplitudes also demonstrated a relationship to learning, but recognition and late positive potential (the explicit measures) were unrelated to these variables. Thus, explicit learning and implicit learning both occurred but were orthogonal to one another. They seem to have occurred in parallel. That most tasks require a combination of conscious and unconscious processes is a position we have seen before (e.g., Jacoby, Begg, & Toth, 1997; Merikle, 1992; Merikle & Reingold, 1992). As Frensch and Runger (2003) put it when reviewing implicit learning studies: "tests are rarely process pure" (p. 14).

The data seem to indicate that conscious processes can help in the learning of artificial grammar. But are conscious processes necessary for the learning of artificial grammar? They may not be. As is the case for implicit memory, people with brain damage that affects explicit learning show intact performance in artificial grammar studies (implicit learning). Knowlton, Ramus, and Squire (1992) reported that amnesiacs showed unimpaired performance on an artificial grammar task. This performance deteriorated when they were asked to make their judgments on the basis of explicit comparisons. Atas, Faivre, Timmermans, Cleeremans, and Kouider (2014) found implicit learning when the respondents were not even aware of the stimuli they were being presented with, let alone the pattern of their presentation. In this study, subjects had to fixate on a central point (a cross) while patterned stimuli were presented in the periphery of their visual fields. These patterns signaled either a potential monetary gain or loss. When the cross turned into a question mark, the respondents had to decide whether they expected a reward or not by pressing the space bar if they believed that a reward had been signaled. If they did not press the bar, the trial did not count. Thus, they could gain money or lose money by pressing the space bar, or nothing would happen to them if they did not press the space bar. Even though subjects were unaware of the pattern (whenever a respondent's fixation point moved from the center, the data were discarded), they displayed a quicker reaction time to reward than to loss. This result showed that sequences can be learned even when the stimuli making up the sequences are outside of awareness. Thus, the respondents demonstrated implicit learning for stimuli they were not aware of having seen.

People even show a mere exposure effect for grammatical strings. Thus, Gordon and Holyoak (1983) found that, after the usual training period in an artificial grammar study, participants preferred novel grammatical strings to novel nongrammatical strings. Apparently, they had abstracted out the underlying relations between the letters and demonstrated a mere exposure effect to them. McAndrews and Moscovitch (1985) obtained similar results. And, finally, as we saw for memory, implicitly acquired knowledge can be retained for far greater periods of time then can explicitly acquired knowledge (see, e.g., Allen & Reber, 1980; Kihlstrom et al., 2007).

An offshoot of artificial grammar has been termed *probability learning*. It too was innovated by A. Reber (A. Reber & Millward, 1968, 1971) and the results parallel those of artificial grammar. In this paradigm, participants implicitly learn about the stochastic structure of a sequence of stimuli. In a typical study, an individual observes a sequence of rapidly presented stimuli. The rate is about two per second and a session lasts a couple of minutes. The stimuli frequently have a complex stochastic structure. Following this "learning" or training session, participants are asked to make predictions about an upcoming sequence of stimuli. Individuals are able to acquire and make use of surprisingly complex probability structures. Millward and Reber (1972) showed that people could successfully track events whose probability structure shifted over a 50-trial period. Participants were also able to predict an outcome when it was stochastically dependent upon another event that occurred up to seven trials earlier. Millward and Reber (1968) had previously shown that people lack explicit memory for stimuli that preceded the target event by more than five trials. Thus, unconscious (implicit) memory can apparently deal successfully with more complex information than can explicit memory. Far from being inferior to conscious processes as Greenwald (1992) averred, unconscious processes, at least in this regard, are more sophisticated than are conscious processes (cf. Dijksterhuis, 2004, on the superior unconscious). Moreover, people can learn even when they are unaware of the stimuli they are learning about (Atas et al., 2014) and come to like repeated patterns even when they cannot identify their nature (Gordon & Holyoak, 1983; McAndrews & Moscovitch, 1985). Finally, Sanchez and Reber (2013) reported that providing pretraining explicit information had no salutary effect on an implicit learning task.

Jiang and colleagues (Jiang, Swallow, & Sun, 2014; Jiang, Won, & Swallow, 2014) demonstrated that implicit learning guides attention even when there are explicit instructions to distribute attention evenly. Jiang et al. asked participants to identify a target (letter) that was more likely to appear in a specific quadrant of a screen depicting a natural scene. During subsequent testing, the monitor or the participant's position was rotated so that he was viewing the scene from a different angle (90° rotation). Moreover, in some experiments, participants were explicitly told that the cue was likely to appear in a new quadrant. The participants implicitly, and quickly, learned to prioritize a specific quadrant during the initial phase of the study, which carried over to the testing phase, regardless of explicit instructions to prioritize a different quadrant. Further, this attentional bias was egocentric, not focused on the environment. That is, attention was likely to be directed to the same spatial quadrant relative to the participant's position rather than to the position of the scene's details after rotation. Because spatial attention is particularly important when details of our environment are processed and responded to, it is important to understand that attentional biases, contingent upon implicit learning, exist and can impact our readiness to perceive different attributes of the environment. In other words, implicit learning can influence not only how we respond to stimuli, but also which stimuli we perceive in the first place. Moreover, this occurs completely outside of awareness.

COVARIATION LEARNING

Another early avenue of studying implicit learning—covariation learning—is most closely associated with Pawel Lewicki (e.g., 1986). Although this work is usually categorized as social psychological because much of it employs social stimuli, it is really about implicit learning—social learning that takes place implicitly. In the basic experimental paradigm innovated by Lewicki, participants are exposed to stimuli that covary lawfully with one another. After some distraction task, the participants are asked questions or required to perform some act that will indicate whether they have internalized this covariation. In study after study, performance was clearly influenced by the previously presented covariations. Sometimes, induction from presented covariations to more abstract categories was demonstrated. In virtually all of these studies, participants seemed totally unaware of, let alone capable of describing, the covariations they had just been influenced by.

The most systematic listing of these studies is contained in a book, which is essentially a compendium of covariation experiments (Lewicki, 1986). In one set of studies (Chapter 4), participants were presented with descriptions of people in whom certain characteristics covaried. In one of these experiments (Experiment 4.2), participants were presented with covarying concrete behaviors. Their subsequent task was to rate the likelihood that certain personality traits would go together. The covarying concrete behaviors and the judged traits were both related to intelligence and to introversion–extraversion. In one condition, intelligence was positively related to introversion and negatively related to extraversion. In a second condition, the direction of the relations was reversed. The concrete behaviors were things like going to parties, having friends, doing well in school, and having challenging hobbies. The later task was to rate 10 people (known to the participants) on 12 scales. Several of the scales referred to introversion–extroversion and several referred to intelligence. The ratings were generally in accord with the previously covarying behaviors. In the first condition, introverts were rated as more intelligent than were extroverts, as predicted. In the other, there were no differences in the ratings. The difference in ratings between the two conditions was statistically significant and in accord with the initial covariations. Unfortunately, the meaning of these findings is not as clear-cut as it could have been. Lewicki did not run a control condition in which there were no covarying behaviors prior to the rating task. As a result, there was no baseline against which to compare the results of the two experimental conditions. It may be that introverts are generally thought to be more intelligent than extroverts so that one set of covariations (Condition 1) added to this difference whereas the other set (Condition 2) diminished it. That seems to be the conclusion that Lewicki came to, and the data are consistent with it. But without a baseline, it is impossible to be certain. What is certain is that prior covariations differentially affected later ratings. Moreover, this was the case even though the earlier and later descriptions were at different levels of abstraction (concrete behaviors vs. trait terms).

A second study (Experiment 4.7) provided similar general support but was also weakened by the absence of a control, baseline condition. Instead of level of abstraction, the focus of this experiment was on whether arbitrary covariations could be internalized. Participants were exposed to auditory self-descriptions, varying in pitch. Pitch covaried with statements relating to personal warmth and capability. Participants then listened to and rated new self-descriptions that varied similarly in pitch but contained no information concerning warmth and capability. There was a general tendency to assign ratings of warmth to higher-pitched voices; the opposite was the case for capability. This was more pronounced when it matched the covariation of the initial presentations than when it did not. These findings are not as arbitrary as the author may have believed. Women's relatively more high-pitched voices tend to be related to ratings of warmth, whereas men's relatively low-pitched voices tend to be more related to capability (Oleszkiewicz, Pisanski, Lachowicz–Tabaczek, & Sorokowska, 2016). The findings therefore parallel the introversion–extraversion and intelligence findings of Experiment 4.2. Covariation in line with preexisting tendencies enhanced those tendencies whereas covariations opposed to these tendencies weakened them. But without a baseline, we cannot be completely certain of this interpretation. Nonetheless, the covariation manipulation clearly had effects.

A more clearly arbitrary connection was demonstrated in another experiment in this series (Experiment 4.9). Here, participants engaged in a shadowing task and were also presented with visual stimuli (pictures of a letter, an umbrella, or a jug) that they were asked to ignore. The attended (shadowed) channel contained neutral words. The unattended (nonshadowed) channel contained both neutral and threatening words. One of the visual stimuli (depending upon experimental condition) covaried with the threatening words on the nonshadowed (unattended) channel. Participants were then asked to rate some pictures of people. Each picture also included one of the objects previously seen. Pictures of people with objects that had previously covaried with threatening words were rated as more threatening. Thus, the study participants had processed, stored, and employed arbitrary connections in their evaluations. Moreover, these connections were used to rate the dangerousness of an unknown individual. This occurred outside of awareness and was unreflective. The relevance of these findings to stereotyping and prejudicial beliefs are both obvious and important.

Covariations can be established quite rapidly. Lewicki (1986—Experiment 7.7) had an experimenter interact with participants in a friendly fashion. They were then asked to rate the friendliness of two people depicted in photos. One of the people in the photographs remotely resembled the experimenter. Sixty percent of people saw this person as more friendly before engaging in the interaction with the experimenter. But 85% chose the more similar person after the friendly exchange—a difference that was statistically significant. In this experiment, Lewicki provided a genuine baseline and so the results are easily interpretable.

In another experiment in this series (Experiment 7.8), participants also engaged in an interaction with an experimenter. In one condition, he acted as though he was irritated about their answer to a question. In another, the interchange was neutral. Participants were then asked to go to another room for the "real" experiment and hand a coded paper to whomever was available there. There were two experimenters in the room and both were free. One bore a slight resemblance to the previous experimenter; the other did not. Fifty-five percent of the people in the neutral condition approached the person who resembled the original experimenter. Only 20% of those who had experienced a negative interaction did so. This kind of finding has enormous implications both for social interactions and for clinical issues. We elaborate on these later in this chapter.

Not only can processed covariations be arbitrary, they can be quite complex as well. Studies by Hill, Lewicki, Czyzewska, and Boss (1989) and by Lewicki, Hill, and Czyzewska (1994) showed that people can learn transitive relations implicitly. A transitive relation is of the form: If A = B and B = C, then A = C. Hill et al. and Lewicki et al. exposed their participants to videotapes of schematically presented people performing some simple actions. They also told them that these individuals possessed certain personality characteristics. Unbeknownst to the participants, there was a relationship (covariation) between some of the personality information and the distance between two dots representing the legs of the schematically presented person. Participants then viewed a second video in which the distance between two dots representing the arms of another schematically presented figure covaried with the distance between the dots representing that figure's legs. No information concerning personality was offered. In a final video, only the dots on the arms of a schematic person were presented. Participants were asked to make intuitive judgments concerning the schematic person's personality. The judgments turned out to be based on the distance between the dots on the arms. These results indicate that these people picked up the notion that personality was based on distance between dots on legs, which in turn was related to distance between dots on arms. Participants then inferred that the distance between the dots on the arms was also related to personality. Despite this apparent knowledge, no participant evinced any conscious understanding of these relationships when questioned about them. Participants did not even consciously notice that the dots on the arms varied in distance from one another, let alone that the distance was related to other distances between dots (on legs), which, in turn, was related to personality. This complex knowledge was truly implicit.

Gross and Greene (2007) had their subjects learn an abstract transitive patterning task where the stimuli were faces. They then presented another unrelated stimulus set also consisting of faces. The participants applied what they had learned to the new set of faces. The authors concluded that this kind of learning may underlie the apparently intuitive knowledge of experts. That is, experts apply what they have abstracted in one situation to another apparently unrelated situation (cf. P. Reber, 2013). But if this is the case, it seems reasonable to assume that people also misapply abstract relationships to areas that are not appropriate for them. This can lead to mistakes and perhaps to pathology. A person can accurately abstract a relational pattern from an important other and then apply it to a different person for whom it does not hold. This has been shown experimentally (Andersen & Przybylinski, 2012). Clinicians see this all of the time. In psychoanalysis, it is termed transference. Perhaps, just as important, the clinician is not immune to misapplying these processes to her patients. This is termed countertransference (Racker, 1988). Similarly, in trauma survivors, we often observe how an innocuous stimulus in the environment, like a sound or a place or a personality characteristic, can be paired up with a sense of being in danger. We have often heard survivors of domestic violence state that they cannot move on to dating other people because of seemingly innocuous reminders of their ex-spouse (e.g., one of our [VS] patients shared that she ended a date early because the man she was talking to stated he enjoyed country music, just like her ex-husband; liking country music had become so powerfully associated with the traits of being controlling and aggressive that she experienced panic automatically).

IMPLICIT LEARNING IN THE LIFE SPAN

There are also data showing that the ability to process covariations begins very early in life (Roter, 1985, cited in A. Reber, 1992). Czyzewska, Hill, and Lewicki (1991, cited in Lewicki et al., 1992) reported that 4- and 5-year-olds learned a covariation between the color of the clothing worn by children depicted on a poster and the nature of their physical activity. Moreover, the covariations children can learn can be quite complex and superior to their conscious ability to process covariations. In one experiment by Lewicki (1986; Experiment 5.2), children age 5 were shown to be capable of managing two covariations simultaneously. They were exposed to matrices of colored squares containing pictures of objects. Certain objects covaried with certain colors. These color–object matches differed on the right and left halves of the matrices. The matrices were then covered, and the task was to guess the location of the previously presented objects. The covered matrix was brought to the child by an experimenter who approached either from the child's left or right side. The direction of approach covaried with whether the correct object–color match was predicted by the left or right half of the previously viewed matrix. The children were more accurate at guessing the location of the target then would be expected by chance. Thus, they were able to combine knowledge about the matrix with the direction of the experimenter's approach. (We can barely follow the sequence when writing about it, yet children could do so in a dynamic, *in vivo* environment.) Saffran, Aslin, and Newport (1996) reported implicit learning in even younger children. Infants were exposed to simple auditory sequences and later preferred listening to sequences that had the same underlying structure (mere exposure effect). (Also see Saffran, 2003).

Implicit learning does not only appear early in life; it lasts well into old age. Frensch and Runger (2013) report that another task often used to assess implicit learning, the Serial Reaction Time Task (SRTT), is relatively unaffected by age.[1] Verneau, van der Kamp, Savelsbergh, and de Looze (2014) also reported that whereas explicit learning declined in old age, implicit learning was relatively stable well into old age.

Summarizing some of his research findings, Lewicki (1986) argued that social cognition is particularly likely to be affected by implicit processes. This is because social stimuli are often ambiguous and therefore more open to alternative interpretations than is objective reality. In addition, covariations in the environment will be learned implicitly regardless of whether they are sensibly connected or not. This conclusion has significant implications for understanding biases, stereotypes, and other social phenomena. In fact, a recent study shows that this kind of learning of bias can be modeled artificially. That is, AI machine learning can pick up human biases by simply looking at co-occurrences of language on the Internet (i.e., covariation learning ala implicit learning in humans). Caliskan, Bryson, and Narayanan (2017) reported that having an AI program statistically parse ordinary language on the Internet resulted in exactly the kinds of biases identified by tests of association like the implicit attitude test (IAT; Banaji & Greenwald, 2013; Greenwald et al., 1998). This may be a good model for how implicit learning works in humans. It is largely amotivational and arational. It simply picks up, within limits, regularities in the environment. Since our culture provides regularities that reflect our biases, that is what an empirical program or empirically based implicit learning will pick up. Finally, it is likely unconscious just as the AI learning does not betoken awareness. (See below.[2])

IMPLICIT LEARNING IS UNCONSCIOUS

There are quite a lot of data that directly and convincingly show that the knowledge demonstrated in these studies is not in awareness (i.e., is unconscious). Lewicki, Hill, and Bizot (1988) had participants learn covariations that enabled them to efficiently locate a target. The participants in this study were faculty members of a psychology department who knew that the experiment involved nonconscious processes. Despite their motivation and their best efforts to determine what was going on, none identified the relevant covariation. In fact, they were not even able to determine that a covariation lay at the bottom of the study and explained their improved performance. Most guessed that subliminal stimulation was involved. Lewicki, Czyzewska, and Hoffman (1987) allowed their participants (college students in this case) unlimited time to figure out the nature of the covariations they had been exposed to and learned. As an added incentive, they were promised $100 if they could identify any systematic feature of the stimuli they had just been exposed to. Some spent hours trying to solve the problem but none succeeded. In fact, no one even came close.

Finally, there are data showing that what is learned implicitly can be orthogonal to conscious knowledge. That is, although behavior is clearly altered, conscious knowledge and attitudes remain unchanged. Hill, Lewicki, Czyzewska, and Schuller (1990) had people implicitly learn a connection between a facial feature and a personality characteristic. Although they later behaved as though they had made this connection, participants reported that they did not believe that the two variables were related in any way. This supported an earlier finding by Lewicki (1986, Experiment 4.1) in which half of the participants were presented with covariations between traits that disconfirmed their conscious views of the association between those traits. The other half of the participants viewed covariations consistent with their conscious views. All participants were then asked to rate various stimulus people (some fictitious and some known to them). Individuals in the disconfirming condition were more likely to violate their conscious beliefs in their ratings than were individuals exposed to covariations consistent with their conscious views. Explicit, conscious views remained unchanged in both conditions. And no one recognized the covariation that had been experienced. Finally, Musen and Squire (1993) reported that amnesiacs could learn color–word associations but denied having any knowledge of those covariations. All together, these studies show that implicit and explicit learning are separable phenomena (i.e., they can be orthogonal to one another). Additionally, explicit learning seems to be related to awareness whereas implicit learning is not (i.e., it is unconscious).

STRATEGIC BEHAVIORS AND IMPLICIT LEARNING

Some work on covariation learning examined strategic behaviors. Ghinescu, Schachtman, Sradler, Fabiani, and Gratton (2010) used a version of the flanker paradigm, in which participants viewing a computer screen focus on a central target item "flanked" by symbols such as letters and arrows serving as distracters, or "noise." Participants have to categorize a target stimulus as quickly as possible, ignoring the distracters. The distracting symbols can be congruent (compatible) or incongruent (incompatible) with the target. The usual result of this kind of study, termed the "flanker effect," is that participants have a shorter reaction time and more accurate performance on congruent than on incongruent trials. Immediately before each trial in the Schachtman et al. study, a cue (a letter—either A, B, or C) was shown that predicted whether the stimulus would be congruent, incongruent, or equally likely to be either. There were three conditions: (1) explicit instructions (what each cue meant and that they should use the cues to help them respond), (2) partially explicit instructions (only that the cues were predictive and that after several trials they would be able to use them), and (3) no instructions about the significance of the cues. The researchers found no effect of group on the participants' performance (i.e., the flanker effect occurred equally strongly in all three groups), indicating that even participants without explicit knowledge about the cues used them to make strategic adjustments. The authors concluded that strategies can be implicitly learned and implemented. Atas et al. (2014), reviewed above, showed that the flanker effect can take place even when the stimuli being presented are out of awareness.

A type of implicit strategy formation was also observed in a study investigating a rock–paper–scissors (RPS) game (Wang, Xu, & Zhou, 2014). In this study, the researchers challenged the common game theory assumption that people's action decisions are based on consciously constructed strategies. If that were true, they argued, rational RPS players would attempt to completely randomize their action choices so as to render them unpredictable. Instead, they found that when participants won, they tended to repeat the same action (rock, paper, or scissors). Wang et al. also demonstrated a clear cyclical (and hence predictable) pattern of responses to losing actions, suggesting that participants developed implicit strategies for playing RPS. This continued even when the opponent was changed. Although the researchers did not specifically assess whether or not the players could verbalize their cyclical patterns of play, this investigation suggests that implicit learning may take place in developing response strategies to complex situations, involving multiple individuals, in changing dyads. Because the RPS game is typically played in rapid sequences, it can be argued that the simplest form of implicit learning that occurs is attempting to play the same action after winning a round, gradually morphing into a more complex cyclical response pattern (i.e., operant conditioning takes place, resulting in something closely akin to what Skinner, 1974, termed "superstitious behavior").

This behavior, a result of implicit learning, may then be transferred or generalized from one social context to another. What this means is that people repeat strategies even when they are no longer valid and that they have no idea that they are doing so. Covariation learning has also examined the implicit learning of social cues. Heerey and Velani (2010) had participants engage in a computerized version of RPS with an avatar portrayed as another participant. On certain trials, the avatar displayed a nonverbal social cue that could be used to predict his move (poker players call this a "tell"). When the avatar expressed this cue, participants began to win more over time. Although they were not explicitly aware of the predictive social cue, they were able to use it to predict the avatar's behavior. It is important to note that this social learning took place within a single, multiple-round game. Finally, Gross and Greene (2007) showed that not only can complex learning occur implicitly, its lessons can be applied by analogy to another situation. These findings have important implications for the learning of behavior patterns in relationships. It suggests that we may, very quickly and imperceptibly, engage in relationship patterns based on cues from others that we cannot identify. This harkens back to the classic work of Ambady and Rosenthal (1992, 1993) who showed that very brief observations (under 5 minutes and as quickly as 30 seconds) could predict outcomes in classes and even in psychotherapy. Lieberman (2000) has in fact gone as far as to suggest that implicit learning is the very basis of social intuition. Malcolm Gladwell (2005) popularized this kind of finding in his bestselling book *Blink*.

UNDERSTANDING IMPLICIT LEARNING

What are we to make of implicit learning? As with implicit memory, the debate seems to be over whether there are two distinct systems of learning: explicit and implicit. Presumably, each has different neurophysiological underpinnings. Or is there a single learning system that can be addressed in multiple ways? Once again, it seems that explicit learning is easier to locate in the brain than is implicit learning. We refer the interested reader to P. Reber (2013), reviewed in our discussion of implicit memory (see Chapter 11), for more on this topic. Rather than repeat the evidence and counterevidence, let us state that we come to the same conclusion as we did in that review. The best understanding of the data, in our opinion, follows Reber's theorizing. Recall that he argued that there is an identifiable and localizable system for explicit memory and learning housed in the medial temporal lobe (MTL). Implicit memory and learning, on the other hand, have no specifiable location but are due to the general plasticity of the nervous system. Implicit learning is a by-product of the way our neurons form connections with one another. Implicit learning is a function of brain plasticity. These connections are distributed throughout the brain and therefore cannot be identified as a localized system.

In the case of implicit learning, the neuronal connections that are strengthened as experiences are repeated leads to the extraction of the underlying statistical structure of the information contained in those experiences. That which gets repeated becomes more strongly connected than that which is idiosyncratic. This naturally comes to reflect the underlying structure of the information as irrelevant aspects drop out and critical aspects become strengthened. This then generalizes to other experiences to the extent that they share a similar stochastic structure. So the general tendency of neurons in the brain to become more strongly connected the more often they fire together comes to reflect the regularities of our experiences and allows for categorization of them. And virtually none of this goes on consciously. Additionally, the huge number of possible connections allows for efficient storage of much more information than the explicit system is capable of. So there is much more capacity for implicit than for explicit learning. The brain, in this analogy, "learns" just as did the AI system set up by Caliskan et al. (2017). Again, we describe this idea in more detail and derive more implications of this kind of model when we review PDP.

CLINICAL IMPLICATIONS OF IMPLICIT LEARNING

The research on implicit learning, taken as a whole, indicates that people can, and normally do, analyze the covariations in their environment. These analyses are often conducted outside of awareness; their results are also often not available to consciousness. Moreover, these unconscious or implicit processes seem to be able to process covariations more quickly and to grasp more complex covariations than can conscious processes. And implicit capacity is far greater than explicit capacity. Analogically, implicit learning functions much like the AI described by Caliskan et al. (2017). Calling upon conscious processes may interfere with these abilities. And implicit learning is not limited to the concrete covariations encountered in the environment; unconscious inferences act on these covariations to produce more abstract learning (i.e., unconscious inductions are performed upon the covariations encountered). All of this does not always occur effortlessly. Demands on attention may interfere with implicit learning. Alternatively, conscious, explicit processes may play some role in the learning process. Regardless, implicit learning is not what we would typically refer to as "conscious." As we did when discussing implicit memory, we would argue against separate implicit and explicit learning systems that are orthogonal to one another. We would also argue against a single system that underlies them both. Instead, we believe that there is probably an explicit system that can be identified but that implicit learning represents the plasticity of the entire nervous system rather than a specific system having a specific location and with its own set of rules.

Implicit learning affects behavior in easily demonstrable ways. It begins early in life; shows little variation in capacity across individuals; weakens little, if at all, with age; and is robust with respect to brain damage. Its effects are not related to conscious awareness of having learned something; responses feel intuitive or at the "gut" level. The influence of implicit learning is probably ubiquitous in our daily lives. Further, since it begins very early in life, its ultimate impact could be far reaching. This is central to the study of attachment (Bowlby, 1969), for example. Attachment processes begin when a child is very young before he is capable of learning from explicit instruction; therefore, learning and encoding of experiences occur implicitly. As Cortina and Liotti (2007) put it: "Experiences coded implicitly are not lost but have powerful adaptive and non-adaptive consequences for development. These experiences are carried forward as a series of unconscious 'procedural' expectations" (p. 205). These authors cite the behaviors of 1-year-olds in Ainsworth's (Ainsworth, Blehar, Waters, & Wall, 1978) Strange Situation as an example of how unconscious expectations are played out in early childhood. The child's attachment history leads to implicit learning of what to expect from the mother. The end result is an unconscious mental model of attachment, which can be characterized as relatively secure, avoidant, or resistant. That unconscious mental model predicts the child's behavior in the Strange Situation. Moreover, a review article by Dykas and Cassidy (2011) found substantial evidence that early attachment style predicts not only behavior but also perceptions of others many years later. These authors found that securely and insecurely attached individuals literally "see" the world differently, with insecure individuals defensively excluding painful information from further processing. Further, unlike securely attached persons, those who had insecure attachments were more likely to perceive even innocuous information through a negative lens congruent with their early attachment experiences. All of this takes place unbeknownst to the perceiver, likely because experiences and events that occur in the initial 3 to 4 years of a child's life cannot be consciously recalled (due to inadequate brain and language development) but are stored implicitly (implicit memory). As Cortina and Liotti (2007) put it, "Early, implicit, preverbal experience is important. . . . It forms the basis for prototypes of models of interpersonal relating" (p. 209).

One major clinical implication of all of this information and evidence is that a patient may be approaching relationships and interests with a model based on implicit learning that contradicts what the patient consciously espouses and believes to be true. Because the model was likely formed many years before a therapist sees a patient, it may also be at odds with current environmental contingencies and therefore maladaptive. Implicit learning is not some higher form of wisdom that consciousness can only obstruct or intrude upon. This is not the unconscious of the Romantics. It has strengths but it also has limitations. It is radically empirical. That is, it is almost entirely based on experiences but lacks reflection (like AI). Although the ability to form connections unconsciously is powerful, the ability to evaluate the meaning or relevance of these connections can be weak to nonexistent. By virtue of being amotivated, implicit learning processes are uncritical and lack the capacity for self-reflection or judgment. Whatever covaries in the environment (within limits) will be learned, whether sensibly related or not. And this learning will not be restricted to concrete instances. The person will unconsciously generalize them to conceptually related stimuli. Sometimes (mostly) this results in adaptive understanding of the world. But sometimes it results in maladaptive expectations of and reactions to events. This too is automatic and unreflective. This means that beliefs, phobias, maladaptive behavior patterns, and other psychological occurrences may not be motivated or, at least, not entirely motivated. This could explain some of the neurotic beliefs people seem to live their lives by but deny, seem oblivious to, or find themselves unable to change. Take, for example, a process that may be operating in survivors of chronic or intense trauma. The PTSD symptoms of hypervigilance, dissociation, or avoidance can be understood as a normative, implicitly learned response to abnormal and threatening conditions. They are initially adaptive, assuring survival, but later on, when the environment they were learned in is no longer operative, these coping mechanisms become maladaptive. This is well illustrated in patients whose trauma occurred at a very early age and was not verbally encoded; they may exhibit seemingly inexplicable visceral and affective reactions to innocuous cues such as particular sounds, tastes, or textures. It is also evident in the kind of PTSD we see in war veterans whose expectations and reactions were well suited to a dangerously unpredictable environment but are not adaptive in civilian life. Moreover, once such covariations are abstracted out of the environment, they tend to have long-term effects through biasing future responding. They become "self-perpetuating" as Hill et al. (1989) and Lewicki et al. (1989) put it. (Also see Lewicki, 1992, 1997.) Similarly, we know from our clinical practices that many patients with a history of abandonment may struggle when we leave for vacation. Although consciously they may realize or "know" that we will return, the implicitly learned connections between physical absence (albeit very temporary) and feelings of abandonment are strong. With some patients even the physical distance throughout the week can be overwhelming, and so they call us, for example, to confirm the day and time of their appointment. Explicitly, they forgot the exact time and wish to be certain of it. Implicitly, calling and hearing the therapist's voice is reassuring and thus helps manage the anxiety or fear of abandonment/disappearance.

The ease with which complex covariations are learned, along with their early appearance, robustness, and self-perpetuating bias, have profound implications for the way people understand their worlds and live their lives. Consider that implicit learning begins and matures before explicit learning. This means that much of our early learning is entirely implicit. Self-perpetuating biases can maintain such learning. Behaviors based on this learning can become automatic. Problems are especially likely to arise when implicit learning, originally based on relationships with significant others, is inappropriately applied to current relationships (see Andersen & Przybylinski, 2012). The earlier the learning takes place, the more automatic and unconscious it can become. The person will be unaware of having these biases. She may even deny having them. In these ways, they can be maintained into adulthood even if the environment ceases to support them. If the learning represents reality well, the person will display good gut instincts and intuitions and will therefore generally react adaptively to events. If the learning leads to a distorted view of reality or if reality has changed with no commensurate change in learning, the person will show poor judgment and maladaptive reactions to life's challenges. She will act as if something is so when it is not or as if something is not so when it is. In neither case will the person be able to explain her mode of operation or why she acts as she does. If adaptive learning predominates, she will be mentally healthy; if maladaptive learning predominates, she will be neurotic or even personality disordered. Most people can be expected to show a mixture of these outcomes.

If the above scenario is accurate, implicit learning may account for some of the apparently unconscious pathology so often encountered by clinicians. In this account, pathology is not solely a consequence of defensively walled-off ideas, affects, and conflicts. It is not entirely due to maladaptive, automatic thinking. It is also and perhaps largely attributable to implicitly learned modes of reaction and behavior. It is resistant to change because of the robust nature and self-perpetuating bias of implicit learning as well as the resistance of automatic behavior to change, not because of motivated resistance. Jurchis and Opre (2016) say something of this sort and conducted an experiment to support this view. They found that their subjects were able to learn complex cognitive structures that associate neutral and emotional contents. Further, these subjects employed these structures without being aware of doing so (much as Lewicki, 1986, showed). Jurchin and Opre concluded that unconscious processes and contents may be partly responsible for dysfunctional affective responses.

If the above is accurate, the therapist should keep in mind that patients are not necessarily resisting knowing what they have learned about the world and about what to do about it; they really do not know. They have arrived at all sorts of unconscious conclusions about the world. Some will be accurate; some may be wildly off. Some may even blatantly contradict strongly held conscious beliefs. If events covaried in a nonsensible or maladaptive fashion, that is what the patient will have learned. And the patient will often be unable to report it. When therapists help people make these connections, when they make the unconscious conscious, make transference interpretations, examine automatic thoughts, challenge assumptions, or engage in Socratic dialogue, they are not always breaking through resistances or defenses to make the person realize something that she already knew. Instead, they are helping people make wholly new connections that allow them to understand their experiences. They are making patients aware of implicitly learned assumptions and beliefs (see Stolorow & Atwood, 1989). So an important lesson to be learned from implicit learning is for the therapist to focus on what has been learned and to try to build new, adaptive learning on top of it to compete with and ultimately supplant it. Finally, what has been termed "transference" can be a product of implicit learning. The patient has learned how to relate and applies that learning to others whether it fits reality or not. The therapist can infer what that learning may have been like, what the patient's interpersonal interactions may have been like early in life, by attending to the way she relates to her. Likewise, the therapist would do well to attend to how she relates to others and how that may affect the patient. Rather than being steeped in conflict, much of this is normative. Nonetheless, it is clinically diagnostic and critical to understanding the functioning of the patient and how the therapist's functioning may impact her.

NOTES

1. In the SRTT, a visual cue appears in one of four positions on a screen. The task is to press a button representing the correct position. Unbeknownst to the subject, the cues have a stochastic structure that the subject implicitly learns.

2. This study demonstrates that common everyday language is so biased toward race and gender (and probably a host of other things) that a machine, operating in a purely statistical manner, easily picks it up (Greenwald, 2017).

CHAPTER 13

Implicit Motivation

Another line of empirical research, that of implicit motivation, began in the late 1940s and was inspired by the pioneering work of Henry Murray (discussed in Winter, 1998). The innovators here were David McClelland and John Atkinson. (See McClelland, 1987, for a review of the early work.) Early on, the researchers (McClelland & Atkinson, 1948) experimentally manipulated a basic motivational need (hunger) and measured its activation via a version of Murray's Thematic Apperception Test, thereby employing imagery and narrative to empirically tap into people's implicit motivational needs. McClelland (1984) believed that people were largely unaware of the values and needs guiding their lives. He therefore was skeptical about how well self-reported goals reflect individuals' true values or behavior (McClelland, 1972). Later, he (McClelland et al., 1989; Weinberger & McClelland, 1990) saw implicit and explicit motives as both relating to behaviors, albeit in different ways.

BEGINNINGS AND THE ACHIEVEMENT MOTIVE

McClelland soon focused his efforts on a motivational need that he saw as focal for success: the need for achievement (nAch). Overall, the achievement motive is about deriving pleasure from mastering challenging tasks. People high in achievement motivation strive to accomplish for accomplishment's sake (Schultheiss, Patalakh, & Rösch, 2012). A person high in nAch wants to challenge herself for the purpose of testing her abilities and, ultimately, improving. The nAch is an intrinsic need and, as such, it can be negatively impacted by the presence of extrinsic incentives (Spangler, 1992). Although succeeding at challenging tasks is motivating for people high in *n* Achievement, tasks that are too difficult—and therefore have a low probability of being mastered—are less likely to be pursued. This is because success at such a task is likely attributable to luck rather than to ability. Tasks that are too easy are equally unlikely to be pursued since anyone could succeed at them. In essence, a high-nAch individual is in competition with himself, and only a moderate level of risk or a task of moderate difficulty can provide useful feedback that can then facilitate improvement. Success at such a task provides the "kick" that someone high in nAch seeks. Warren Buffett is probably an example of someone high in achievement motivation. Although he has amassed huge wealth, he seems to care little about using it for the finer things in life. For example, he lives in a modest home, owns a nonluxury car, and drives it himself. He had to be talked into purchasing a private jet. The money he makes just seems to be a way he keeps score of his personal achievements. And he plans on (and has already begun) giving it all away (Schroeder, 2008).

McClelland's exploration of the achievement motive soon moved beyond the experimental laboratory setting to the workings of nAch in society. The most remarkable example of this work may be his historical analysis of the workings of nAch, as reflected in literature from ancient Greece up through the 1950s. McClelland (1961, 1978) found relationships between high *n* Achievement and economic growth. McClelland was able to trace the economic rise and fall of societies to their collective motivation for achievement and even to cultural/religious values (i.e., the Protestant work ethic) that reflected achievement motivation. Thus, he was able to show that changes in nAch affect history. McClelland then applied these findings to affecting personal entrepreneurial success (McClelland & Winter, 1969). He demonstrated that people with higher motivation for achievement are happier and more satisfied in entrepreneurial roles, which consequently affects the prosperity of society as a whole. Further, he could intervene in this process. He was able to increase the achievement motivation of local entrepreneurs in several villages in India and then demonstrate that this increase in nAch led to increased economic productivity. He later conducted longitudinal studies that showed that *implicit motives* (need for power, to be described below) predicted the performance of executives in a major international corporation (see Winter [1991]).

EXPLICIT AND SELF-ATTRIBUTED MOTIVES

McClelland's line of inquiry into human motivation led to some confusion and discord in the field. Many researchers ignored the central principle on which McClelland built his theoretical framework, namely, that people cannot accurately describe their implicit motives (for a detailed review, see Schultheiss & Brunstein, 2010). Some tried to tap into motives using self-report measures, only to discover that their results were discrepant from those of indirect, projective, assessment tools. To organize and make theoretical sense of this disorder, McClelland et al. (1989) and Weinberger and McClelland (1990) posited the existence and differential mode of operation of two separate motivational systems, which they termed "self-attributed" motives and "implicit" motives. The former was conscious and accessible through self-report; the latter was relatively unconscious and accessible through analysis of stories and other spontaneous verbal productions (see Smith, 1992, for detailed scoring systems for several of the implicit motives). In this new model, both conscious and unconscious motives were important but represented different psychological systems and operated in qualitatively different ways. As a result, they predicted different behaviors and were predicted by different child-rearing practices. The implicit motivational system, measured via projective stories, was said to be largely preverbal and developed through early affectively charged experiences (McClelland & Pilon, 1983). It is therefore usually inaccessible through self-reflection and self-report. In their work on the achievement motive, for instance, McClelland and Pilon found that scheduling of feeding and severity of toilet training in young children was significantly correlated with *n* Achievement 20 years later. Other research (McClelland, 1961; Veroff, 1969) has suggested that the parents of high-achievement individuals encouraged and rewarded their children for mastering tasks that are challenging but age-appropriate. Explicit motives, on the other hand, represent one's conscious beliefs and self-concept about what one's motives are. Importantly, they are thought to develop later in life through experiences that are verbally encoded (Rawolle, Schultheiss, & Schultheiss, 2013). For instance, in their review of the literature, McClelland et al. (1989) noted that people were more likely to self-report high achievement motivation if they have already formed or heard an opinion of themselves as having achieved something concrete. In other words, if I praise you for passing your licensing exam, you are more likely to rate yourself as motivated by a need to achieve.

The two types of motivational systems also predict different behaviors. Explicit motives are more likely to relate to short-term behavior and verbalized goals in situations that can be easily identified with the person's conscious values and motives. In contrast, the implicit system of motives is more likely to predict spontaneous and long-term behavior (i.e., when the person is not actively focused on the motive and/or situation). In adults, high *n* Achievement has been associated with overall academic performance, consistently and over time (O'Connor, Atkinson, & Horner, 1966), whereas self-attributed high achievement predicts concrete choices, for example, setting a goal to obtain a high score on a specific test (Ajzen & Fishbein, 1970).

Weinberger and McClelland (1990) elaborated theoretically upon these explicit and implicit motivational systems. They argued that the two systems are not only associated with distinct types of behavior but are also relatively independent of one another (i.e., orthogonal) and responsive to different incentives. In other words, what we believe we are motivated to do and what we implicitly strive for may be (and often are) two separate things. As a result, the two systems are also not always in alignment, which has significant implications for a person's functioning as well as the person's mental and physical health (more on that below). McClelland et al. (1989) hypothesized that "implicit motives . . . might provide a general orientation toward certain types of goals but that self-attributed desires often reflect social norms that help define more narrowly the areas in which those goals are to be accomplished" (p. 692). Overall, McClelland et al. (1989; see also Weinberger & McClelland, 1990) found that self-attributed motives respond to social–extrinsic incentives (e.g., a parental instruction to finish a task). In other words, people who described themselves as high achieving accomplish more when responding to social demands to do so. In contrast, implicit motives appear to respond to task-oriented incentives, such as, for instance, the pleasure of mastering a challenging task. This is a finding that has been replicated and expanded upon (e.g., Brunstein & Maier, 2005; deCharms, Morrison, Reitman, & McClelland, 1955; Koestner, Weinberger, & McClelland, 1991; Schultheiss & Brunstein, 2001). The two types of motives have been shown to differentially predict performance (Biernat, 1989; Brunstein & Maier, 2005) as well as personal goal commitments (Rawolle et al., 2013; Schultheiss, Jones, Davis, & Kley, 2008).

TYPES OF IMPLICIT MOTIVES

Implicit motivation is not restricted to achievement. Originally, three implicit motives were examined and garnered a great deal of theoretical and empirical support: achievement (discussed above), power (*n*Pow), and affiliation (*n*Aff). Intimacy motivation (*n*Int) was developed later by

Dan McAdams (see McAdams & Vaillant, 1982, and McAdams, 1992) to capture a different aspect of affiliation and has also been strongly empirically supported. More recently, oneness motivation (OM) was developed to capture the need to be part of something beyond oneself (Siegel & Weinberger, 1998; Weinberger, 1992; Weinberger & Smith, 2011).

The Power Motive

Satisfaction of the *n* Power and the *n* Affiliation motives, unlike *the n* Achievement motive, in which one competes with oneself, require the presence of others. Study of power motivation was largely innovated by David Winter (1973, 1992, 1999). In a series of studies, Winter (1973) linked high *n* Power in college students to participation in competitive sports and holding office in student organizations. Unlike leaders high in *n* Achievement, who may display task-related micromanaging tendencies (Schultheiss et al., 2012), high-power leaders seek to and derive pleasure from influencing other people. Winter applied these insights to major political leaders (see Winter, 2005, 2010). He studied these figures through their speeches, interviews, and spoken or written texts, examining the relationship between their motivational profiles and large-scale political events. He found that not only can implicit motivation be measured without direct access to the person being assessed but that it may be possible to predict political behavior from these motives (see Winter, 2005, 2010). For instance, he found that the degree of *n* Power evident in U.S. presidents' inaugural speeches correlated with future ratings of their greatness given by historians. Through detailed studies of John F. Kennedy and Bill Clinton, Winter further illustrated that higher *n* Power, relative to *n* Achievement, predicted successful political performance, presumably because high power motivation allows individuals to navigate the complex bureaucratic networks of politics, which frequently require negotiations and putting energy into maintaining power dynamics. There is a negative aspect to power motivation as well. Leaders high in power motivation show less consideration for moral imperatives in making decisions (Fodor & Smith, 1982) and respond to negative feedback with a reduction in creativity (Fodor, 1990).

The power motive has two aspects to it: to influence others, be it through controlling or impressing them, and to receive recognition for doing so (Fodor, 2009). Power-motivated individuals can often be found in professions where they can influence, inspire, or overpower others (e.g., teachers, athletes in highly competitive sports, politicians, corporate executives). Power-oriented individuals are also susceptible to behaviors that increase a sense of power, even if that sense is illusory, as in drinking. Thus, McClelland and colleagues wrote of the relationship between power motivation in men and consumption of alcohol (McClelland, Davis, Kalin, & Wanner, 1972). A high need for power is not inherently positive or negative. Rather, it is how it is expressed that matters (Schultheiss & Brunstein, 2010), as illustrated by the professions it is linked to. Winter (1973) compared the motivational need for power to fire—having the potential to accomplish a lot of good, but also needing constant monitoring due to its destructive potential. As Schultheiss et al. (2012) have pointed out, the desire to influence others is not often viewed positively in society. As a result, many individuals high in *n* Power seek socially accepted avenues of motive satisfaction. For instance, high-power leaders may seek to impact others by empowering and inspiring them. On the other hand, high-power people can be heavy-handed and express the motive by trying to dominate others. In one of his early studies, Winter (1973) found that college students who exhibited high power motivation often associated with classmates who were relatively unpopular. These classmates then enjoyed an increase in self-esteem and status through their association with a high-power individual. On a larger scale, the power motive can be expressed through social activism and leadership (e.g., Mahatma Gandhi or Martin Luther King). A number of highly charismatic U.S. presidents, for example, Jefferson, Lincoln, the two Roosevelts, Truman (Winter, 1987), and Kennedy (House, Woike, & Fodor, 1988), have been found to possess high power motivational needs. On the flip side, individuals high in power motivation, like President Woodrow Wilson, for example, have also been found to be particularly susceptible to flattery and ingratiation and, consequently, to the influence of people willing to provide them with such blandishments (Fodor, 2009).

Developmentally, power motivation is predicted by parental permissiveness of sex and aggression in their infants (McClelland et al., 1989). In this context, permissiveness in sex and aggression means that the parents do not punish or strongly discourage the expression of anger (I know you are angry at me, that's OK) or infantile sexuality (e.g., masturbatory activity). The power motive has also been related to biological phenomena. McClelland et al. (1989) reported that a high implicit need for power is associated with an increased stress response and overall impaired functioning of the immune system. More recently, it has been determined that gonadal steroid changes (in testosterone for men and estradiol for women), as well as cortisol levels, can be impacted by satisfaction or frustration of power motivation in high-power individuals (Wirth & Schultheiss, 2006; Wirth, Welsh, & Schultheiss, 2006; for a review, see Schultheiss, Rösch, Rawolle, Kordik, & Graham, 2010). It appears, then, that the implicit power motive is related to the individual's experience of stress and, as a result, has an impact on overall health. McClelland and Jemmott (1980) argued that the greater activation of the sympathetic nervous system in individuals with a high need for power may have an immunosuppressive effect, thus rendering them more vulnerable to illness (Segerstrom & Miller, 2004).

The Affiliation, Intimacy, and Oneness Motives

Affiliative motivation, at its inception, was defined by Heynes, Veroff, and Atkinson (1958) as a need for relatedness with others, be it a concrete person or a group (Weinberger et al., 2010). Overall, individuals high in *n* Affiliation are thought to seek and derive pleasure from social connections, avoid confrontation, focus on people rather than performance, and experience a need for being liked by others (Schultheiss et al., 2012). Earlier studies of Affiliation motivation demonstrated that people high in this need tend to find jobs that are people-oriented (Exline, 1960), value interpersonal peace (Rokeach, 1973), and will change their behavior so as to avoid conflict (Walker & Heyns, 1962). They also tend to avoid and often do poorly at competitive tasks (Karabenik, 1977; Terhune, 1968). All of these behaviors serve the purpose of maintaining a positive interpersonal environment.

To achieve this goal, individuals high on *n* Affiliation have been found to more readily initiate social interactions (Lansing & Heyns, 1959), read social cues and faces (Atkinson & Walker, 1956), and learn social networks (McClelland, 1985). In addition, fulfillment of the need for Affiliation seems to bring about stress relief and has health-promoting effects (McClelland, 1989). More recent studies (Schultheiss, Wirth, & Stanton, 2004; Wirth & Schultheiss, 2006) have attributed these effects to increased progesterone in high-affiliation individuals (in their studies, the participants were only women)—a hormone that may have a soothing and mood-stabilizing effect. However, the affiliation motive, as initially conceptualized, appears to have much more complex underpinnings. Early writers (e.g., Boyatzis, 1973; Byrne, 1961) reported that the striving for closeness appears to be fueled by a fear of rejection rather than by a desire for intimacy. In essence, these authors proposed an avoidance model, which suggests that the source of affiliation motivation is avoiding displeasure rather than attaining pleasure. Indeed, McClelland et al. (1989) reported that the most consistent childhood predictor of high affiliation motivation in adulthood was the mother's ignoring of her infant's cries. And although, as stated above, satisfaction of the affiliative motive may bring about stress relief and soothing, frustration has been associated with negative consequences, such as a higher likelihood to overeat when under stress, as well as with poor blood sugar control in individuals with type I diabetes (McClelland, 1989).

Winter (2003) has also significantly contributed to the affiliation literature through his studies of political leaders. He has found, for example, that politicians high in nAff tend to be more vulnerable to scandals and become hostile or defensive under threat. High affiliation motivation predicts orientation toward others and seeking social situations. However, such individuals tend to gravitate toward friends who are similar to them so as to minimize the possibility of rejection. Politicians high in nAff, then, are more likely to take advice from similarly minded individuals or even subordinates who flatter them rather than from experts if such experts differ in opinion from them.

In an attempt to address these seemingly contradictory aspects of affiliation motivation, as well as to understand a more mutual form of social interaction, McAdams (1980, 1989, 1992) developed the concept of intimacy motivation. Intimacy motivation is defined as a consistent readiness and preference for seeking and experiencing interpersonal warmth, closeness, and interactions. In contrast to the earlier displeasure–avoidance connotations of the affiliative motive, intimacy motivation is approach-oriented and mutual. At its core, it involves sharing one's life, experiences, and inner reality with another person (Weinberger et al., 2010). Several differences have been established between affiliative and intimacy motivation. Most notably, individuals high in intimacy motivation tend to talk about others in dyadic terms and focus on close dyadic relationships, as opposed to high-affiliation persons, whose general orientation is toward any kind of social or group contact. Overall, high-intimacy individuals tend to be happier and better adjusted, friendlier, more cooperative, and more popular than their low-intimacy counterparts (McAdams, Jackson, & Kirshnit, 1981; McAdams & Powers, 1981). High intimacy motivation appears to predict not only well-being, but also job satisfaction and marital happiness (McAdams & Vaillant, 1982). Unfortunately, relatively little work on these motives has been conducted in recent years, and the interpretation of the existing findings is complicated by manipulations and measurements that may not be accurately distinguishing between nAff and nInt (cf. Weinberger et al., 2010).

Lastly, based on psychoanalytic tradition (Silverman, 1976; Silverman & Weinberger, 1986), one of us (Siegel & Weinberger, 1998; Weinberger,1992; Weinberger & Smith, 2011) has proposed the existence of the oneness motive, conceptualized as the need to belong to or become part of a larger whole (Weinberger et al., 2010). This motive is similar to the affiliation and intimacy motives in that it is implicit (i.e., people are not customarily conscious of its operation) and also manifests in interpersonal relationships. Weinberger et al. have argued that this motive is instrumental in developing and maintaining a therapeutic relationship, contributing to what has extensively been studied as a crucial factor in people's improvement in treatment: the therapeutic alliance (Weinberger, 2014).

The beginnings of the work on the oneness motive can be traced back to the subliminal psychodynamic activation (SPA) experimental work on wishes for merger with the good mother of early childhood innovated by Lloyd Silverman (e.g., Silverman & Weinberger, 1985, described in Chapter 7). Unlike the SPA studies, which experimentally primed hypothesized oneness wishes, Weinberger (1992) conceptualized these wishes as an unconscious personality/individual difference variable akin to an implicit motive. What this means is that wishes for oneness are fairly universal but vary in strength across individuals. SPA research, through priming, creates an acute sense of oneness, but one can also see it as a trait that can be measured without being primed. Weinberger (1992) termed this variable Oneness Motivation (OM) and defined it as an unconscious need to become part of, at one with, or belong to a larger whole. It is mostly, but not exclusively, manifested in interpersonal settings, and can be impacted by the qualities of those settings, including psychotherapy. Weinberger and colleagues (Siegel & Weinberger, 1998; Weinberger, 1992; Weinberger, Kelner, & McClelland, 1997; Weinberger & Smith, 2011) also conceptualized some crucial differences between the oneness motive and intimacy and affiliation motivation. Similarly to the intimacy motive, and unlike the affiliation motive, OM does not contain the negative aspect of avoiding rejection but can be seen as only containing positive attributes when activated. But OM differs from *n*Int in that it need not involve a dyadic relationship.

Krass (1997) investigated the relationship between oneness and creativity. Creativity was measured via a battery of tests and the ratings of professors of fine arts students. Krass then divided the students into relatively creative and relatively uncreative. He used the Tellegen Absorption Scale (TAS; Tellegen, 1982) to measure conscious and OM to measure unconscious oneness. Both the Tellegen and OM differentiated the groups but were uncorrelated with one another. Trevouledes (2003) examined the relationship between hypnotizability and oneness. She used the Stanford Hypnotic Susceptibility Scale—Form C to assess hypnotizability and the TAS and OM to measure oneness. Again, both measures were related to hypnotizability but not to each other.

Weinberger also applied the system to therapeutic interventions to determine whether they increased oneness and whether this increase was related to outcome (Siegel & Weinberger, 1998; Weinberger & Smith,

2011). One such study involved a mindfulness intervention (Kabat–Zinn, 2005) designed to help patients cope with chronic pain and/or medical conditions. Higher OM scores led to better outcome at the end of treatment and at 2-year follow-up. Weinberger, Bonner, and Barra (1999) measured OM in inpatients with character disorders receiving psychodynamic psychotherapy. They found that OM increased over the course of treatment. Further, OM at the end of treatment was related to low neurotic behavior, low psychotic behavior, and low negative interpersonal interactions on the ward at the end of the treatment year, as assessed by floor nurses who were blind to OM scores. It therefore seems that an unconscious desire to be part of something beyond the self may underlie some of the oft-cited (e.g., Weinberger, 1995, 2014) value of the therapeutic relationship to psychotherapy outcome. (See Weinberger and Rasco, 2007, for more discussion on this possible connection. Weinberger and Smith, 2011, offer more possible processes that may underlie these effects.)

CLINICAL IMPLICATIONS: THE INTERSECTION OF IMPLICIT AND EXPLICIT MOTIVES

Some research has focused on the alignment, or lack thereof, of explicit and implicit motives (for a review, see Schultheiss et al., 2010). Overall, results show that certain personality characteristics, like self-determination (Hofer et al., 2010), ability to regulate negative affect (Baumann, Kaschel, & Kuhl, 2005), and referential competence (Schultheiss, Patalakh, Rawolle, Liening, & MacInnes, 2011), contribute to greater congruity of the two types of motives. Other personality traits, like extroversion/introversion, have been found to predict the way in which a motive may get expressed in terms of pursuing a particular occupation (Winter, John, Stewart, Klohnen, & Duncan, 1998). Winter et al., for instance, discovered that extroversion/introversion did not correlate with either the Affiliation or the Power motive. However, a combination of high nAff and extroversion predicted engagement in volunteer work, as well as a tendency to combine work and family roles. In contrast, introverts who were high in the Affiliation motive were more likely to be experiencing stress in their intimate relationships, to be divorced, or to be separated. Presumably, such individuals both fear rejection/abandonment (high nAff) and find social interactions overly stimulating (introversion), creating an internal conflict. Extroversion and the Power motive, on the other hand, were predictive of entering high-impact careers, where one has the opportunity to influence a lot of people (Winter et al., 1998).

The lack of overlap between implicit and explicit motivational needs has also been connected to goal pursuit and progress (e.g., Rawolle et al., 2013). Pursuit of explicit goals that are incongruent with implicit motives may interfere with satisfaction of motive-congruent goals and/or lead to apparently inexplicable dissatisfaction ("I achieved my goal, how come I'm not happy?"), thus causing the individual to experience a diminished sense of well-being (Brunstein, Schultheiss, & Grassmann, 1998). Schultheiss et al. (2008) reported that attainment of goals consistent with one's implicit motives can lead to lowered depression scores, whereas failure to attain such goals can have the opposite impact. Overall, it appears that the pursuit and satisfaction of implicit motives is consistently linked to increased happiness and well-being, as well as decreased depression, whereas the pursuit and satisfaction of explicit motives may not be so linked. As Schultheiss et al. (2010) have argued, commitment to goals that are incongruent with implicit motives can impair emotional well-being, especially if it is preventing the individual from working toward the attainment of motive-congruent ones (see also Brunstein et al., 1998). Similar results have also been obtained cross-culturally (Hofer & Chasiotis, 2003).

Kuhl (2000) has proposed that when the implicit and explicit motivational systems are aligned, they can, so to speak, communicate with each other and "agree" on which goals are to be pursued. As a result, the individual will experience minimal stress. This is a model that builds upon the premise that stress compromises the individual's capacity for emotional regulation and, as a result, posits that incongruence of the motivational systems will be associated with increases in negative affect. In an experimental study, Baumann et al. (2005) demonstrated that motive alignment was linked to both the ability to decrease negative affect and to the ability to increase positive affect. These findings have important clinical implications. All too often, clinicians may see patients who express that they want something but are implicitly motivated to pursue something else. For instance, a person may have the expressed desire to become a high-ranking executive with many subordinates (high explicit power motive) but not be particularly implicitly motivated to do so. For example, let us assume that this person's most prominent implicit motive is affiliation. The person will then have the verbalized desire to dominate others, which often means running the risk of engaging in confrontations, being feared, disliked, or criticized. Implicitly, however, a high need for affiliation means that the person is terrified of being rejected and abandoned. That would make for increased stress and internal turmoil, whereby the person may end up failing at both his explicit goal of assuming more power over subordinates and his implicit need for approval and affiliation.

Should clinicians address disparities between the implicit and explicit motivational systems? If so, how would they lessen these disparities? These seem like worthwhile clinical pursuits in light of empirical data supporting the notion that better alignment leads to better mental health outcomes and life satisfaction. It is important for clinicians, on the one hand, to be familiar with the literature on implicit and explicit motivation and, on the other hand, to be attuned to clients' overtly expressed and implicit motives. As was demonstrated in the works of McClelland and of Winter, individuals' verbal productions and narratives contain valuable information about their implicit motivation that can then be compared to their self-reported motives and concrete goals. This is a natural fit for therapists. They can help bring implicit motives to light through listening to and making motivational sense of the stories their patients tell. The ultimate goal would then be to assist the patient to align those motives with expressed motivation and goals. As we highlighted earlier, implicit motives are general and can be satisfied through any number of avenues (a modified form of primary process). An individual high in implicit power motivation can fulfill that need through being a teacher, a competitive athlete, a leader in a company, a politician, or a stay-at-home parent. Similarly, someone with high nAch or nAff may also feel fulfilled in any number of roles. One of the clinician's tasks thus becomes helping a patient determine how her identified goals may align with or contradict her implicit motives and then assist her in paving pathways toward amending those goals to fulfill implicit needs as well. Similarly, as in the case of introversion/extroversion, personality traits can aid in or hinder the expression of implicit motives. Again, therapists can help their clients identify explicit goals that are congruent with their implicit needs as well as in alignment with other personality characteristics.

CHAPTER 14

Automaticity

In Chapter 6, we briefly reviewed early work on the nature and operation of automaticity—a normative unconscious phenomenon that goes back at least to William James (1890/1950), who discussed something like it in his chapter on habit. As explicated earlier in this book, the predominant theory of automaticity was that once mental processes have been sufficiently rehearsed, they begin operating autonomously, circumventing intentionality and awareness (Schneider & Shiffrin, 1977; Shiffrin & Schneider, 1977). Automatization ensures efficiency—once learned, mental processes can operate without the intervention of intentional thought. This leaves willful mental capacities open to attend to new, as yet unprocessed, information. We also reviewed control processes—the conscious, more effortful, but also more flexible, counterpart to automatic processing. Control processes allow us to digest and respond to new information in novel ways. They can become automatic (and unconscious) with rehearsal and practice. (This was one of the central tenets of functionalism, as discussed in Angell, 1907, reviewed earlier in this book; see Chapter 3.) Automatic and control processes evolved as concepts within the information-processing model (see Chapter 6), popular in the 1960–1970s.

THE CURRENT VIEW OF AUTOMATICITY

A great deal of work has been done over the last three decades that broadens our understanding of the process of automatization, addresses the question of why automatic processes are so difficult to change, and explores the clinical implications of automaticity. This work has revolved around two major developments. The first (e.g., Bargh, 1994; De Houwer, 2006; De Houwer & Moors, 2007) concerns the nature of automatic processes. It reflects a shift in how we think about and understand automaticity, from an all-or-nothing process (i.e., a process is either all automatic and implicit or all controlled and conscious) to a focus on the aspects of automaticity that various mental processes display (i.e., controllability, efficiency, intentionality, consciousness—see below). It turns out that an automatic process need not evidence all of these aspects. They can be independent of one another so that one process may evince one or two of them and another could be characterized by a third and so on. The second major development (see Bargh, Schwader, Hailey, Dyer, & Boothby, 2012) concerns the assumption that all automatic processes begin as initially consciously learned skill acquisitions, later on becoming automatic and no longer requiring conscious input. Both of these developments have significant implications for understanding the interplay between conscious and unconscious characteristics of higher-order mental processes and behavior.

We begin with the early conception that automatic processes develop through conscious repetitive practice (e.g., Angell, 1907; James, 1890/1950; Shiffrin & Schneider, 1977). Bargh et al. (2012) argued that this was not necessarily the case. They divided automatic processes into two categories: preconscious (not requiring any initial conscious thought or prior rehearsal) and postconscious (a result of repeated rehearsal and, at least initially, some conscious thought or intention). According to Bargh et al., it is the postconscious automatic processes that are developed through skill acquisition. Much like the early models of automaticity, these processes require prior or concurrent intentionality and conscious repetition in order to become automatic. Such goal-dependent automaticity is present in decision making, cognitive skill acquisition, motor performance, and even in maintaining relationships.

As stated above, Bargh et al. (2012) also highlight what they termed preconscious automatic processes. These phenomena, they argue, are not consciously learned or rehearsed until becoming automatic. Instead, they result from sensory or perceptual input, which then implicitly and effortlessly impacts conscious higher mental processes. Bargh et al. argue that many social-cognitive processes, including behavior contagion, consumer behavior, embodiment (discussed next in this book), emotional regulation, moral and social judgments, motivation, and goal pursuit can be attributed to preconscious automatic processes. They see these processes as being directly influenced by the environment, without the person having any awareness of this influence. For instance, in the domain of embodiment, our judgments of others have been shown to change as a result of sensory experiences (e.g., Williams & Bargh, 2008a, 2008b). We think we are making a judgment based on consciously available information, which then results in conscious decision making. However, empirical evidence suggests that even seemingly unrelated sensory perceptions can exert significant impact implicitly.

Sensory stimulation affects our social interactions without our realizing it. Facial appearance affects our judgment of others' character traits, much as we may not want to admit it (Todorov, Mandisodza, Goren, & Hall, 2005; Willis & Todorov, 2006). We engage in unconscious mimicry when we make new acquaintances, which increases social bonding and cohesion (Bargh, 2017; Chartrand & Bargh, 1999; Lakin, Chartrand, & Arkin, 2008), unless these others are perceived to be a member of an outgroup (Leander, Chartrand, & Bargh, 2012; Leander, Shah, & Chartrand, 2011). We walk more slowly when primed with stimuli related to the elderly (Bargh, Chen, & Burrows, 1996; Hull, Slone, Meteyer, & Matthews, 2002) but mostly when we have a positive disposition toward the elderly (Cesario, Plaks, & Higgins 2006). What is more, Bargh et al. (1996) also review a body of research demonstrating that such social judgments can be observed as early as infancy (e.g., Hamlin, Wynn, & Bloom, 2007, 2010). These findings are of great significance in trying to understand moral judgment, biases, ingroup and outgroup attitudes, and a wide variety of other social attitudes and behaviors. Some even suggest that a number of these effects may either be hard-wired or acquired very early in life (see review of embodied cognition later in this book). These results suggest that higher-level automatic processes can be activated without being initially conscious and without consciously mediated repetition. Moreover, this kind of automaticity is especially likely when the stimuli are synchronous with the individual's self-perception. This is even more true when the synchronous stimuli have positive valence ("positive affect plays an important gatekeeper role in allowing perceptual activation to flow automatically to behavioral tendencies" Bargh et al., 2012, p. 595).

Because relational patterns are also carried out automatically, lacking intentionality or controllability (Bargh, 1994), they are likely to persist unless conscious effort is put into overriding them. A large body of literature suggests that attachment patterns remain relatively stable across the life span (e.g., Cozolino, 2014; Fraley & Shaver, 2000), as do other automatically activated implicit sequences of mental events, such as stereotyping (Monteith, Ashburn–Nardo, Voils, & Czopp, 2002). Once a stereotype becomes associated with a particular racial or societal group, it is activated upon perception of a characteristic of the group (e.g., skin color), regardless of the individual's conscious attitude or judgment. One of us (VS) recently worked with a patient who experienced significant conflict and distress around being biased against a particular social group. He knew that those biases were based on his mother's repeated complaints about that social group during his childhood. Not only did this patient recognize the prejudice of his mother, he even condemned it as untrue and corrosive. Nonetheless, he was unable to shift his emotions or control the physiological reactions triggered by interactions with representatives of that group.

More than 30 years ago, Devine (1989) found that most people tend to share the knowledge of racial stereotypes prevalent in their culture, even when they do not consciously endorse them. Fiske and Tablante (2015) showed that this is still the case. Devine also found that subliminal presentation of a racial stereotype led to a more hostile interpretation of the motives of a character in an ambiguous story. A large body of research has supported Devine's findings. Bargh et al. (1996), for example, found that subliminal priming of faces of young African American males caused European American participants to express more hostility upon mild provocation than did presentation of European American faces. In another study, Chen and Bargh (1997) found that participants not only manifested higher levels of hostility themselves, but also perceived their partners in a game as more hostile. Although this perception was accurate, the partners' hostility was a reaction to the participants' own hostile behavior. The participant had no awareness of her own culpability, however. That is, participants created the hostility of their partners and then attributed it to that person's character while holding themselves blameless. (This is closely akin to the *correspondence bias* of attribution theory discussed in the next chapter.)

Preconscious automaticity was not the only change in conceptualizing automatic processes. De Houwer and Moors (2007) argued that it is wrong to conceptualize automaticity as a unitary construct that necessarily possesses all of the features described by Bargh (1994): unconscious, efficient, unintentional, and uncontrollable. In other words, Bargh's "four horsemen of automaticity" can exist in any combination. They do not all have to appear together in every automatic process, as the early models of automaticity seemed to assume (see Bargh, 1994). To describe a particular automatic process, then, we must specify which features of automaticity are present in it. A process can be called automatic, De Houwer et al. conclude, if it possesses *any* of those features but cannot necessarily be assumed to possess all of the other features of automaticity as well. So there are a multitude of properties and combinations of properties that an automatic process can have.

De Houwer and Moors (2007) call this approach "decompositional" in that the concept of automaticity is decomposed into nonoverlapping features (i.e., autonomous, unconscious, uncontrollable, goal-directed or goal-independent, unintentional). De Houwer and Moors (2007) then assert that, in order to describe a mental process as automatic, we must specify which automaticity features are present. For instance, these authors see automatic processes as goal-related or goal-independent. They further assert that there are many automatic processes related to goals. And, in these varied goal-related processes, some automatic features are more general than others. Further, some features of automaticity are subordinate to others, whereas some features are independent of one another. For example, unintentional processes are postulated to be a subset of uncontrolled processes, such that uncontrolled processes may be intentional or unintentional, whereas an unintentional process will always be uncontrolled. Processes unrelated to goals, on the other hand, can be purely stimulus-driven as long as the stimulus can be registered (the implicit activation of the preconscious phenomena discussed above). And lastly, effortlessness or efficiency, as a feature of automatic processes, does not necessarily overlap with the other features.[1]

CAN AUTOMATIC PROCESSES BE REVERSED OR CHANGED?

One important avenue of research and theorizing concerns the reversibility of automatic processes. Shiffrin and Schneider (1977) initially demonstrated that it took many trials, many consciously driven repetitions, to make a process automatic. Similarly, once automaticity had been achieved, they found it very difficult to reverse. More recent studies, cited above (see Bargh et al., 2012), indicate that repetition of conscious behavior may not be necessary for the creation of automatic processes (preconscious automaticity). That does not mean that it is easy to reverse them, however. In fact, it may be even more difficult to reverse a concept or stereotype that was not created through conscious practice than to undo a behavior created through conscious repetition. The stereotype, concept, or behavior might not be noticed. The person might not know where it came from. There would therefore be no conscious incentive to change it or even conscious knowledge of what needed to be changed. And no matter what, automatic processes are difficult to undo without constant attention being paid to them. Wegner (1994) offered an empirically derived explanation as to why corrective control processes require such constant attention and monitoring if they are to override an automatic process as well as why automatic processes often return with a vengeance. In order to extinguish an unwanted automatic behavior, a conscious controlled process must be in place to override the possibility of that behavior. But there is a second, unconscious, process taking place at the same time. This unconscious process monitors the environment and the individual's mental state for the unwanted behaviors, thoughts, or desires, thereby priming them. Wegner wittily termed this outcome "ironic" because the very process of monitoring for unwanted behavior increases the risk of engaging in that behavior by priming it. As soon as motivation or attention to the conscious control processes flags, which it often does because they require more mental resources than do automatic processes, the action of the unconscious ironic process leads right back to the undesired behaviors or thoughts. Wegner's theory has significant implications for clinical work (discussed below) and offers an understanding of the phenomenon of relapse—one of the most challenging problems in psychotherapy generally and substance abuse recovery in particular.

A possibly more interesting question is whether change can be achieved without conscious practice of controlled behavior overriding automatic behavior. Some research suggests that this is possible. Weinberger, Siegel, Siefert, and Drwal (2012) were able to reduce avoidance behavior in spider-fearful people through exposure that was out of awareness. Insight and awareness are bypassed in such a scenario. Perhaps this could also be applied to other automatic behaviors. The finding has obvious clinical implications. But no matter how change is achieved, it cannot be expected to be easy nor can we be confident that it will last.

CLINICAL IMPLICATIONS OF AUTOMATIC PROCESSING

Automaticity seems to be an area that has not escaped the notice of clinical theorists. Beck's (1972, 1976) cognitive theory of emotional disorders argues that very complex mental sequences that reinforce these disorders can be set in motion by stimuli that do not typically produce the same reaction in healthy individuals. For example, depressives may exhibit a selective bias toward seeking and perceiving stimuli that maintain a negative self-concept. In this context, bias is defined as preferentially processing disorder-confirming information, regardless of how accurate or inaccurate it is (Teachman, Joormann, Steinman, & Gotlib, 2012). This has been empirically supported in a number of studies (e.g., Hogarth, 2011; Matthews & Wells, 2000; McCusker & Gettings, 1997), whose findings suggest that automatic processes partly underlie various mental disorders. In this case, automatic processing serves to maintain a negative self-image. Beck even indexes it by what he termed "automatic thoughts" and showed that depressed patients are typically not aware of engaging in them until it is explicitly brought to their attention.

Matthews and Wells (2000) proposed a stage model of processing stimuli, which implicates automatic attentional biases in both anxiety and affective disorders (see also Williams, Watts, MacLeod, & Mathews, 1988). Further, automaticity of cognitive biases has been shown to impact obsessive and addictive behaviors. Hogarth (2011) found that automaticity plays a distinct role in the etiology of substance dependence, independent of impulsivity and hypersensitivity to reinforcement. McCusker and Gettings (1997) tested the automaticity hypothesis with gamblers and found that they show "automatic, non-volitional, attentional and memory biases" (p. 543) for information related to gambling. Specifically, they found that gamblers showed pronounced selective and automatic attention to gambling-related words on a Stroop task. Simply put, substance abusers and gamblers process information related to the abused substance and to gambling, respectively, differently from controls. Simple exposure to a stimulus related to their addiction is sufficient to prime an automatic behavioral reaction that bypasses conscious thought.

The above priming effect can help account for the prevalence of relapse. Recall that Wegner's (1994) ironic processes predict that the controlled act of trying not to engage in a behavior automatically primes that behavior. If we apply this conception to the clinical phenomenon of relapse, said relapse can be seen as a product of the interaction between automatic and control processes. In the absence or temporary abeyance of willpower and conscious overruling of already automatized behaviors, ironic processes can lead right back to the undesirable behavior. This understanding also suggests a possible solution, along with a caveat. The solution is to make the desired state automatic. Thus, what we are proposing, to turn an adage on its head, is to make the conscious unconscious (cf. Newirth, 2003).[2] The caveat is that even if we succeed in doing this, the old learning and therefore the old behavior is not eliminated but exists as a parallel alternative and can reemerge. In effect, the patient will have two alternative ways of reacting. The one chosen should depend upon the relative strength of the alternative automatic behaviors in interaction with context. That is, one set of behaviors, say the more adaptive one, may be prepotent in one context, whereas the other, the maladaptive one, may be more likely in another context. Additionally, because the old maladaptive behaviors are operating unconsciously, one may not even be able to notice them and thus have no incentive to change or even understand that they lead to undesirable outcomes. The person may therefore not realize that anything needs to be changed.

Another implication of automatic processing concerns the optimal length and frequency of psychotherapeutic treatment. A great deal of data show that socially constructed biases, such as prejudices and stereotypes, are automatic and can implicitly have great impact upon people's attitudes and behaviors (Greenwald & Pettigrew, 2014). It is reasonable therefore to hypothesize that the unconscious influence of automatized relational and thought patterns, including those stemming from intergenerationally transmitted traumatic responses, should also be powerful. Moreover, if prejudice takes years (if not generations) to uproot, it only follows that changing automatic mental events and behaviors in patients might require long-standing and concentrated effort. As Shiffrin and Schneider (1977) observed, it takes many trials and failed attempts to extinguish an automatic behavior, even a post-conscious simple one, acquired in a laboratory setting. More modern views of automaticity would also seem to suggest that reversals would prove difficult. Moreover, preconscious, entrenched, automatic behaviors might be even harder to change than postconscious automatic behaviors. And there is also the problem of context wherein a person could behave adaptively in some contexts (e.g., in the therapy room) but not in others (e.g., at home with the family). Moreover, under stress (a subcategory of what is termed "cognitive load" in the research literature), people tend to revert back to previously learned automatic means of responding (Wilson, Lindsey, & Schooler, 2000). So change, operationalized here as control processes regularly overriding automatic processes, can be expected to be difficult and may take a long time. This, in turn, suggests that psychotherapy may have to be long term or, at least, require periodic returns to treatment.

Consistent with De Houwer and Moors's (2012; see also Moors & De Houwer, 2006) argument that automaticity can be deconstructed and that each automatic process can possess a combination of features, Teachman et al. (2012) propose that discrepancies between different symptom presentations and types of emotional dysregulation can potentially be explained by looking at different features of automaticity and their accompanying information-processing biases. From their review of the literature, they conclude that such distinctions may differentiate between anxiety and depressive disorders. Major depressive disorder was only found to involve uncontrollable processing of emotionally meaningful stimuli (but not necessarily unconscious or efficient processing of said stimuli). Anxiety disorders, on the other hand, do not merely involve uncontrollable, but also unintentional and unconscious processing of fear-relevant stimuli. Teachman et al. also suggest that an ability to disengage from negative material (which would require intention and consciousness) can result in improved mood and may be impacted by treatment. So it is possible to reverse automatic processes (in this case for depression), but it may be useful for clinicians to know which features of automaticity are more prevalent in various clinical profiles so that they can focus on those. Moreover, the concerns about treatment length and frequency, described above, would still hold.

We propose that, from the very nature of automaticity and of ironic processes, it follows that long-term therapy may be best for achieving lasting changes in automatic behaviors. Alternatively, we may have to resign ourselves to the necessity of periodic booster sessions or multiple therapeutic interventions. Even when the patient recognizes his problem and knows what needs to be done (e.g., to discontinue certain self-injurious or compulsive behaviors, to modify interpersonal patterns), change is problematic and introduces additional stress into his life. It is our belief that precisely because some complex mental event sequences are created and operate implicitly and become automatic (preconscious automaticity), their impact on a person's functioning can be so pervasive that any attempt to eliminate them can cause a significant amount of discomfort and even psychic pain. These difficulties contain exactly the recipe for the reemergence of the problematic coping the patient is trying to change. Additionally, the new therapeutic means of coping that has been developed in the course of psychotherapy may be restricted to certain contexts, whereas the original maladaptive means of coping may be more general or, at least, more contextually connected to situations the patient typically encounters outside of the therapeutic setting. We believe that all of these factors may call for long-term treatment or built-in periodic booster sessions in contrast to the short-term therapies often investigated empirically and promoted by managed care. These findings may further explain why follow-ups so often reveal a return of the problematic behavior (Steinert, Hoffman, Kruse, & Leichsenring, 2014a, 2014b; Weinberger, 1995, 2014; Weinberger & Eig, 1999; Westen, Novotny, & Thompson–Brenner, 2004).

Being mindful of findings in the area of automaticity can help clinicians better understand the recalcitrance of their patients' difficulties. Our patients are not always—or at least not entirely—motivated to engage in maladaptive actions by self-denigrations or dynamic unconscious issues. It appears that identifying automatic thoughts or making the unconscious conscious may not be sufficient to successfully treat patients engaging in automatic behaviors or acting in accord with ironic processes. Another step is needed. Corrective control processes, which require constant monitoring, motivation, and effort, may have to be practiced over and over again until they themselves become automatic and override or at least successfully compete with previously automatized maladaptive behavioral or thought patterns. And this practice may have to be repeated in multiple contexts. For example, based on studying automatic processes in individuals with anxiety disorders, McNally

(1995) asserts that anxious patients can benefit by cultivating attentional biases typically found in healthy controls.

NOTES

1. These authors argue that according to this new understanding of automaticity, the terms "automatic" and "implicit" mean the same thing.
2. Newirth (2003) proposes something very much like this for psychoanalytic treatment.

CHAPTER 15

Attribution Theory

Attribution theory evolved from the classic work of Fritz Heider (1958). It posits that people continuously monitor themselves and their environment, inferring causes of their own behaviors, of the behaviors of others, and of the events taking place around them. These causal attributions are processed (sometimes distorted) in accordance with preexisting causal beliefs (Weiner, 1986, 2000). The earliest attribution theorists (e.g., Kelley, 1967; Thibaut & Riecken, 1955) believed that the connection between antecedents (beliefs, information, motivation) and attributions was largely conscious. Later attribution theorists, however, held that although they can be made conscious with focused effort, attributions take place outside of awareness (i.e., implicitly—see, e.g., Weiner, 1986). Many current models employ dual-processing (independent conscious and unconscious processes) models to understand attributions (Strack & Deutsch, 2015).

At a basic level, attribution theory states that people tend to understand behavior as either dispositionally or environmentally caused. This choice, however, is often not based on the conditions actually underlying the behavior but on whether the individual is personally engaged in the behavior or viewing it in others. Two early attribution researchers, Jones and Harris (1967), found that people are generally inclined to attribute the actions of others to inferred personality characteristics (dispositions) rather than to situational factors (environment—see also Jones & Nisbett, 1972; Ross, 1977). This tendency to prefer dispositional explanations when observing the behavior of others was originally called the "fundamental attribution error" (Ross, 1977) but now is less dramatically termed "correspondence bias" (Gilbert & Malone,

1995). Additionally, Baumeister, Bratslavski, Finkenauer, and Vihs (2001) reported that when judging others' motivation, people tend to weigh negative information more heavily than they do positive information. They named this type of attributional bias the positive–negative asymmetry effect. Schyns and Hansbrough (2008) reported that this effect is particularly prominent in organizational settings (companies, corporations, political institutions), where followers tend to interpret errors as the direct result of leadership incompetence, regardless of the error's origin. That is, this negative evaluation prevails even if followers/ subordinates are consciously aware of situational factors underlying the error. The data therefore show that people tend to attribute the behaviors of others to their character, are especially likely to do so when negative outcomes are involved, and even more so when an organization is involved. This is important for clinical work, as detailed below.

People tend to make very different inferences when judging the causes of their own behaviors. Under these conditions, they are much more likely to understand behaviors in terms of environmental contingencies and circumstances beyond their control: they behaved as they did because it made the most sense given the conditions they faced (e.g., you yell at a driver who cuts you off not because you are an angry person but because the circumstances made you frustrated, as would be the case for anyone). One exception is the attributions people make for their own successes and failures. Success tends to invoke stable and internal dispositional attributions, whereas failure is more likely to be blamed on environmental factors (Campbell & Sedikides, 1999; Sedikides, Campbell, Reeder, & Elliot, 1998). This has been termed the self-serving bias, and it too has important implications for clinical work. Below, in the section on clinical implications of attributions, we discuss negative self-bias, wherein a person tends to attribute negativity to himself and positivity to outside factors. This would seem to contradict the self-serving bias. We will see that this is not necessarily the case.

These findings make phenomenological sense. People tend to attribute causality to whatever is most salient in their experiences. Consider the problem of interpreting another's behavior. One cannot observe motives, nor is one typically aware of environmental contingencies unless they are very powerful. What is most salient is the behavior itself. The simplest and most obvious explanation is that the behavior is a result of who the person is. Thus, a dispositional attribution becomes likely. A person is seen yelling; he is then judged to be an angry person. Now consider understanding one's own behavior. The person is well aware of how the environment is impinging upon him and what he is consciously trying to achieve. His disposition is not perceptually salient to him, however, as it is always there. He therefore attributes his behavior to the environment: He is yelling because the other is being absurdly unreasonable and because his efforts to work it out have failed. And if he yells frequently, well, that is because there have been a lot of frustrating circumstances. And this is just how early attribution theorists saw it. For example, Jones and Nisbett (1971) and Ross (1977) assumed that the correspondence bias occurs because the perceiver—the person judging another's behavior—does not see, and therefore fails to appreciate, the full impact of environmental factors on the actor's behavior.

Recent theoretical and research contributions have implicated dual-processing models in accounting for attributional biases. Strack and Deutsch (2015) review these models. The basic point common to all dual-process explanations is that we have two information-processing systems that operate in parallel. One is more impressionistic, automatic, and unconscious. The other is more reflective, controlled, and conscious. The former operates as the default; the latter requires effort and can over-ride the former (if you recall, this was discussed above as we reviewed automatic and control processes). According to this conception, it is the impressionistic system that has the initial interpretive say. It is in its nature to be biased toward features present in the situation. That is, it treats perceptions (impressions) as immediate and unmediated. Only if the reflective system is engaged can we "unbias" it. So if a person is act-ing in a hostile fashion, we are more likely to assume she is a hostile or angry person because we are *perceiving* the hostility. Only if we attend to enough salient information that indicates otherwise, and we are moti-vated to make use of it (e.g., we saw another person offending the indi-vidual and we must render a judgment), is the reflective system likely to be used to correct for the initial bias.

Dual-processing models provide an empirically based explanation for systematic differences in attributional-processing outcomes. But the dual-process explanation can be challenged in that the conscious versus unconscious distinction is not absolute; mental processes can carry char-acteristics of both. (We have just encountered this kind of mix of pro-cesses in our discussion of automaticity above; see Chapter 14.) This is significant in that, if we assume that attributions contain both conscious and unconscious elements, we might be able to utilize the conscious elements to bring the unconscious and automatic ones to light. This is important in exploring and gaining insight into our biases, beliefs, deci-sion making, and behaviors. Nonetheless, even though all processing may be a mix of conscious and unconscious features, some judgments may be more in line with what we would term unconscious processes, whereas others may be more consciously influenced.

There is a model that can account for attribution results with-out positing qualitatively different dual processes and that also takes automaticity into account. Bar–Anan et al. (2010) argued that people attribute actions to what seems to them to be accessible, plausible, and/or self-promoting. This can account for all of the attribution results we have presented thus far. The correspondence bias is therefore due to what is plausible and accessible, namely, the behavior of the actor (accessible) and our implicit theories of personality (plausible). Likewise, the positive–negative asymmetry effect is due to what is accessible (the organizational failure) and plausible (mistakes are due to inherent problems in management and authority). In terms of accessibility, no one notices when an official does the right thing (it is said that if no one comments on or notices a sports official, he is doing a good job), but mistakes are salient and accessible since we must react to them (a sports official makes a bad call and there are endless replays and criticisms). There are no accolades for getting it right. In terms of plausibility, we have an inherent distrust of decision makers and systems. When there is a miscarriage of justice, we do not usually see it as a random, chance event. Instead, we believe that there is something fundamentally wrong with the system. The bias toward attributing our own actions to the environment can be understood similarly. What is accessible is the situation; what is plausible is that we behaved sensibly. This also falls under the self-promoting factor posited by Bar–Anan et al. Finally, the self-serving bias is an obvious case of the self-promoting factor. But it is also consistent with what is accessible to the person at that time. This reasoning is closely akin to that of Nisbett and Wilson (1977) reviewed in Chapter 8.

Bar–Anan et al. (2010) have also provided empirical support for their model. In a study reminiscent of Nisbett and Wilson (1977), they conducted five experiments. In all of them, they primed a goal that influenced behavior but offered an alternative, incorrect, plausible, and accessible explanation. Subjects chose the incorrect explanation each time. In the first two experiments, men were primed with the goal of interacting with a female tutor and chose to be taught by a woman over a man. However, they stated that their choice was based on their intrinsic interest in the topic being taught. In Experiment 3, subjects were primed with the goal of helping others and then asked to choose a game. They chose the helping over the nonhelping game. But they stated that the game they picked was the more interesting one. In Experiment 4, subjects were primed to earn money and chose a game that allowed for such earning over one that did not. They stated that it was the challenge level of the game that drove their choice, despite the fact that they were not told of the differential difficulty of the games until after they chose. Experiment 5 replicated the results of Experiment 4 but added a condition in which the subjects were reminded that they did not know of the difficulty level until after they had chosen. This eliminated the effects. Bar–Anan et al. explained these results as having two stages. In the first, the person was primed unconsciously. This automatically activated a goal. Because the subjects were unaware of this activation, they did not know why they behaved as they did. As a result, they attributed their behavior to whatever was accessible (not the real reason), plausible (depending upon what they were told), and self-serving (what made them look good in their own eyes). The authors argue that this occurs quite frequently in real life. Further, once people have come to an incorrect conclusion about why they behaved as they did, it is self-perpetuating. After all, they do not wish to see themselves as irrational, mistake-prone, and out of conscious control. The clinical implications of this are obvious.

CLINICAL IMPLICATIONS OF ATTRIBUTION THEORY

In general, it follows from attribution theory that patients will tend to see their own behavior as dependent on situational constraints, whereas therapists may be more likely to attribute their patients' behaviors to their enduring personality characteristics. This will be especially so when dealing with negative outcomes, which are often the focus in psychotherapy. The data support this conclusion. Therapists appear prone to understanding their patients dispositionally, whereas patients are generally likely to understand their behaviors as situational (Hunsley, Aubry, Verstervelt, & Vito, 1999; Kendall, Kipnis, & Otto–Salaj, 1992; Murdock, Edwards, & Murdock, 2010). This is not necessarily an expression of resistance on the part of the patient or a lack of empathy on the part of the therapist. Instead, it is the work of normative implicit attributions. Only by focusing our attention on them and consciously making an effort to bring them to awareness can we counteract their influence. Oftentimes, patients relate events to which they responded angrily, passively, or in a rather disorganized fashion. As the literature suggests, a clinician's interpretation may not necessarily include an appreciation of the particular circumstances that the patient encountered. Rather, a dispositional attribution bias may lead the therapist to infer that her patient is generally angry, or passive, or emotionally disorganized. Conversely, patients may persistently attribute their behaviors to situational factors, thus failing to notice their own behavioral patterns and their consequences. This may be seen when patients show a strong bias toward blaming others, including the therapist, without taking personal responsibility or even entertaining the idea that they may behave in a similar fashion across diverse situations. To top it off, much of this takes place outside of awareness.

The literature on success and failure attributions also has important clinical implications. It is not necessarily resistance or narcissism when a patient attributes successes to herself and failures to outside forces. And then, what do we make of findings that seem to go against some of the tenets of attribution theory, such as patients who readily make negative stable self-attributions rather than positive ones? Research studies on normative processes are often focused on the general population and not on individuals with emotional difficulties or disorders. Such patients often suffer from depression, anxiety, or the aftermath of trauma and have been found to possess certain preferential biases toward negative information in the environment (see the section on Affective Salience below). It is possible, then, that early implicit learning has taken place (as discussed earlier; see Chapter 12) or that early pre- or postconscious automatic processes have resulted in these biases (see above discussion on automatic biased processing; see also Chapter 14). In this case, the patient's negative attributions are accessible (they have learned them and/or heard them repeated for much of their lives, originally by others but eventually by themselves so that they have become automatized), plausible (it makes sense to them given their history and learning), and/ or self-promoting (furthering their image of themselves). So far from contradicting the *self-serving bias*, both are examples of accessible, plausible, and/or self-promoting attributions as discussed by Bar–Anan et al. (2010). It is imperative, then, to examine the roots of these negative self-beliefs and attributions in treatment. It is also important to understand how they acquired certain qualities of automaticity, which qualities they have acquired, and under what conditions these qualities are manifested, in order to successfully treat the disorders. Additionally, Gilbert and Malone (1995) reported that people find it difficult to modify previously made inferences, even after they have been proven wrong (whether by insight or by focus on and challenging of automatic thoughts). Thus, resistance to change and to accepting issues within oneself is normal, not pathological. It still must be dealt with, of course, but this knowledge provides a different view as to how.

Therapists are not immune to attribution biases either. Hunsley et al. (1999) reported that therapists are more likely to view early termination as the result of patient improvement or environmental factors rather than as attributable to client dissatisfaction. They (therapists) did not fail, circumstances were such that the patient terminated. Or they were so effective that the patient improved earlier than anticipated. Practically speaking, it behooves the therapist to be aware of these potential biases and to take them into account in her work with her patients. This may be something that the therapist can share with her patient to help him become aware of his own biases as well as the potential biases of the therapist. In addition, it could help the patient to understand why others may react to him as they do (i.e., they make dispositional attributions concerning the patient's behaviors especially when they turn out badly). Finally, the therapist may want to alert the patient to his human tendency to stick with old ways of thinking even when they patently do not work (and be aware of this in herself). These are areas crying out for research. As far as we know, no systematic empirical work in these areas, as they relate to psychotherapy, has been conducted.

CHAPTER 16

Affective Primacy

We first addressed the concept of <u>affective primacy</u> in Chapter 7's discussion of mere and subliminal exposure effects. As we stated there, affective primacy was proposed and systematically investigated by Zajonc (1980, 1984, 2000; Murphy & Zajonc, 1993), who posited that affectively charged information is processed more readily and more quickly than is cognitive information. He also argued that affective processing requires less stimulation and fewer resources than does cognitive processing. Finally, he averred that there were separate cognitive and affective systems in the brain/mind. LeDoux (1990, 1995) presented evidence for the existence of the latter in the form of two pathways of processing information in the brain—an emotional-processing channel through the amygdala and a cognitive-processing channel through the hippocampus. LeDoux (1996) argued that the faster, emotion-processing pathway goes directly from the thalamus (an information-relay structure in the brain) to the amygdala, circumventing the neocortex. As a result, we are able to quickly categorize a stimulus, for example, as likable or unlikable, without consciously recognizing it. LeDoux termed the pathway through the neocortex the "high road" and the path directly to the amygdala the "low road." Here we focus on affective primacy on its own terms rather than as part of the literature on priming. Additionally, we bring it more up to date.

As one might expect, with further research, the picture has become more complex and nuanced than the one we presented earlier. First, as did the early work on automatic and controlled processing, the early work on affective primacy seems to have confounded several distinct areas that ought to be considered separately (cf. Bargh, 1992; Bargh et al., 2012). One is the issue of whether affective information is processed more rapidly than are other kinds of experiences. Next is whether there are separate cognitive and affective systems in the brain/mind. Third is whether affect has pride of place in our processing such that experiences automatically elicit an affective reaction to a greater degree than they elicit cognitive reactions. That is, given both possible ways of processing stimulation, is affective processing favored? Finally, regardless of whether affective processing is faster, separately housed, or initially preferred over cognitive processing, are affective aspects of our experiences more salient to us than are other kinds of experiences? Do we notice them more than we notice nonaffective aspects of our experiences? Zajonc (1980, 2000) and LeDoux (1996) argued that all of these things are true and are part and parcel of affective processing. Subsequent work seems to indicate that these are separate issues, with separate data bases. Moreover, different researchers have come to different conclusions concerning them.

SPEED OF AFFECTIVE PROCESSING

We begin with the issue of speed. Is affective processing more rapid than is cognitive processing? The work of LeDoux (1996, 2012) seems to provide the strongest evidence in favor of this hypothesis. The aforementioned low road from the thalamus to the amygdala versus the high road from the thalamus to the neocortex explains this difference. The former is unconscious, subcortical, and crosses fewer synapses than the latter, which is cortical, more conscious, and neuronally longer. Also see Zajonc (2000) and Murphy and Zajonc (1993). (The low vs. high road paths also relate to the idea of separate cognitive and affective systems discussed below.) Tamietto and DeGelder (2010) reviewed neurophysiological data that support faster emotional than cognitive processing. So did Rolls (2018), whose model is very similar to that of LeDoux. But LeDoux's model is based on nonhuman organisms, mostly mice. Although LeDoux (2012) argues that the model can be applied to humans as well, he himself admits this evidence base to be a shortcoming. And, in 2015, LeDoux backtracked a bit by saying that this may be a problem with his model. So this view is not without issues.

On the other side of the ledger is what has been called the "cognitive primacy hypothesis," which argues that people have to know what something is before they can respond affectively to it (Lazarus, 1984; Storbeck & Robinson, 2004; Storbeck, Robinson, & McCourt, 2006). Therefore, cognitive processing must be quicker than affective processing. Nummenmaa, Hyona, and Calvo (2010) conducted six experiments comparing the speed of affective and semantic judgments in response to visual scenes. In all six, the semantic judgments were quicker. Calvo, Avero, and Nummenmaa (2011) compared affective and cognitive judgments of stimuli in the periphery of vision, thereby making the decisions less conscious. They too obtained cognitive primacy. These authors interpreted their findings as definitively debunking affective primacy and strongly supporting cognitive primacy.

The data of Nummenmaa and colleagues would seem to have dealt a powerful blow to affective primacy in its "affect is faster" form. But all is not as clearcut as their findings might have us believe. Lai, Hagoort, and Casasanto (2012) argued that neither cognitive nor emotional processing is faster. Instead, the speed of processing of either depends upon the context in which it is embedded. They conducted two experiments to test this hypothesis. The first was essentially an extension of Nummenmaa et al. (2010). In addition to assessing speed of cognitive and affective responding, they created an affective context (asking respondents to categorize words as positive or negative) or a cognitive context (asking respondents to categorize words as human or animal) before categorizing complex scenes. They found that affective judgments were faster than cognitive judgments in both conditions, although the difference was greater in the affective context condition. Thus, they partially supported their hypothesis in that context affected speed of processing. But they also failed to replicate the Nummenmaa et al. cognitive primacy findings. In fact, they obtained the opposite results (i.e., affective primacy for complex scenes). In their second experiment, they looked at judgments of words in the context of affectively or cognitively judged complex scenes. Now, they obtained the context effects they predicted. That is, an affective context (Are the scenes positive or negative?) led to faster affective responding to words, whereas a cognitive context (Are the scenes indoor or outdoor?) led to faster semantic (cognitive) processing of the words. This result fully supported the authors' context-dependent hypothesis. Overall, the studies indicated that affective processing is quicker in an affective context no matter what, whereas cognitive processing for words but not for complex scenes was quicker in a cognitive context. Thus, the data are unclear about whether cognitive or affective processing is faster. We must tentatively conclude that it depends, but we do not yet know what the relevant moderators and/or mediators are. Speed is therefore not a way to differentiate cognition from affect at this time.

PRIMACY OF AFFECTIVE PROCESSING

What about the nature of affective evaluation? How fundamental and automatic is it? Cacioppo and Bernston (1994) as well as Eagly and

Chaiken (1993) define evaluation as a differentiation of experiences into good and bad. Bargh (1994) argued that there is an initial evaluation of all experiences as good or bad, approach or avoid, and that this evaluation takes place outside of awareness. Doré, Zerubavel, and Ochnser (2015) came to a similar conclusion two decades later and identified the brain structures that their review suggested underlies this automatic evaluation. (We identify these brain structures and discuss their neuronal model below.) There are evolutionary and neurophysiological reasons that support this point of view. In terms of evolution, it makes sense for an organism to react with approach or avoidance before it has any certainty about what is out there. If our ancestors waited too long, they could end up hurt or worse if what was out there was dangerous. Alternatively, they could have lost an opportunity if what was out there was potentially edible (see Norman et al., 2011). Bernston, Boysen, and Cacioppo (1993) as well as Norman et al. showed that evaluation is linked to approach and avoidance at a neurophysiological level. In fact, it is a fundamental property of both high- and low-level neural circuits. Thus, evaluation, conceptualized as a precursor to approach or avoidance, is a fundamental aspect of our functioning. And since it is literally built into our nervous system, it also operates outside of awareness (i.e., unconsciously).

There are also data concerning the relative strength of affective versus nonaffective processing. De Gelder et al. (1999), Tamietto et al., (2009), and Tamietto and de Gelder (2010) have all reported that an emotional facial expression can be correctly identified and appropriately reacted to by patients with blindsight, who nonetheless deny having seen the face, let alone its expression. Recall also that Murphy and Zajonc (1993) reported that a subliminally presented affective facial expression is more easily processed than is a subliminally presented gender of face in non-brain-damaged individuals.

Perhaps the strongest evidence in favor of this aspect of affective primacy is the work of Fazio and his colleagues on evaluative priming. Fazio, Sanbonmatsu, Powell, and Kardes (1986) used an evaluatively evocative prime (e.g., spider or saint) prior to an evaluatively congruent or incongruent target (e.g., repulsive or appealing). Participants responded more quickly when the evaluations were in sync than when they were not. There have been dozens of studies investigating these effects and most have found them to be present. Herring et al. (2013) list many of these. The reader interested in pursuing this area in detail is also referred to De Houwer, Teige–Mocigemba, Spruyt, and Moors (2009), Spruyt, Gast, and Moors (2011), and Wentura and Degner (2010) for reviews. Herring et al. (2013) also conducted a meta-analysis on this literature, focused on studies that asked participants to evaluate a target stimulus as good or bad. (These studies generally employ what is called the evaluative decision task; EDT.) Herring et al. identified 125 outcomes and found strong confirmation of the effect. The affective valence of the prime influenced the speed with which people responded to a subsequent valenced target. Matched valences are quicker. Further, making a good/bad judgment resulted in stronger effects than other kinds of judgments. Critically, these effects were only statistically significant when respondents were told to just respond. When additional instructions, rewards for correct responding, or feedback concerning responses were given, the effects vanished. This is a finding we have seen many times now in relation to unconscious processes. Efforts to focus attention or to bring a task into consciousness weakens and often destroys said effect.

On the other hand, some studies have shown that semantic priming dominates over affective priming (Calvo & Nummenmaa, 2008; Nummenmaa et al., 2010; Storbeck et al., 2006). So the data are not unequivocal concerning the superiority of affective over cognitive processing. We reviewed some of this above. Relevant to the Fazio evaluative priming task, many studies have also demonstrated semantic priming. We have reviewed these earlier in this book (see Chapters 5–7). Also see McNamara (2005) for a review. Thus, we have evidence of primacy for both kinds of priming. As far as we know, there are no studies pitting one kind of priming against the other. If the literature on speed of processing is any guide, the results can be expected to be equivocal with semantic priming dominating in some situations and affective priming dominating in others. So, although we can state with certainty that affective priming occurs, occurs rapidly, and seems ubiquitous, we cannot say that it is superior to or has prime of place in comparison to cognitive processing.

So what can we conclude? Bargh's (1994) decades-old review stating that there is an initial automatic good/bad evaluation of all experiences appears to be correct. This aspect of affective primacy can be said to have solid empirical support. We do evaluate stimuli in a basic and automatic way, categorizing them as good or bad in the service of approaching or avoiding. What we cannot say is that affective processing always supersedes or overrides cognitive processing. Nor can we say that affective processing is always the default or earliest sort of processing when we encounter a new experience. It is our guess that both cognitive and affective processing occur with one or the other dominating depending upon circumstance or both occurring simultaneously. Again, this parallels the findings on automaticity in which several properties were thought to always covary but turned out to sometimes be independent of one another (see Bargh, 1992).

SEPARATE AFFECTIVE AND COGNITIVE SYSTEMS

That brings us to the issue of whether or not there are two separate systems, one cognitive and the other affective. Recall that LeDoux (1996) said that there were two such systems, which he referred to as the high road and the low road. Support for this view has since been supplied by Vuilleumier (2005) and by Tamietto and de Gelder (2010). According to this model, the cortical high road provides detailed sensory information and results in conscious perception. It relies on cortical processing. In the visual system, this processing starts in the primary visual cortex (V1), projects through V2 and V4 on its way to the inferotemporal cortex, and then proceeds to the amygdala. The subcortical low road, on the other hand, analyzes information in a rudimentary way, assessing the emotional significance of an experience before that experience is consciously recognized. Its functioning is unconscious. In the visual system, low spatial frequency information is sent to the amygdala by a subcortical pathway through the superior colliculus and the pulvinar (see Milner, Goodale, & Vingrys, 2006).

This view has been challenged, however. As we stated earlier, the model is based on lower animals. Pessoa and Adolphs (2010) found no low road in primates. That is, they could not identify a functionally independent subcortical route to the amygdala in subhuman primates. They reported that the visual input from the superior colliculus ended in the inferior nucleus of the pulvinar but that connections to the amygdala come from the medial nucleus of the pulvinar. And these two regions of the pulvinar do not seem to be connected neuronally. According to these authors, this means that the pulvinar does not process visual information subcortically; it is part of cortical visual circuits.

LeDoux (2012) argued against this interpretation of the data and in favor of separate roads to affective processing. He cited data from animals other than mice, including primates (Kalin, Shelton, Davidson, & Kelley, 2001; Kalin, Shelton, & Davidson, 2004; Antoniadis, Winslow, Davis, & Amaral, 2007) to bolster his case. (But LeDoux, 2015, was a bit less certain later on.) Rolls (2018) also posits two systems and explicitly ties his model to that of LeDoux. In his view, the high road involves language circuits. This allows for conscious decisions and planning. He posits three branches to the low road. There is a goal-oriented branch that involves the anterior cingulate cortex, there is a branch involved in habitual reactions that involves the striatum and the basal ganglia, and there is a branch focused on autonomic reactions that is dependent upon the orbitofrontal and anterior cortices and the amygdala. All of these operate unconsciously.

Similarly to Rolls (2018), Doré et al. (2015) tried to identify the main brain sites for evaluative processes. Their review implicated the amygdala and ventral parts of the striatum as receiving sense and autonomic information. They also concluded that the ventromedial prefrontal cortex, orbitofrontal cortex, the insula, the dorsal anterior cingulate cortex, and the periaqueductal gray are also important to evaluation. The amygdala was seen as critical for recognition of threat, just as LeDoux (1996) argued. But in contrast to LeDoux (1996), Doré et al. (2015) also saw the amygdala as responsive to other dimensions of experience, including positive aspects of affective experience. So the amygdala is not simply involved in negative or threat evaluation, it is rather a system that monitors affective stimuli generally. However, it is especially sensitive to negative stimuli. The insula is more balanced and responds to both positive and negative experiences equally. In combination with the dorsal cingulated cortex and the periaqueductal gray, the insula is also part of a brain pain system, with the periaqueductal gray also focused on negative affect.

For now, as with speed, the literature on whether or not there are distinct pathways for conscious and unconscious affective responding is not definitive. There seem to be valid arguments both ways and no way to choose between them.

There is a third alternative, however. Instead of separate cognitive and affective pathways, perhaps the difference is in the interconnections of overlapping neuronal networks. Thus, there are no separate cognitive and affective brain systems; instead, there are complex interconnections that sometimes result in cognitive and sometimes result in affective processing. Additionally, also depending upon the nature of these interconnections, sometimes the output is conscious and sometimes it is unconscious. The trick would be to identify the nature of these interconnections and the interactions between brain circuits that reliably produce these results. Dehaene and his colleagues (Dehaene, 2008, 2014; Dehaene, Charles, King, & Marti, 2014) suggest something of this sort to differentiate conscious from unconscious processes. van Gaal and Lamme (2012) also propose a model of this sort. We will come across the work of Dehaene again when we cover computational neuroscience models of the brain/mind. There we will review his neural reuse model of the mind, termed "neuronal recycling," wherein he posits a co-opting of neuronal circuits originally created for one purpose to perform new, novel functions (Dehaene & Cohen, 2007). For now, we will have to say that the status of separate cognitive and affective circuits versus no such differentiation versus some sort of neural reuse model is moot at this time.

THE SALIENCE OF AFFECTIVE EXPERIENCE
AND ITS CLINICAL IMPLICATIONS

Finally, we come to the question of whether affective experiences are generally more salient to us than are other kinds of experiences. Belief in such salience does not need to have a position on speed, ontology of separate systems, or primacy of processing. The question is whether such experiences are more easily noticed than are their nonemotional counterparts.

Binocular rivalry studies present a different stimulus to each eye to determine which stimulus dominates our perception. The stimuli are systematically varied. Several such studies have shown that emotional content predominates over nonemotional content. That is, when an emotional stimulus is presented to one eye and an alternative nonemotional stimulus is presented to the other, the respondent tends to be aware of the emotional over the nonemotional. More specifically, aversively conditioned stimuli predominate over neutral stimulation (Alpers, Ruhleder, Waltz, Mulberger, & Pauli, 2005); emotional scenes predominate over nonemotional scenes (Alpers & Pauli, 2006); emotional facial expressions predominate over neutral facial expressions (Alpers & Gerdes, 2007; Bannerman, Milders, De Gelder, & Sahraie, 2008; Yoon, Hong, Joormann, & Kang 2009); and faces that were associated with affective social information predominate over faces not conveying such information (E. Anderson, Siegel, White, & Barrett, 2012). It is possible to argue that these findings simply show that more informative stimulation is more noticed than is less informative information. One would have to compare cognitive with affective information in this paradigm to address such a criticism. As far as we know, such a study has not been conducted. However, Murphy and Zajonc (1993), reviewed earlier in this book, demonstrated that subliminal affective information in the form of facial expression predominated over subliminal gender in the form of male and female faces. Here is a direct test, and it favored the saliency of affect over the perceptually critical variable of gender. It is only a single study, but it seems to offer a powerful argument for affective salience in terms of what is noticed more, even at a nonconscious level.

There are also studies that have focused on investigating the salience of affective information when presented with more complex stimulation. For instance, Sharot and Yonelinas (2008) and Riggs, McQuiggan, Anderson, and Ryan (2010) showed that the more affectively arousing a scene is, the more viewers fixate on the details of its affective subregions. Niu, Todd, and Anderson (2012) reported more fine-grained results. Like Sharot et al. and Riggs et al., they found that when looking at complex scenes, it is the more affectively salient stimuli rather than other information-bearing details that first attract and hold our attention. Niu et al. also found that when people were presented with a series of positive, negative, or neutral photographs, they allocated their attention to details in accordance with the affective charge of the image. That is, individuals tended to fixate their gaze on the most affectively salient details over visually salient ones. Finally, they found that differences in attention were related to the quality of affective valence. Negatively valenced regions in the image elicited more fixations than positively valenced regions. People seem drawn to emotionally charged stimuli, especially if they have negative valence. Or, as many drivers have noticed, we can't tear our eyes away from car crashes. And as clinicians may have noticed, patients often seem to report negative over positive experiences and over positive interpretations of events. Perhaps this is not simply a function of the fact that our patients come in because of negative issues and difficulties they are hoping to address in therapy. Perhaps it is also a function of normative information processing that favors the salience of affect, especially negative affect.

Affective Organizing of Experience

Affective stimuli are not only unconsciously salient in the environment; affect also can be used to categorize experiences. That is, emotion not only captures attention, it serves an organizing function. In 1999, Niedenthal, Halberstadt, and Innes-Ker proposed the theory of "emotional response categorization." They argued that it is normative to group together stimuli that elicit the same emotional response and to treat such stimuli as "the same kind of thing" (p. 338). They further argued that experiences are affectively organized and that stimuli are characterized and categorized based on the perceiver's emotional response to them (as opposed to perceptual or linguistic features of the perceived objects or events). These authors found that emotional arousal can increase the likelihood of emotional categorization of any sort. In other words, regardless of what emotion they elicited in the participants, the results were the same: increased emotional categorization. Kernberg (1987, 2004) says something very much like this. He has argued that people initially organize their experiences into good and bad, which he terms "splitting." Only later do they categorize perceptually (cf. Weinberger & Weiss, 1997).

The Niedenthal group applied their model to clinical issues and found that dysphoric individuals categorize emotions in a biased fashion, based on their mood. These data suggest that the ability of dysphoric individuals to process stimuli is strongly biased by their chronic negative feelings—a bias many clinicians have likely observed in such patients. As we saw in the section on Automaticity (see Chapter 14), individuals who suffer from psychological problems (e.g., depression and anxiety) not only process affectively laden information differently, but also show bias in what they see as affectively laden. Stimuli that may appear neutral to others may idiosyncratically be given preferential processing because they are seen as affective by these individuals.

To summarize: patients may be more likely to categorize emotionally when emotionally aroused, when they evidence a chronic mood which then influences the particular emotion they use to interpret their experiences, and/or when they suffer from a psychological condition that biases them to misinterpret neutral information as emotionally meaningful. This is a fruitful area for research and has important clinical implications as a general principle for understanding individuals seeking help.

Finally, recent work seems to indicate that affect-based attention can be seen as a component of emotion regulation (for a detailed overview, see Todd, Cunningham, Anderson, & Thomson, 2012). We may not only be unconsciously drawn to affectively arousing experiences and then use affect to categorize these experiences, we may also regulate consequent responses to those experiences by fine-tuning emotional filters. What all of this adds up to is that emotions are primary in much of our functioning. We are quickly and powerfully drawn to emotionally laden stimuli, and we are also influenced by our affective responses to the onslaught of stimuli encountered in our daily lives. These affective reactions can bias our processing and influence our behavior, and they can be even more powerful when we are not aware of them. In a nutshell, *emotions grab our attention, help us organize our experiences, and play a major role in regulating those experiences.*

Conclusions about Affective Primacy

What can we conclude about affective primacy? First, affect and its influence is not a unitary event. Like automaticity, there are many aspects to it. And the data for some are more persuasive and consistent than are the data for others. Our review indicated mixed evidence for separate affective and cognitive systems. We can therefore not come to any definitive conclusions about them at this time. Likewise, the data for affective processing occurring more rapidly than cognitive processing are also mixed. We therefore cannot say that affective processing is quicker (or slower).

Our best guess is that affective processing is quicker in many situations, but cognitive processing is quicker in others. Future research will need to pin down when and where this is true. Here is what we believe we can say with a reasonable amount of confidence. There is a powerful tendency to categorize experiences as good or bad. This seems to take place outside of awareness and involuntarily. It makes sense in terms of adaptation and is probably tied to approach-and-avoidance tendencies. Neurophysiological evidence seems to back this up. We can also say with some confidence that emotional experiences are generally more salient to people. They are more likely to be noticed, to grab attention, and to serve an organizing and regulatory function than are other kinds of experiences. Some clinical theorists seem to have noticed this and made it central to their thinking (e.g., Kernberg, 1987, 2004). However, we have to admit that we do not yet know with any certainty how this happens. The possibility of these effects being due to separate systems and greater speed of processing has not been proven (or disproved).

The finding that affect tends to attract people's attention and is salient in their experiences probably sounds like an obvious truism to many clinicians. But it is important. Many, if not most, of the problems brought in by patients can be traced to emotional experiences (e.g., trauma). There is also specificity of emotional organization for those suffering from chronic mood disturbances (e.g., depression or anxiety disorders). The affective findings reviewed above indicate that we can expect patients to automatically categorize experiences positively or negatively, to be more likely to notice such experiences, to especially note negative experiences, and to organize themselves around such experiences. Finally, most of this occurs outside of awareness (i.e., unconsciously).

It may be beneficial for therapists to remember that their patients are configured so as to be drawn to affective experiences, whether they consciously want to or not, and that they will attend more readily to negatively than to positively toned information (again, whether they consciously want to or not). People's tendency to "fixate" on negatives is, at least partially, determined by a normative implicit process rather than being a result of a learned emotional bias, as many theorists from various schools of therapy seem to argue (e.g., Beck, Rush, Shaw, & Emery, 1979; Rogers, 1959; de Roten, Drapeau, & Michel, 2008). It may be beneficial for patients to know this about human functioning so that it does not seem so pathological to them (or to the treating clinician). The therapeutic task then may not only be to demonstrate the errors and logical inconsistencies of this organization (although this is a useful first step) but to help provide new emotionally tinged experiences that can counteract the normatively developed way of reacting to the world our patients come in with.

CHAPTER 17

From Metaphor to Embodied Cognition

"Knowledge is only a rumor until it lives in the muscle" (a proverb of the Asaro tribe of Papua New Guinea, as cited in Brown, 2015, p.7). The physical world, our interactions with it, and the nature of neuronal networks has a much more significant impact on our thought process than previously believed, in that we are constantly using our bodies and the information stored in them to make sense of our experiences, to understand abstract concepts, and to guide our behaviors. This phenomenon is clearly instantiated in metaphors. The first ones to study this in a systematic way, from the 1970s on, were Lakoff and his colleagues (Lakoff, 2012, 2014; Lakoff & Johnson, 1980a, 1980b, 1999). They noted the role of metaphors in shaping our reality and argued that metaphors are much more than linguistic structures or poetic vehicles (Lakoff & Johnson, 1980a). Rather, the human conceptual system is itself structured metaphorically (Lakoff & Johnson, 1980b)—that is, many concepts are represented and understood through other concepts or systems of concepts. This is pervasive in our everyday lives.

WHY METAPHORS WORK

Metaphors not only help us understand complex and abstract concepts, they are central to our own personal narratives. They determine whether we see ourselves as a victim or a survivor of a tragedy, for example. Metaphors are touching! (Yes, this is a metaphor.) And it is precisely because of their groundedness (another metaphor) in bodily experiences (their embodiment) that they are capable of conveying or evoking a stronger and more meaningful experiential reaction than descriptions or adjectives alone (Levitt, Korman, & Angus, 2000).

Metaphors and abstract thought are understood through the ways in which they are embodied. Think of the many metaphors we all use in thinking about ourselves and our lives: we travel through the journey of life, categorize people as warm or cold, feel distant or close to them, feel weighted down by stress, put too much on our plates, and feel our heads spinning. All of these examples illustrate the ways in which we construct our life's narratives through bodily experiences (i.e., through metaphors). The body, in this sense, is inextricably linked to cognitive processes, guiding and shaping our thought formation. This realization led to the study of embodied cognition, now such a major part of social psychology, cognitive science, and neuroscience.

EMBODIED COGNITION

Embodied cognition is the theoretical proposition, now backed by a broad foundation of empirical research, that cognitive states are embedded in the body, that is, embodied. In other words, higher-level mental processes are grounded to some degree (have parallels) in the body's sensory and motor systems. Although this notion of embodiment can be traced back to William James's (1890/1950) views on emotions (we are afraid because we run; we do not run because we are afraid), the last two decades have seen a proliferation of research in the area. In this chapter, we review some of the more important findings; we then discuss their clinical implications.

A vast body of research has shown that the mind does not work independently of the body, but rather is grounded in the body's physical interaction with the environment. There are several theories of brain and mind functioning that lead to this conclusion, and there is much debate over which explains the data best. We review what we consider the best such model, namely, neural reuse (M. L. Anderson, 2010, 2014) in the next part of this book. For now, what is important is the argument that bodily states can not only be seen as metaphors for mental states, but are often concretely tied to those mental states. Our cognitions, as we will see, are often, if not invariably, tied to our orientation in time and space, as well as to our sensory experiences. That is, when we say that someone is "cold" or "warm" or we feel "distant" or "close" to someone, these expressions actually reflect the physical dimensions they refer to. In other words, there is a strong correlation between the physical and psychological states these words signify. Importantly, these embodied cognitions can, and often do, take place unconsciously, without necessarily involving a "full-blown physical episode" (Winkielman, Niedenthal, Wielgosz, Eelen, & Kavanagh, 2015, p. 152). To illustrate this notion, we examine recent findings in several areas of embodiment research. These data show links between psychological phenomena (e.g., perceptions and attitudes toward self and others, affective processing, and psychological relatedness) and physical properties of objects or of the environment (e.g., temperature, spatial positioning/properties, and taste).

Temperature

Focusing on what Asch (1946) called the most powerful personality trait—warmth—Williams and Bargh (2008a) demonstrated that the experience of physical warmth promoted increased feelings of interpersonal warmth. They asked participants to hold a hot or cold beverage. In their first experiment, participants had to judge the personality of a target person along 10 bipolar dimensions, half of which were related to the personality trait of warmth/coldness. As hypothesized, the participant group who held a cup of hot coffee, in comparison to the cold beverage group, rated the target person as higher in characteristics related to the warm end of the warm/cold dichotomy, but not on any nonwarmth-related characteristics. In Experiment 2, they found that holding something warm promoted prosocial behavior. The participants in Experiment 2, which was framed as a product evaluation (of a therapeutic pad), were asked to choose compensation for participating in the study. They could either be compensated with a reward for themselves or with a gift certificate for a friend. An overwhelming 75% of the participants primed with a cold therapeutic pad chose a gift for themselves. The effect was reversed for a warm pad, where 54% chose the prosocial gift. The participants in both experiments were not aware of the impact that the physical experiences of warmth or coldness had on their social evaluations and behavior. In fact, they were completely unaware that the experimental manipulations had anything to do with the subsequent evaluations or decisions they had to make, suggesting that a simple experience of temperature may have a significant yet unconscious impact on how conscious social appraisals are constructed and, indeed, on how we interact with others.[1]

Similar findings have been reported by other researchers who examined the experience of warmth/coldness and its relation to feeling socially connected. Zhong and Leonardelli (2008) asked participants in two groups to recall an experience where they felt socially included or socially excluded, respectively. They found that the group who recalled an inclusion experience estimated the room temperature to be higher than the group who recalled an exclusion experience. In a second experiment, the authors induced feelings of social inclusion or exclusion through a virtual interaction. The dependent variable was the likelihood of seeking warm food or drink (hot coffee or soup) versus cold food or drink (apple/ crackers or a cold Coke). Consistent with Williams and Bargh's (2008a) findings, these authors found that the experience of social exclusion led people to seek out warmth, in the form of hot coffee or soup, more than did the social inclusion group. These authors titled their paper, "Cold and Lonely: Does Social Exclusion Literally Feel Cold?," highlighting the embodied nature of the experience. The participants literally equated social rejection with coldness. Kang, Williams, Clark, Gray, and Bargh (2011) had their subjects handle either a warm or a cold pack. They then had the participants play a game involving willingness to invest money. Those primed with warmth invested more than those primed with cold. They interpreted this difference as due to warmth being connected to trust and coldness to mistrust. Story and Workman (2013) conceptually replicated Kang et al. (2011). They found that priming with warm versus cold objects predicted cooperation in a Prisoner's Dilemma game. (But see Dermot et al., 2014, for a failure to replicate Williams and Bargh.)

These findings have also been replicated cross-culturally, suggesting that temperature embodiment is universal. Ijzerman and Semin (2009) conducted three studies at the University of Utrecht in the Netherlands. Their experiments found that holding a hot beverage or increasing the temperature in the room induced participants to feel socially closer to others (greater social proximity). These researchers then expanded their investigation to language use. They found that placing participants in a warmer room elicited more concrete language and a more relational conceptual focus, signifying that when people feel warmer, they tend to focus more on details and patterns of interdependence. Thus, feeling "warm" led to more intimate (warmer) interactions. All of these temperature studies have implications for psychotherapy. They suggest that when patients feel "warm," and when they perceive the therapist as "warm," they are more likely to discuss intimate issues to cooperate with and to feel more trusting of their therapist.

Time and Space

The properties of the space we occupy and how we position ourselves in that space have been found to impact our appraisals of self, others, and the world in a variety of ways. Meier and Robinson (2006) demonstrated that people who scored relatively high on neuroticism and depressive symptomatology tended to favor lower regions of physical space, that is, to spot targets more quickly when they were in the lower visual field.

Distance is another property of space that has been related to our perception of social relationships. Williams and Bargh (2008b) demonstrated that simply asking participants to place dots closer or farther apart (thus priming the concept of physical closeness/distance) led them to evaluate their emotional bond with family as stronger or weaker, respectively. Other researchers have demonstrated links between the concepts of physical expansion and greater self-actualization or self-growth (Landau et al., 2010).

Boroditsky and Ramscar (2002) demonstrated that the abstract concept of time may be at least partially grounded in the more concrete, more easily grasped concept of space. These researchers showed that priming participants with the concept of forward or backward motion (by showing a figure either riding a chair forward or pulling a chair on a rope) significantly impacted how they thought of events temporally. After the prime, participants were told that "Next Wednesday's meeting has been moved forward two days" (p. 186). The group exposed to a forward motion tended to estimate that the meeting was moved to the upcoming Friday, whereas the group exposed to backward motion tended to think of the meeting as moved to the earlier Monday. These results were behaviorally replicated in a second study, in which the authors interviewed participants actually standing in line (for food), asking them the same question about a meeting being moved to Friday or Monday. They found that people who were further along in the line were more likely to assume a forward motion and perceive the meeting as having been moved to Friday. This result was also replicated at an airport, where people who had just flown in were significantly more likely to pick Friday over Monday. Thus, these authors demonstrated that people actively moving through space (moving forward in line for food or just having flown in from another airport) also tended to perceive themselves as moving through time versus thinking of time as coming toward them. Thus, in order to understand a complex abstract concept like time, we defer to a concept—space—that we can physically relate to due to its groundedness in physical experience. This is perhaps why we have such a difficult time understanding and, at the same time, such a great fascination with science fiction movies where time is presented as a nonlinear concept.

Additional research has shown that the perception of how far or close we are (positioned on a physical drawing of a timeline) to past successes may have a significant impact on how favorably we assess our current self. In a series of studies, Wilson and Ross (2001) demonstrated that people tend to evaluate distant past selves less favorably than they do their current self. They also tend to evaluate their trajectory of improvement as faster (steeper) than that of others. In addition, these authors had participants fill out questionnaires about their perceived personality characteristics. They were then asked to think back to the beginning of the school term (approximately 2 months earlier) and rate how they perceive themselves to have been then. The researchers manipulated the wording of the question to convey that the beginning of the term was either in "the recent past" or "all the way back," thus verbally influencing participants to think of the beginning of the semester as a recent or more temporally distant event. As hypothesized, participants tended to describe themselves less favorably, especially on traits that were deemed important, when the same point in time was qualified as "way back" than as "recent." This finding is important because it indicates that people tend to change how they retrospectively evaluate themselves based on how far temporally they perceive themselves to be from a particular point in time, a finding that may be clinically significant. The further back a memory, the more negatively the person may judge herself as having been. Conversely, the more recent an event, the more favorably the person will seem to herself. This is not because of actual change over time but because time is embodied that way naturally.

Taste

Exploring the relation of taste perception to emotional processing and interpersonal appraisals has also provided fertile ground for studying the embodiment of thought. A number of recent studies have connected various taste sensations with people's appraisals of self and others. Meier, Moeller, Riemer–Peltz, and Robinson (2012) reported that sweetness was associated with more positive self- and other ratings. Respondents perceived strangers who liked sweet foods as more agreeable. They also found a relationship between personality and preference for sweet foods. Participants who indicated higher preference for sweet foods not only scored higher on a measure of agreeableness, even after controlling for other taste preferences (bitter, salty, spicy, sour), but also were shown to report higher prosocial intentions and to engage in more prosocial behaviors. Meier et al. (2012) also asked participants to savor a candy or a piece of chocolate (vs. control conditions of no taste savoring or savoring a nonsweet taste). They found that tasting a sweet treat (but not a nonsweet treat or no treat at all) increased both their self-reported agreeableness and helpful behaviors (spontaneously agreeing to participate in another study without compensation).

   The connection between sweet taste and positive feelings toward others has been expanded to include feelings of love and romantic attraction. Chan, Tong, Tan, and Koh (2013) induced feelings of love in their participants by having them write about such experiences, and then asked them to rate a variety of foods (i.e., bittersweet chocolate or sweet-sour candy). As predicted, the induction of feelings of love increased ratings of sweetness (interestingly, no such effects were obtained in other hypothesized taste-feeling pairs, like jealousy-sour/bitter or happiness-sweetness). Similarly, Ren, Tan, Arriaga, and Chan (2014) found that participants exposed to a sweet taste evaluated a hypothesized romantic relationship more favorably than participants not exposed to that taste prime. Moreover, these authors also demonstrated that, compared to controls, participants who drank a sweet drink (Sprite or 7-Up) reported a significantly higher interest in initiating a romantic relationship. This may also relate to the terms people use to address those they are in an intimate relationship with (are sweet on): honey, sugar, sweetheart, sweetie, and the like.

Bitterness, on the other hand, has been associated with hostility (Sagioglu & Greitemeyer, 2014). These authors examined participants who had been asked to consume a bitter beverage and compared them with a control group who consumed a nonbitter drink. The experimental group showed higher self-reports of hostility, aggressive affect, and aggressive behavior than the control group. Importantly, the authors of these studies point out that they varied the intensity of the bitterness and measured participants' aversion to it, but neither of these variables impacted the results.

Interestingly, studies have also discovered some unique mechanisms mediating the influence of embodiment on the formation of cognitions, highlighting the role of the ambiguity of the evaluative situation (Ren et al., 2014) as well as the role of culture (Gilead, Gal, Polak, & Cholow, 2015). After consuming a sweet prime in the study conducted by Ren et al. (2014), participants tended to rate a hypothetical relationship more positively when they were asked to imagine it or when a target person was described to them. Interestingly, these results were not obtained when participants rated existing relationships. In our view, this may be because the respondents knew what their actual relationships were like and this knowledge overrode the effects of the sweet prime. The authors of these studies came to a different conclusion. They speculated that their results were due to the ambiguity of the evaluated targets (relationships). They propose that embodied cognition comes more strongly into play when we are in ambiguous situations and thus relying more heavily on embodied information to interpret vague stimuli. This proposition may have implications for how we understand the role of embodied cognition and metaphoric thinking in clinical situations.

Gilead et al. (2015) not only confirmed that the embodiment of cognition is a normative process that takes place across cultures, but also uncovered some specifics about how culture impacts it. Their study took into account the fact that sweetness in Israeli culture is not associated with the positive characteristics discussed above but rather is used as a metaphor of inauthenticity. Similarly, spiciness is a verbal expression of someone's intellectual capacity (again unlike in Western culture where it may be more closely associated with intensity, interest, or passion—"spice things up"). The researchers had participants perform a computer task in which they read a story about a woman who was described in a way that portrayed her as both intelligent/competent and possessing some characteristics of inauthenticity. Participants were split up into two groups; one was instructed to eat spicy snacks during the task, and the other was given sweet snacks. The study found that participants in the sweet condition rated the hypothetical woman as more inauthentic, whereas those in the spicy condition rated her as more intelligent and overall gave more favorable evaluations of her. These results were obtained despite the fact that participants reported enjoying the sweet snack more than the spicy one. Gilead et al. (2015) concluded that embodiment can be significantly influenced by verbally transmitted cultural meanings and is not only dependent on preverbal mechanisms. This also suggests that embodiment is not simply connected to physical, evolutionary-based networks. Culture and learning matter too.

There are dozens and dozens more studies that relate to embodied cognition. We cannot review all or even most here. We have chosen a selection that we believe demonstrates the phenomenon and that can be related to psychotherapy. We review several more when we discuss neural reuse in the next section of this book. The reader who wants additionally examples can peruse Lakoff (2014) who cites and summarizes many more such studies.

CLINICAL IMPLICATIONS OF
EMBODIED COGNITION—BACK TO METAPHORS

The findings just reviewed are critically important to the practice of psychotherapy. Metaphor was important from the beginning in psychoanalysis (e.g., in dreams—Freud, 1900). A later review of the varying uses of metaphors in several psychoanalytically oriented therapeutic modalities (Welch, 1984) reveals that metaphors are seen as useful because they have the capacity to introduce and resolve paradox, thereby providing a new frame of thinking: evoking feelings, images, and concepts that were previously hidden from awareness and blending old elements into a new whole. Even transference in psychotherapy can be seen as a metaphor— understanding one concept through another, examining one relationship through another (to transfer, as if to move from one place to another).

Metaphors promote new learning. Welch (1984) discussed all of these benefits of using metaphors in treatment without reference to embodied cognition, which as a framework and an empirical line of study was still in its nascent years. This is changing as psychoanalytic thinkers become more aware of this work (e.g., Vivona, 2009; Bornstein & Becker–Matero, 2010). Cognitive therapy also enjoined the therapist to engage in metaphor in the therapeutic work (Otto, 2000), again, without mention of embodied cognition. This too is changing (e.g., Mathieson, Jordan, Carger, & Stubbe, 2015).

The experiential approach to psychotherapy has also recognized the value of metaphor as an important catalyst of change. Martin, Cummings, and Hallberg (1992) examined what they referred to as the *"mnemonic, epistemic,* and *motivational* functions of metaphor"* (p. 143; italics in the original). They analyzed 29 audiotaped therapy sessions from four therapies, where the therapists had been instructed to make intentional use of therapeutic metaphors. The authors then investigated the memorability of therapist-introduced metaphors, their impact on patient ratings of the session's helpfulness, and the patients' understanding of the metaphors' epistemic and motivational functions (why they were remembered). The results demonstrated that, overall, patients remembered therapist-introduced metaphors about two-thirds of the time (66%) and that sessions for which metaphors were remembered were rated significantly higher in helpfulness than sessions for which the patients did not remember the use of metaphors. When they analyzed patients' answers to the question of why they believe they recalled the metaphors, Martin et al. concluded that metaphors "enhanced emotional awareness and understanding" and provided "conceptual 'bridging'" (p. 145). In addition, they appeared to enhance connection with the therapist and help participants clarify their goals.

Although the Martin et al. (1992) study does not directly address the embodied nature of metaphors, it is important in three ways. First, it highlights the finding that metaphors are indeed useful in treatment and can be clinician generated. Second, it confirms some of the hypothesized functions of metaphors and also suggests that they work on at least three levels: emotional, cognitive, and relational. And finally, it extends the generality of the use of metaphors to a third therapeutic modality, experiential (the first two being psychodynamic and cognitive). As the authors suggest, metaphors may be uniquely suited to access and evoke experiential content—a characteristic that points to their embodied nature.

Other authors have conducted more in-depth analyses of the uses of specific metaphors in treatment. Levitt et al. (2000) examined the use and evolution of the "burden" metaphor in two experiential treatments of depression. They not only looked at the relationship between metaphor use/change and therapy outcome, but also at the patients' emotional involvement in therapy (operationalized as "experiencing" in therapy—the degree to which the patient is focused on internal experiences) as well as the degree to which their narrative conveys a focus on external, internal, or self-reflective processes. The results they obtained highlight the embodied/experiential nature of metaphors as well as their role in therapy outcome. In the good-outcome therapy, the burden metaphor was found to evolve into a metaphor of unloading, of shedding a burden; in contrast, in poor-outcome therapy, no such shift was observed. More curious, however, were the findings about the relationship between the use of metaphors and the patients' "experiencing" or involvement in therapy and the therapeutic focus of reflection. Levitt et al. (2000) found that, in the poor-outcome treatment, metaphors were mostly used when the patient was not in a highly experiential state. In good-outcome therapy, on the other hand (yet another metaphor), patient and therapist use of metaphors happened at the same time and when the patient was in a heightened emotional state and more attuned to his emotions. In this therapy, the patient was in an experiential state more frequently than the poor-outcome patient, both in the treatment overall and in interactional sequences involving the "burden" metaphor. In other words, the patient was fully emotionally engaged in transforming the metaphor of "burden" to a metaphor of "unloading," involving embodiment in the transformation of a pervasive narrative of himself in the world. As Levitt et al. (2000) point out, it may be the case that patients in successful treatments more effectively develop a core metaphorical theme, and that theme becomes related to the major issues they are struggling with. Metaphors, in such treatments, are used to represent internal embodied experiences (depression as a physical burden; relief as lifting the burden and thereby lifting depression) and to connect such experiences with cognition and language to facilitate expression and restructuring. One of our patients (VS), after a year-long treatment for posttraumatic stress and depression, succinctly put it, "Now I finally can switch to neutral." He was finally able to experience the calming of his nervous system, which had been taxed by the vigilance following his traumatic experiences. Switching to neutral represented an ability to feel carefree in the moment, mindful but unburdened.

Overall, embodied cognition can contribute much to a broadening of our understanding of how therapy works in a variety of therapeutic modalities (Faranda, 2014) and may constitute a common factor in psychotherapy (Weinberger, 1995, 2014).

WHAT LIES BEHIND METAPHOR AND EMBODIED COGNITION?

If we accept the idea that our conceptual apparatus is indeed embodied and structured metaphorically, as Lakoff and Johnson (1980b) argued, then we are faced with the questions of when and how did such embodiment take place. Evidence suggests two possible means: the first is environmental and argues that these phenomena develop through experience. In this account, language and thought become formed through physical interactions during the first few years of life. This has been termed scaffolding (Garcia-Marques & Ferreira, 2009; Niedenthal & Alibali, 2009; Williams, Huang, & Bargh, 2009). Take the affection is warmth metaphor, for instance. Young infants are soothed by their parents through touch and holding. Hugs are warm and convey affection, care, and support. No wonder, then, that we characterize affectionate people as warm and prefer interacting with them over interacting with "cold" people. The metaphors of depression as a burden and trauma as loss of control are also predicated on early experiences. Sadness can feel like a heaviness in one's chest or a lump in one's throat that dissolves into tears, and children learn at a young age to connect extreme circumstances with loss of bodily functions (e.g., enuresis). The second explanation of embodiment is more nativist and is evolutionarily based. In this conception, we understand embodiment in terms of exaptation of neurons whose workings originally evolved for other purposes (e.g., motor and sensory activity) but were co-opted (along with other neurons) to also serve cognition and emotion (M. L. Anderson, 2010, 2014; Dehaene & Cohen, 2007; Gallese, 2007; Gallese & Lakoff, 2005). We develop this idea when we review computational neuroscience models generally and neural reuse specifically, later in this book. For now, let us simply say that this conception posits that the networks underlying physical functions and processes also underlie cognitive and emotional experiences.

Embodiment of trauma has been of particular interest to both clinicians and researchers due to its significant implications for therapeutic work, which we are now just beginning to understand. Tay and Jordan (2015) taped, transcribed, and studied interviews with survivors of the 2010–2012 earthquakes in New Zealand and examined how metaphors were used to express a sense of a loss of control. The participants were all survivors who had sought help for clinical or subclinical posttraumatic stress disorder. Tay and Jordan observed that whereas some participants discussed a physical or concrete loss, many also talked about loss of control in an abstract way. A particularly interesting group of transcript excerpts pointed to a transfer of sorts, in which physical and abstract loss of control were discussed in consecutive turns. One participant's metaphor of "sitting at the back of a jumbo jet" evolved into "not being able to get a hold" of her loved ones, conveying an overall sense of lack of anchors—in the air at the back of a jumbo jet and metaphorically not being able to hold her family, interpersonal contact being described in terms of physical contact. Another participant described how the earthquake left her with an overall sense of fear and uncertainty about her future, her relationships, even her professional aspirations, using the metaphor "the whole ground had shifted" (p. 562). Yet another used similar visual and kinesthetic markers to describe an inner sense of lack of safety and fear of the unknown. As in the last example, she used literal descriptions of the earthquake as metaphorical descriptions of their psychological aftermath: "the ground was still moving" and "we were in the dark" (p. 563).

On a more general level, the therapeutic relationship, which we know to be a critical aspect of successful psychotherapy (Weinberger, 1995, 2014), may owe a part of its effectiveness to embodied feelings of warmth, trust, and so on. Whether these are based on scaffolding (i.e., early physical experiences that have become central to thought and feeling) or on overlap of neurons is for future research to decide but does not change the relevance of these connections to psychotherapeutic outcome. The same holds for transference, which can be seen as understanding one relationship through another, and to metaphorically moving forward.

Finally, as we stated above, metaphors promote new learning. This maps very well onto therapy. Successful therapeutic work requires new learning, as well as the formation of new behavioral patterns. An important role of metaphors in psychotherapy may be to "shake up" old embodied cognitions and supplant them with new, more adaptive ones. In embodied cognition, thought patterns are seen as (metaphorically speaking) written in the flesh. Thus, meaningful change has to be experiential too in order for new knowledge and insight to lead to long-term symptom reduction. Or, as one of our (VS) patients pointed out, "I have to now make it part of my cells." She too, like the Asaro tribe, had discovered the importance of making new knowledge part of your muscle.

NOTE

1. See Bargh (2016) for a review of the development of his work and how he thinks about it. Also see Bargh (2017) for a high-level popular review of his and others' work on unconscious processes.

PART IV

COMPUTATIONAL
NEUROSCIENCE
AND THE UNCONSCIOUS

We have argued for the existence and importance of unconscious processes. In support of our argument, we reviewed a great deal of empirical evidence and applied that evidence to clinical work. And we have described some attempts to provide an overall understanding of these processes, from grand theories like those of psychoanalysis to more empirically based and narrow theories like those of Dixon (1981), Spence (1964), Marcel (1983a, 1983b), and Shevrin and Dickman (1980). These were historically important and helped make the study of unconscious processes respectable and even took it into the mainstream. They also led to what we believe are important psychotherapeutic implications. None of these models can account for all of the findings and psychotherapeutic implications we have put forward, however. Moreover, the most recent of them is decades old. Are there more current models that can aspire to this goal? Is there now a better way to conceptualize the findings, to provide an undergirding for them?

There have been recent attempts to understand the mind, and therefore unconscious processes, that we believe represent major contributions toward achieving this goal. They are not in complete alignment at this time; in fact, there are serious disagreements among them. The field is in a productive ferment, but there may be some commonalities across models that can help us to better understand unconscious processes. Most of

239

these recent attempts can be said to fall under what have been termed computational models of the mind/brain (Sun, 2008). Computational models focus on describing mental knowledge structures and how they operate (our cognitive architecture). They are attempts to empirically address questions of epistemology. The goal is to understand cognition (defined broadly so as to include motivation and emotions) dynamically, that is, in a process-oriented fashion. The early models were based on computer functioning. Of special note was the groundbreaking work of Newell and Simon (e.g., Newell & Simon, 1972, 1988; Simon & Newell, 1971; also see Gigerenzer & Goldstein, 1996, for a discussion of the computer metaphor of mind). Although we allude to them, we do not review these computer-based models in any detail since they seem to have been superseded. Correctly so in our view. For example, Newell and Simon propose a serial model of cognitive functioning, whereas all modern models assume parallel functioning.[1] The models we do review here are based on biological properties of the brain. This type of model is sometimes termed "computational neuroscience" to capture the effort to model the brain in the theorizing. The computations in these models refer to the actions of neurons, groups of neurons, networks of neurons, and/or relatively highly organized and independently operating systems of neurons termed "modules." We describe a few of the main models and try to determine how some of the findings we reviewed and implications we have drawn can be derived from one or more of these models. We also speculate on how the apparent disagreements between them might be reconciled so as to provide a modern, tentative model of unconscious processes that explains the findings we have discussed and the therapeutic implications we have derived from those findings. Based on those implications, we offer a model of psychotherapy, normative implicit psychotherapy (NIP), that we believe to be more based on our current knowledge of unconscious processes than are the schools of psychotherapy currently extant. We realize that our integration is speculative and preliminary, but we believe it can help to organize the material and fruitfully move the enterprise forward.

NOTE

1. As we detail in subsequent chapters and alluded to earlier in this book, the mind functions in parallel. That is, many operations occur simultaneously. In a serial model, such as that proposed by Newell and Simon (1972, 1988), one operation occurs at a time. This is the way computers work, and it is the model Newell and Simon adopted. It was also the prevailing model of the mind at the time that they wrote. (Also see Erdelyi, 1974, who was ahead of his time in pointing out the assumption of serial processing was probably wrong.)

CHAPTER 18

Computational Models of the Mind

The main models we review here are massive modularity, connectionism (as operationalized by parallel distributed processing [PDP], and neural reuse. The latter flows into embodied cognition and metaphor, which have particular relevance for psychotherapy. One major way to differentiate these models is in terms of how general a processor the brain/mind is said to be. These range from almost completely general PDP to consisting of largely separate and independently operating processors (massive modularity), and one in between (neural reuse).

This thinking about thinking has a long history. The general processing approach can be traced to James's (1890/1950) chapter on habit, Hebb's (1949) work on the organization of behavior, Lashley's (1950) equipotentiality model of brain functioning, and Pribram's (1970) distributed coding. James wrote that the units in the brain become more and more strongly connected the more often they act together. Similarly, Hebb argued that when neurons fire together, they become connected so that they are increasingly likely to fire together on subsequent occasions. Lashley held that the brain is relatively undifferentiated, that is, it is a general processor. PDP, as we will see, makes similar (albeit more sophisticated) arguments. The notion that the brain consists of specialized structures goes back even further, to phrenology (Gall, 1822–1825/1835). The idea here is that the brain contains myriad separable parts. Every function carried out by the brain/mind can be localized to a specific part of the brain, which deals exclusively with that function. The phrenologists thought that measuring protrusions and indentations in the scalp could identify these brain modules. Later on, neurologists seemed to locate specific brain areas that controlled sensory and motor functioning (Fritsch & Hitzig, 1870) and language (Broca, 1861/2011;

Wernicke, 1885/1989). Modern massive modularity is a more recent, sophisticated, and empirically based version of this basic belief. Contemporary computational models are the descendants of both the general-processing and specialized structure views. And all of it can be said to have started, in our modern era, with the seminal work of Fodor (1983).

MODULES: THE GROUNDBREAKING WORK OF FODOR

In 1983, Fodor published a book entitled *Modularity of Mind*. The title implies that Fodor was on the side of specificity of function and location in the brain. This title can be misleading, however. Although he did introduce an original, computational model of modules, Fodor did not assert that the brain was a collection of such modules. In fact, he argued that these kinds of modules performed specific and limited functions and that the rest of the mind/brain was more or less a general processor where "it all comes together." Carruthers (2006, p. 4) described Fodor's view of the brain/mind "as a general-purpose computer with a limited number of distinct input and output links to the world (vision, audition, etc.)." As Prinz (2006) put it, he might better have called his book "The Modularity of Low-Level Peripheral Systems." According to Fodor, high-level perceptual processing and cognition are avowedly nonmodular. Massive modularity crossed this boundary to aver that virtually the entire brain/mind is composed of modules, albeit defined somewhat differently from the account put forward by Fodor.

Fodor (1983) defined modules as having many, if not most, of nine specified properties. In the order he presented them, they are:

1. *Domain specificity:* A module deals with very specific inputs and only those inputs, that is, a module only processes very specific information. This is the "what" of the functioning of the module. What kind of information does it process? Practically, this should show up as certain brain regions exclusively dedicated to very specific functions and only to those functions.

2. *Mandatory operation:* This means that a module operates in a very specific way and cannot deviate from that mode of operation. Modules are therefore not under voluntary control and cannot be turned on or off. They operate in an automatic fashion. Not so incidentally, this means that modules operate unconsciously; we are not aware of their operation nor can we be.

3. *Limited central accessibility:* The operation of a module (which is only concerned with very specific inputs—i.e., domain-specificity) is

inaccessible to the rest of the mind/brain. The other systems/modules in the brain/mind have no access to another module's internal functioning. All they are presented with, all they can deal with, are the results of this internal information processing, that is, its outputs. These internal operations must therefore be unconscious. This will be reinforced when we define encapsulation and shallow output below.

4. *Fast processing:* Because modules are specialized and constructed to process a particular form of information in a particular way, automatically, they can do so very quickly and efficiently. After all, they do nothing else and are designed for this specialty. Thus, their output is generated quickly and efficiently relative to nonmodular functioning.

5. *Informational encapsulation:* In later writings, Fodor (2000) identified this property as the most critical characteristic of a module. In fact, he declared it to be the central, defining feature of modules. Modules are isolated from the rest of cognition. They operate independently, with no access to the operation of other modules. This means that a module only has access to a limited database of information (it is encapsulated). When a module processes its inputs, it cannot access information stored elsewhere nor use such information as part of its operations. It is restricted to the information contained in its inputs plus whatever information might be stored within the modular system itself. This is the flip side of limited central accessibility. Modules cannot obtain information from other modules or brain processes (encapsulation) nor can other modules or brain processes obtain access to the inner workings of a module (inaccessible). Encapsulation refers to the fact that the flow of information into the module is heavily restricted. Inaccessibility refers to the restriction of the flow of information out of the module.

Thus, modules are enclosed systems, which do not let much information in or out. Since they cannot exchange much information with other systems/modules, most of the information potentially available in the brain is not used in the operations of any one isolated module. According to Fodor (2000), these are the sine qua non of modules. They must be present if one wishes to identify something in the mind/brain as a module. If domain-specificity refers to the "what" of modular functioning, inaccessibility and encapsulation refer to the (very limited) communication between modules. This also means that the output must necessarily be rudimentary or "shallow." (See property #6 below.)

6. *Shallow outputs:* Modules are said to produce relatively simple, basic, and nonconceptual outputs. This flows from the automatic, encapsulated, and inaccessible processing of modules. It means that the information generated by a module is not high level like a thought or

belief. Higher-level processing requires the operation of a nonmodular, central system.

7. *Fixed neural architecture:* Modules can be identified with circumscribed neural structures in the brain, dedicated to the realization of that module and that module only. This can also be called localizability. Modular functioning can be localized to specific areas in the brain. The finding, reviewed earlier, that focal damage to specific parts of the brain results in specific mental deficits is adduced as strong support for this property of modules, as well as for their existence. This feeds into the next criterion below, specific breakdown patterns. Additionally, neuroimaging studies seem to show that specific brain areas are active when people perform certain mental tasks. We will see shortly that this is not as neat as it seemed (Prinz, 2006).

8. *Characteristic and specific breakdown patterns:* This is the necessary consequence of fixed neural architecture or localization and refers to the idea that when there is a lesion or other kind of breakdown in a module, the effects are very specific to the functioning of that module and do not result in impairments in other systems/modules. The impaired functioning is restricted to the specific domain of the module. We can infer the purpose and functioning of the module by its distinctive pattern of breakdown. This is sometimes referred to by saying that the system is functionally dissociable. We reviewed some of these data in our section on brain damage (see Chapter 9).

9. *Characteristic ontogenetic pace and sequencing:* Modules are innate and develop according to a set pattern laid down by genetics and in response to proper stimulation (input) from the environment. That is, modules are part of our evolutionary inheritance and "develop according to a specific, endogenously determined pattern under the impact of environmental releasers" (Fodor, 1983, p. 100). Learning has virtually no role to play in this conception.

In the next three chapters, we examine work that followed but often disagreed with Fodor's modular model. First is massive modularity, which modifies Fodor's view of modules and extends modular functioning to higher cognitive processes. Next, we discuss connectionism in the form of PDP, which essentially denies the existence of modules. Finally, we consider neural reuse, which, in our view, can serve as a bridge between massive modularity and connectionism.

CHAPTER 19

Massive Modularity

Massive modularity crosses a line in the sand laid down by Fodor. Whereas Fodor argues that modules are limited to noncentral basic and elementary functions, those championing massive modularity aver that the brain/mind is mostly, if not entirely, modular and that this modularity includes sophisticated central processes (see, e.g., Carruthers, 2006; Kurzban, 2010; and Pinker, 2005). According to proponents of this view, the brain/mind is a collection of such independent units, each with its own anatomic (neurophysiological) structure. In order to make the case for central modules and a brain/mind that is almost if not totally modular, proponents of massive modularity must alter and even jettison some of the properties of modules that Fodor laid out. That is, a module for those proposing massive modularity is not the same as a module proposed by Fodor (cf. Carruthers, 2006). Below we describe the basic history of this movement, its underlying rationale, and the type of modules it postulates. Finally, we draw clinical implications of this view.

Massive modularity is most often connected with evolutionary psychology (e.g., Buss, 1999; Carruthers, 2006; Clarke, 2004; Kurzban, 2010; Pinker, 1997, 2005; Sperber, 1996; Tooby & Cosmides, 1992). Advocates of evolutionary psychology see the brain/mind as a naturally selected system of computational components that evolved to help our ancestors survive and reproduce. These components are largely, if not entirely, composed of specific neurological networks (called modules) that evolved to solve specific adaptational problems that our ancestors encountered during the Pleistocene epoch (about 2 million to about 12,000 years ago—the period of the environment of evolutionary adaptedness for humans). We can infer what these challenges were by identifying the brain/mind's functional capacities. The entire brain/mind system, composed of dissociable subsystems, would have been built up gradually, over evolutionary time, by adding subsystem to subsystem such that the functioning of the whole has redundancy built into it. This would mean the whole is somewhat protected or at least buffered from damage to any of its parts. Over a half century ago, Simon (1962) argued that this would be the best way to design any complex system, particularly a biological one. More recently, Marcus (2004) described how such a process could result in the evolutionary development of our nervous system. First, a subsystem or an aspect of a subsystem in the nervous system would be copied, yielding two (or more) instances of that structure (redundancy). Then, one or more of these copies would be modified (through natural selection) so as to address a new, adaptationally important, task. As Carruthers (2006) put it, "Evolution needs to be able to tinker with one function in response to selection pressures without necessarily impacting any of the others" (p. 19). This process would continue over evolutionary time until we end up with the current brain/mind.

Massive modularity was innovated or, at least, first systematized in an ambitious series of papers by Tooby and Cosmides (e.g., 1992, 1995). (See Clarke, 2004, for a cogent summary of Tooby and Cosmides.) These thinkers argued that there are universal aspects to human nature that cut across cultural differences (i.e., are hardwired in our brains). The underlying structure for this shared humanity is instantiated by neurophysiological mechanisms, or modules, that evolved through natural selection. This means that we inherit most of our cognitive architecture in the form of these modules. Finally, this innate structure did not evolve to help our species adapt to modern exigencies but to the circumstances faced by our Pleistocene hunter–gatherer ancestors. Thus, our minds evolved and are designed to help us survive and procreate in an environment that no longer exists. This has important implications for our reactions to the circumstances that currently confront us and our conspecifics (i.e., members of the same species). It also provides a unique solution to questions of epistemology. How we know, how we gain knowledge, and what we are capable of knowing is attributable to and constrained by the operation of the modules making up our brains. Thus, how we know and the nature of what we know are based on empirically discoverable modular functioning (see Clarke, 2004). This has important implications for both normative and clinical functioning in our modern (non-Pleistocene) world. It also provides empirical backing for Kant's ideas of a priori (innate) knowledge, intuitions (the ways we orient ourselves in time and space), and categories (through which we understand our experiences), reviewed way back in Chapter 2.

BASICS OF MASSIVE MODULARITY

Steven Pinker (1997) wrote a best-selling and very well received book entitled *How the Mind Works* that, among other things, laid out the basics of massive modularity. Pinker (2005) later reiterated the main points of massive modularity in response to a critical review by Fodor (2000). According to Pinker, there are three main themes underlying massive modularity. The first is that thinking is a form of computation. The second is that the brain/mind is specialized. And the third is that the brain/mind evolved during the Pleistocene epoch. These are interrelated. Below, we explicate what Pinker means.

We have already defined computation as an effort to describe and understand the dynamic operation of mental/neurophysiological knowledge structures. By computation, Pinker means information processing of a particular kind, carried out by evolutionarily developed brain structures and designed to perform certain very specific functional tasks. These brain structures therefore specialize in "computing" the answers to very specific questions. Computation refers to uniquely human (or animal) ways of processing information that follow their own rules and procedures (Pinker, 2005). The computational structures in the mind/brain (modules) are not designed to solve random or arbitrary problems; rather, they evolved to solve those problems that increased the chances of survival and procreation of our Pleistocene ancestors.

Thus, the mind is composed of subsystems (modules) that are dedicated to particular kinds of information processing, that result in particular kinds of reasoning or goal attainment, and that operate in the service of solving Pleistocene-based survival and procreation challenges. There are numerous such modules (Clarke, 2004), each dedicated to a specific problem, which it solves in its own way. So, rather than following a single set of rules, the human mind/brain is organized into several domains that employ different ways of processing information, which result in different ways of understanding different aspects of reality such as physical objects, living things, other minds, and so on. Pinker refers to the different rules and modes of processing in these different domains as "core intuitions" that guide the "reasoning" (computation) in each domain. This is what is meant by specialization and is closely akin to (and Pinker means it to refer to) domain specificity such as we described earlier. To put it all in a nutshell, Pinker (2005) argues that "the mind is a naturally selected system of organs of computation" (p. 22). So massive modularity posits a multitude of independently and/or quasi-independently operating subsystems or modules. The model also describes how these modules would need to function in order to work in the hypothesized manner (the brain being largely, if not entirely, modular, with complex central systems not excluded from this set of modular subsystems). And here is where massive modularity must part company with Fodor, who explicitly argued that modules need to be limited, noncentral, and relatively few in number compared to the rest of the mind/brain. Probably the best source for these descriptions and contrasts is Carruthers (2006).

According to Carruthers, the modules in a massively modular mind/brain cannot be Fodor-like modules. First, and most obviously, as soon as central systems are said to be modular, the model has seriously departed from that of Fodor. Fodor's assertion that modules must be peripheral, basic, and noncentral must be jettisoned. Once central modules are posited, modules also cannot be required to have the shallow outputs posited by Fodor. The outputs of central modules would have to include conceptual thoughts and beliefs. Likewise, speed of processing could no longer be characteristic of modules as Fodor was comparing the speed of his version of modules to central, nonmodular processing speed. Now that central processes are also modular, there is no basis for comparing speeds. It would just be that some modules process information more quickly than others. The one exception might be conscious processes, which might not be modular and might be slower than is even central modular processing. More on that later.

Some characteristics can be retained, however. Thus, mandatory operation would still be characteristic of a module in a massive modularity model. Modules are also still conceptualized as operating automatically, according to built-in sets of rules. (And, not so incidentally to the focus of this book, that would mean that the modules in a massive modularity model of the mind/brain operate unconsciously.) Fixed neural architecture or localization is also retained. Each module is characterized by neural circuitry that is dedicated to that module. Additionally, modules are still a product of evolution and hence innate. Thus, characteristic ontogenetic pace and sequencing are retained. And, finally, characteristic or specific breakdown patterns continue to be an attribute of massive modularity modules. Thus, when there is damage to a module, the effects of that damage are unique to the functioning of that module. Recall that this is also sometimes termed functionally dissociable systems. So, limited central accessibility, fast processing, and shallow outputs are gone, but localization, functional dissociability, innateness, and mandatory operation (and therefore the centrality of unconscious processes) remain.

What is to be done with the remaining characteristics of Fodor's model is less clear and more complex. Domain specificity may or may not have to be eliminated. At the very least, it would have to be redefined. Some modules could be domain-specific in the Fodorian sense.

That is, they would deal with only very specific inputs. This definition would apply to the kinds of elementary processes identified by Fodor as characteristic of modules. But other modules could not function in this way if central processes are to be included. If, for example, there are modules that deal with practical reasoning, they could not be limited to a specific type of input. They would have to be capable of dealing with any belief or desire as input. The fate of encapsulation and inaccessibility is even more complex. These, of course, are central to Fodor's view of modules. Carruthers analyzes the purpose and necessity of these properties. He concludes that what is essential to them is what he terms "frugality." The idea is that a module can only deal with a limited database or it would be overwhelmed with information and be unable to function. Fodor argues that the way the mind/brain achieves this is through encapsulation. That is, a module has a limited and dedicated database and consults no other data. Carruthers argues that frugality does not require complete encapsulation. He differentiates between what he terms narrow-scope and wide-score encapsulation. A <u>Fodor module</u> is narrow-scope. It cannot draw on information outside of its functioning purview. But a module might also be able to draw on outside information as long as it does not draw on all possible outside information. In other words, a great deal of information may be accessible to the module, but only a small percentage of it is accessed on any given occasion. This is wide-scope encapsulation. If this can be said to be the case, then Fodor's case against central modularity evaporates. Central modules are wide scope as are some noncentral modules, whereas basic, elementary modules tend to be narrow scope. The same argument can be made for inaccessibility. A given module cannot have access to the inner workings of all other modules or to the output of all other modules, but it can have access to the workings and output of some, depending upon circumstances. So we have both narrow- and wide-scope accessibility, depending upon the module and its mode of processing. This greatly increases the flexibility of the system and allows for central process modularity. Pinker (1998, 2005) makes similar points.

Massive modularity therefore posits a myriad (literally thousands) of mostly innate, independent processing systems (modules), each with a distinct neural realization. Each of these modules will have a specific task to perform, which it will perform in a myriad of ways. All of this will have developed, due to selection pressures, over evolutionary time. Finally, like all current models of the brain/mind, the components work in parallel rather than serially so that many are operating at once. A convenient metaphor for this conception is a "modular" stereo system. A CD player can be independent of speakers, and both can be independent of an amplifier and a tuner, and so on. The system works together even though the components are dissociable. All components are "on" at the same time to create the sound that we want, and we can remove a component without affecting the others.

Carruthers also posits a global workspace where many of these modules can meet and interact (the place where it all comes together as Fodor put it) that is nonmodular. This is where consciousness would be, and its processing would be slower than that of modules, even central ones. Not all massive modularity theorists agree, however. For example, Kurzban (2010) seems to posit a completely modular mind. For Kurzban, even the self is modular (Kurzban & Aktipis, 2007). This social cognitive interface (SCI) or, as Kurzban and Aktipis colloquially term it, the "press secretary," operates on information that can enhance the person's social standing and/or persuade others to come around to his point of view. This module does not make its own decisions or even have access to what motivated said decisions. That is the purview of other modules. But, like the "interpreter" of Gazzaniga (2009), it will try to explain what the person has done. Unlike the interpreter, it is not concerned with creating a coherent narrative per se. Its job is to create a self-serving narrative, a narrative that puts the person in the best possible light so as to further social interaction. In both the Gazzaniga and Kurzban models, there seems to be no global workspace, only encapsulated modules. This difference between the Carruthers, Gazzaniga, and Kurzban views of massive modularity has implications we discuss below. Carruthers (2009; Engelbert & Carruthers, 2010) has also wrestled with the question of whether we truly introspect or merely come to conclusions about ourselves in the same way that we come to conclusions about others. He leans to the latter; for him and most massive modularity theorists, there is no privileged access and introspection as most of us think of it. It is an illusion, as Ryle (1949/2009) argued decades ago. Carruthers is also open to the possibility that what seems like privileged access is simply another module, like the interpreter posited by Gazzaniga (2009) or the SCI posited by Kurzban and Aktipis (2007). So, although there is consciousness and a global workspace in Carruthers's model of massive modularity, there is no "self" or privileged access. In this, he agrees with both Gazzaniga and Kurzban.

DOES MASSIVE MODULARITY MAKE SENSE?

Evidence for this model is adduced on several levels. First is logic. It is difficult to conceptualize a general learning mechanism that could perform all of the functions that the brain/mind does. A myriad of specialized components makes more sense in both an evolutionary and an engineering sense (cf. Carruthers, 2006; Marcus, 2004; Pinker, 1998; Simon, 1962).[1] There is also evidence from fMRI studies that seem to show local functioning when a cognitive process is occurring (Carruthers, 2006). And the evidence from brain damage studies seems to show that injury to a particular part of the brain affects specific functions without apparently affecting other functions (cf. Carruthers, 2006; Pinker, 1998; also see Laws, Adlington, Moreno-Martinez, Javier, & Gale, 2010). We reviewed some of this evidence in Chapter 9.

Another support for the idea of brain modularity is that there now exist simulation models of a modular brain that seem to work. Investigators working in this area are nowhere near modeling genuinely complex functioning, but the results thus far are promising. Probably the most well-known and sophisticated is ACT–R (adaptive control of thought-rational), innovated by J. R. Anderson and his colleagues. There have been several iterations of this model, the most recent we are aware of being ACT–R 6.0 (J. R. Anderson, 2007). ACT–R attempts to provide an abstract model of brain structure that can explain how it results in mind. ACT–R 6.0 identifies eight specialized, domain-specific, widely encapsulated, independent, and separately modifiable components, or modules, and posits where they may be located in the brain. The ACT–R 6.0 modules and their hypothesized locations in the brain are: a visual module said to be located in the fusiform gyrus; an aural module sited in the auditory cortex; a manual and a vocal module both situated along the motor strip; a retrieval module in the prefrontal cortex; a goal module to be found in the anterior cingulate; an imaginal module in the posterior parietal cortex; and a procedural module in the basal ganglia. These have been operationalized as a set of independent and separately modifiable software components. So it is possible to simulate the mind/brain functioning of these modules. Moreover, there are data supportive of the existence and location of these modules in real brains. These include fMRI and experimental studies (see J. R. Anderson, 2007). Thus, there are data and an ongoing research program that directly seem to support a modular brain.

CLINICAL IMPLICATIONS OF HAVING A MASSIVELY MODULAR BRAIN

There are several ramifications of having a massively modular brain/ mind that are relevant to psychopathology and psychotherapy. One major implication flows from the independence and domain specificity inherent to massive modularity. Since modules process information in their own unique ways, coming to their own conclusions, it is not only possible but also inevitable that we can hold two inconsistent, even contradictory, beliefs or feelings about an issue. We can and do behave inconsistently. We can and do behave one way and profess, honestly, to feel and believe another. Since the brain/mind functions in a parallel fashion, these contradictions can take place simultaneously. And since most functioning is unconscious, we have no awareness, let alone insight, into these contradictions. This is one of the main points made by Kurzban (2010) in his book *Why Everyone (Else) Is a Hypocrite*. This could help explain the myriad things patients do while professing a strong desire not to do them and while holding a value system that would seem to condemn them. Kurzban provides many examples such as ex-New York Governor Spitzer engaging a prostitute, thereby, among other things, violating a law that he had strongly enforced.

Independently functioning modules might partially explain the phenomenon of resistance, wherein a patient professes a desire to change and then resists efforts to accomplish exactly that. The concept of encapsulation, even if it is construed as wide scope, suggests that providing information that demonstrates faulty information processing may not have the desired effects since the modules involved may not have access to that information. This is most clearly demonstrated in phobias and even in normal fear reactions of most humans. For example, Öhman and Mineka (2001) posited and presented evidence for a fear module related to stimuli that were dangerous to our Pleistocene ancestors, such as spiders and snakes. In contrast, torn wires in an electrical outlet, which are objectively far more dangerous, were not feared. This was the case even when images of the stimulation were presented outside of awareness (unconsciously). This effect of encapsulation can be demonstrated by telling a person that a particular snake is harmless without this information having any effect on her fear. People generally are uncomfortable around snakes (and spiders) despite their relative harmlessness, especially in relation to things like guns and frayed wires. This is easily explained by positing a relatively encapsulated fear module for snakes and spiders (see Öhman & Mineka). That module simply does not take in information on the relative harmlessness of particular instances of the fear object. One of us (JW) had this demonstrated to him in a very powerful way at a recent conference. I am afraid of heights. I was hooked up to a virtual reality machine that made it appear as though I was on a ledge high above the ground. I knew that this was not the case, and yet I experienced massive anxiety. Even more telling (and embarrassing), I refused to step off the imaginary ledge that I knew was not there. Thus, I was immune to information that was clearly available to me and that I was conscious of. My fear of heights is pretty strongly encapsulated.

The above formulation offers a naturalistic, normative explanation for many examples of neurotic behavior that resist efforts to change them. It also explains day-to-day normative inconsistencies and conflicts in our cognitive and behavioral lives. What, if anything, does it say about psychotherapy and its efforts to change these cognitions and behaviors? There are two scenarios afforded by massive modularity that we can think of. In one, there is a global workspace where modular output can meet, where, as Fodor said, it all comes together. Carruthers seems to lean in this direction. If this exists, change can occur through the exchange of information that takes place in this area. The idea then would be to get the modules talking to one another in some central medium. In psychodynamic psychotherapy, this is the therapeutic relationship; in cognitive therapy, it is rational discourse. And so on. There is no reason there cannot be several such methods of central, global processing. In all of these cases, there seems to be a need for conscious realization of the problematic issues followed by actions designed to address them. But we must not think that our patients have privileged access to their functioning, even when they are conscious of it. The work would be done as though they were observing the behaviors, thoughts, and feelings of others (see Carruthers, 2009).

There also seems to be a view that there is no modular-free global workspace; the mind is entirely modular. This seems to be the position of Kurzban (2010). This leads to a more pessimistic view of change. To the extent that modules are encapsulated and inaccessible, their functioning cannot be changed. And there is a great deal of evidence that change in therapy tends not to be long lasting, going all the way back to Freud's (1937) paper "Analysis Terminable or Interminable." Many empirical studies since have supported this conclusion (see Weinberger, 2014). Even exposure, largely held to be effective, actually does not work a good half of the time (Craske, Liao, Brown, & Vervliet, 2012; Craske, Treanor, Conway, Zbozinek, & Vervliet, 2014), and its effects tend not to last (Brown & Barlow, 1995; Zbozinek & Craske, 2017). So what are we to do? It would seem that we need to penetrate the modular functioning itself. One possibility is that many modules have wide-scope encapsulation and so can be open to outside information when it is presented in such a way as to be available to the module. The usual way is through consciousness. But Weinberger et al. (2011) presented data that suggested that implicit exposure can be effective in reducing avoidance of spiders. Thus, consciousness may not be necessary to effective psychotherapy. Perhaps more research efforts in this direction, followed by techniques that make use of them, can be helpful.

Overall, the massive modularity model strongly suggests that psychotherapy will not enjoy great success. Changing the functioning of relatively encapsulated, even wide-scope modules is a daunting task. This is made even more difficult by mandatory operation. If modules operate automatically according to built-in sets of rules, change would be extremely difficult. But we know that psychotherapy works even if relapse is stronger than we would like (Weinberger, 1995, 2014; Weinberger & Eig, 1999). How can we reconcile this negative prediction on the effectiveness of psychotherapy with the empirical finding that it is effective and that the size of the effect is meaningful? We believe the answer comes from two other computations models of the functioning of the mind/brain: parallel distributed processing and neural reuse. We review these in turn and then attempt to integrate the models.

NOTES

1. As we will see when we review parallel distributed processing models—PDP—this is not necessarily the case. There are alternatives that work at the conceptual as well as the engineering level.

CHAPTER 20

Parallel Distributed Processing

As we stated in Chapter 19, massive modularity is not the only computational model of the mind. There are others that can seem antithetical to the tenets of massive modularity. Perhaps the most radical alternative is connectionism, whose most well-thought-out version is parallel distributed processing (PDP). Whereas massive modularity posits innumerable, innate, and specialized structures within the mind/brain, each with its own function, PDP posits more generalized and smaller unit processing, which is distributed throughout the brain rather than localized. PDP postulates a radical plasticity in contrast to the domain-specific functioning of massive modularity. Modularity argues for local, semiautonomous functioning via semi-isolated parts of the brain. PDP posits generalized processors that function through massive parallel processing. The two seem so unlike that proponents of one tend to see the other as not viable. After we review PDP, we will see if we can resolve the apparent conflicts between them through a third computational model, neural reuse. This integration will then be shown to have powerful implications for everyday functioning as well as for psychotherapy.

THE NEUROLOGICAL UNDERPINNINGS OF PDP MODELS

Rumelhart, McClelland, and their colleagues (Rumelhart, McClelland, & the PDP Research Group, 1986, Vols. 1 & 2) created a model of information processing based on known properties of the brain and the neurons that make it up. Their strategy was to derive a model of the mind from the structure, functioning, and interconnections of the basic units of the brain, the neurons. The central idea is that thoughts emerge from the interaction of neurons. It was the hope and belief of these theorists that phenomena observed in both brain-damaged and intact-brain individuals would emerge naturally from the operation of these basic units. They termed their model PDP because they posited a myriad of processes occurring simultaneously throughout the information-processing system (the brain/mind). Unconscious processes are a given in PDP; they are taken for granted in the theorizing (Cleeremans, 2014). In fact, the real difficulty is accounting for consciousness (Cleeremans, 2014). The model has exploded in the literature, and there are numerous papers about it and variants of it (see *Cognitive Science*, 2014, *38*(6). It is now one of the central conceptions of human functioning extant (Rogers & McClelland, 2014). We will focus on central tenets and not on differences between versions.

PDP models begin by incorporating some basic facts about the brain into their theorizing. They are the parameters within which the models must work. To begin with, the brain consists of tens of billions of neurons (estimates range from about 70 to about 100 billion). These neurons are highly interconnected through their dendrites and synapses. Each neuron can potentially receive signals from and send signals to anywhere from one to 100,000 of their fellows. This means that each neuron is in potential communication with a vast number of other neurons and that no neuron is very many connections away from any other neuron (Rumelhart & McClelland, 1986, chap. 4). The upshot of all of this is that the brain consists of an extremely large number of highly interconnected elements (McClelland, Rumelhart & Hinton, 1986, chap. 1). All PDP models, therefore, postulate large numbers of highly interconnected units.

Communication between neurons is simple. When neurons fire, they send excitatory and inhibitory signals (called action potentials) to one another. Since neurons are so highly interconnected, a multitude of such excitatory and inhibitory signals impinge on each neuron at any one time. If the sum of these signals is excitatory and exceeds some threshold, the neuron will fire and send off its own action potential. If the sum of the signals is inhibitory, the neuron's firing threshold will increase, effectively preventing it from firing. If a threshold is not exceeded, the neuron will not be affected. This is all that neurons can do; they cannot transmit more complex information. Individually, they cannot send meaningful messages. Somehow, our complex and multifaceted functioning must arise from such simple, apparently uninformative messages (Rumelhart & McClelland, 1986, chap. 4). PDP models attempt to meet this challenge by positing relatively simple units that can only excite and inhibit one another. Then they try to derive complex functioning from this premise.

In addition to being relatively primitive, communication between neurons is relatively slow. Neurons take milliseconds or even hundredths of a second to do their thing. By way of contrast, the units of a computer can perform their operations in nanoseconds (billionths of a second). They are literally a million times faster than the neurons of the brain. Yet, the brain is able to accomplish things in 1 second or less (e.g., perceptual and language processing) that computers are still struggling to achieve. Given the speed at which neurons operate, they can only carry out 100 steps in this time period. If we are to model such processes, we must figure out a way to do so in 100 or fewer steps. Feldman (1985) has termed this the *100-step program constraint*. PDP models are therefore also constrained in this way.

The only way the brain can succeed in so short a period of time is through massive parallel processing (Rumelhart, Hinton, & McClelland, 1986, chap. 3). That is, the 100-step rule can be finessed if many hundreds of thousands (millions?) of highly interconnected individual processes are operating at once, each limited to 100 steps. So, instead of a lot of steps, there are a lot of processes. The massive number of neurons, in combination with their high interconnectivity, means that this solution is feasible for the brain.

Parallelism is further supported by the fact that people perform better on many tasks when a great deal of information is available to them for processing. For example, we can recognize people more quickly and accurately if we both see and hear them than if only one of these sources of information is available to us.[1] The only way this can result in more efficient processing is if both sets of information are processed simultaneously. A sequential computer does not respond more quickly when it is asked to triangulate more and more information. Further, if some of the information is imprecise or ambiguous, as it often is in our environment, the computer is really in trouble (see Feldman & Ballard, 1982). Yet, we get along just fine in such an environment. All PDP models therefore assume massive parallel processing. So the human information-processing system involves the cooperative activity of a vast number of relatively slow and simple processing units, all operating in parallel (Rumelhart & McClelland, 1986, chap. 4).

THE BASIC PDP MODEL

Based on the aforementioned simple facts about brain processing, Rumelhart et al. (1986, chap. 2) proposed a set of characteristics that must be common to all PDP models. First, a PDP system must have a large set of processing units. These PDP units are patterned after the neuron but are not necessarily identical to it. It would take too much to have to build all PDP models from the ground up, so to speak (i.e., from individual neurons). So functional *units*, at a level somewhat higher than neurons, are posited instead. These can be considered groups of neurons that inevitably fire together. The "unit' is analogous to the "node" in the Shiffrin and Schneider (1977) and Schneider and Shiffrin (1977) model reviewed in Chapter 6. Some theorists (e.g., Westen & Gabbard, 2002) have therefore used the terms "node" and "unit" interchangeably. These units are not sophisticated enough or large enough to be considered a module, however. They might be large enough to constitute what has been called a "working" in neural reuse models, which are reviewed shortly. This may be the junction where some computational neuroscience models can meet and be integrated.

Different PDP models posit different units. Specifying the set of processing units and what they represent is usually the first step in creating a PDP model (McClelland et al., 1986, chap. 1). The units in different PDP models can vary from embodying elementary perceptual features like the orientation of a line, to more complex features like a letter (McClelland et al., 1986, chap. 1) or even interpersonal features like an aspect of a tone of voice (Westen & Gabbard, 2002). We will argue below that what neural reuse terms workings can represent a PDP unit. Whatever it depicts, the unit must be sufficiently elementary and general to fit into a very large number of possible representations. No unit is tied exclusively to any particular representation. It is not "used up" when it becomes part of a representation. So it is not encapsulated or inaccessible. In this way, each unit can be involved in representing many different entities. And conversely, the system can employ many different units in each representation it creates. As a result, an extremely large number of units is needed to portray any one feature of a stimulus. This is called "*course coding.*" Specificity is gained through the pattern of units activated rather than by any specialized unit like a module. This allows for a great deal of representational flexibility. An awful lot of simple, barely differentiated units are needed if this strategy is to succeed, but that is one of the givens of a PDP model (since that is one of the givens of the brain). If there is a large and dynamic number of potential events needing to be represented (as there are in the human environment), this turns out to be the most efficient way for a huge number of simple units to be deployed. Course coding is therefore a central aspect of all PDP models.

Each unit in a PDP system is either active or inert at any point in time. This corresponds to the activation or lack thereof of the individual neurons in the brain. Activation of a unit depends upon the overall level of excitation flowing into it from the other units. If the overall excitation exceeds some threshold, the unit will become active and generate an excitatory signal of its own, which will then impinge on other units in the system. If the threshold is not exceeded, the unit will not become active. It may even be prevented from becoming active if the signals reaching it are largely inhibitory.

The effects of excitation or inhibition of a unit (or set of units) depend upon the number of units it is connected to and how it is connected to those units. PDP models posit three kinds of connections a unit can have (Hinton, McClelland, & Rumelhart, 1986, chap. 2). These are termed input, output, and hidden. An input unit receives signals from a source external to the PDP system of which it is a part. This source can be another PDP system (or set of units), or the input can originate in stimulation of a sense organ. An output unit sends signals out of the system. This outgoing signal can be communicated to a motor unit or to another PDP system. Finally, a hidden unit only communicates to other units within the system. That is, its input comes exclusively from other units within the system, and its output goes only to other units within the system. It has no way of directly communicating with any units outside of the system. This sounds suspiciously like encapsulation and inaccessibility and may offer a connection between PDP and modularity (see below). The number of input, output, and hidden units varies across different PDP systems. The organization of their connections to other units within and outside of the system also varies across systems.

The combination of input, output, and hidden units making up a PDP system sounds a lot like a module. The input units represent information entering into and thereby stimulating the activity of the module. The output units represent the information that the module communicates to other parts of the brain (other modules in the brain) concerning the results of its operation. The hidden units represent the modular functioning itself. Recall that a module was defined as a set of highly interconnected neurons with relatively few connections to other sets of neurons (i.e., a relatively circumscribed set of neurons—encapsulated and inaccessible). The more hidden units there are in a system, the more circumscribed it is and the more modular its operation. The smaller the number of hidden units, the less modular the system. Recall also that, in the intact brain, modules communicate with one another. This is the function of the input and output units. The more input and output units there are, the more connected the module is to the rest of brain (or, in PDP terms, the rest of system) functioning. The split brain represents a severing of input and output units (the corpus callosum) between modules so that only hidden units are left. Thus, PDP has a kind of modular functioning built into it. A module is a semi-encapsulated (widescope) parallel distributed process in the brain. The brain is, then, an interconnected series of such subsystems functioning as a meta-PDP system.

It is important to note that the modularity of PDP differs from that hypothesized by Fodor (1983, 2000). PDP systems are far less encapsulated and more connected to other parts of the brain than are the modules described by Fodor. PDP systems are also less encapsulated and more interconnected with other parts of the brain than is posited by massive modularity, as articulated by Carruthers (2006). The brain is far more plastic in PDP models than in any modular conception. PDP is friendlier to massive modularity (Carruthers, 2006; Kurzban, 2010; Pinker, 2005) than it is to Fodorian modularity, but it is still a very different model. It can, however, be reconciled with neural reuse (M. L. Anderson, 2010, 2014), which is another development that arose out of computational neuroscience and (we believe) can serve to integrate the two apparently antithetical models of PDP and massive modularity. (See Chapter 21.)

The pattern of connections among the various kinds of units is one of the parameters that must be specified in any PDP system. This pattern of connectivity constrains what the system can and cannot represent. If the connections are sufficiently numerous and complex, the system should be able to represent just about anything. No currently available PDP model has achieved anywhere near this level of sophistication. In fact, most models are relatively primitive. But it is assumed that this is due to the lack of sophistication and ingenuity of the modelers, not of the model itself. This is to be expected in the beginning of any new enterprise. If a sufficiently complex model could be built, it should, in principle, be able to emulate all of human functioning (see Rumelhart & McClelland, 1986, chap. 27). (But see Fodor & Pylyshyn, 1988, 2015, and Pinker & Prince, 1988, for a different, less sanguine point of view.)

There is one assumption built into every PDP model that enables it to adapt to the environment. This assumption is that when two (or however many) units are simultaneously activated, the activation of one is more likely to lead to the activation of the other on subsequent occasions. That is, their activations become linked to some degree (McClelland et al., 1986, chap. 1). The probability of one unit activating another increases every time the two units are excited in a roughly contemporaneous time frame. In the parlance of PDP models, there is an increase in their *activation weight*, that is, the probability of one unit being activated, given the activation of another unit. It is also sometimes referred to as the strength of the connection. The activation weight or connection strength changes minimally with each co-activation but builds up as co-activation recurs. If such activations occur frequently enough, the activation weight or connection strength can become quite high, all the way up to certainty (a probability of 1.0). This is the PDP understanding of learning. It flows naturally into implicit learning (cf. Cleeremans, 2014; Cleeremans & Dienes, 2008; Rogers & McClelland, 2014). Clark (2013) argued that the mind can be conceptualized as an implicit prediction engine. This accords nicely with both PDP learning rules and implicit learning.

This assumption is called the *"Hebb rule"* because it was modeled after a formulation Donald Hebb (1949) made concerning assemblies of neurons. It could (and maybe should) just as easily have been called the "James rule" after William James (1890) who, in chapter 14 (Association) wrote: "Let us then assume . . . this law: *When two elementary brain-processes have been active together or in immediate succession, one of them, on reoccurring, tends to propagate its excitement into the other"* (p. 566; italics in original). We will therefore refer to this assumption as the James–Hebb rule.[2]

As stated above, the James–Hebb rule is the instantiation of learning in the system. Through past association, units become more likely to become active together in the future. The more often their activation has been associated, the greater the likelihood of their co-activation on subsequent occasions. Whatever they represent will thereby become activated as well. The system has "learned" something in the sense that a new connection has been made. The strength of the connection is analogous to the degree of the learning. The greater the connection strength, the better the learning. Note that volition and translations of signals through complex algorithms are not implicated in this process. This is an automatic, unconscious neurophysiological event.

Let us review what a PDP system consists of. There is a large number of coarsely tuned and intricately connected units. Some groups of such units are connected in a modular-like fashion but without encapsulation (either wide or narrow scope). The connections are weighted as a result of experience. (There are probably also genetically based weights and/or limitations to possible weightings; cf. M. L. Anderson, 2010; Westen & Gabbard, 2002.) This means that certain groupings of units are more likely to fire together or to inhibit one another than are other groupings of units. And the whole system operates in parallel so that huge numbers of units and groupings of units can do their things simultaneously.

That is all there is to any PDP system, in principle. But some pretty remarkable properties can be derived or emerge from these few simple propositions. They have the potential to say a great deal about human functioning. None of these emergent properties depend upon awareness. Everything takes place unconsciously.

EMERGENT PROPERTIES OF PDP

Studies of brain damage have revealed that loss of functioning is proportional to the number of neurons damaged. That is, performance gradually deteriorates as more and more neural units are destroyed. There is no critical unit that controls performance. This has been clearly shown in global degenerative syndromes like Alzheimer's disease (Schwartz, Marin, & Saffran, 1979). PDP theorists call this characteristic of brain damage *"graceful degradation."* In PDP systems, this property emerges naturally from course coding. No unit contains much information or has very much processing power. No unit is unique or indispensable. Instead, the units comprising a PDP system are highly redundant. Loss of a few units, no matter where they are physically located, will have almost no effect at all. Quite a few units would have to be destroyed before performance of the system would noticeably suffer. The more units lost, the worse overall functioning becomes. The deterioration in functioning will be roughly proportional to the number of units damaged. Compare this to the functioning of a computer where loss of a single instruction can send an entire program crashing down. We are all familiar with the effects of mistyping a letter or putting punctuation marks in the wrong place. Computers do not have the property of graceful degradation. The brain emulates a PDP system more than it does a computer in this regard.

Another two emergent properties of PDP systems are the development of schemas and of representations (Norman, 1986, chap. 26). This is a direct result of the James–Hebb rule, which is the basic (really the only) type of learning that takes place in a PDP system. If we assume, in accord with the James–Hebb rule, that co-activation of units increases the connection weights between them, then the units that patterns have in common will develop stronger connection weights than the units that are not common to them. As related patterns are presented repeatedly, the central common core or underlying correspondence between them will be extracted. This will simply be a product of the repeated co-activation of those sets of units common to most of the presented patterns. The result will be a kind of prototype. These PDP prototypes behave similarly to and can be identified with what are usually referred to as schemas or representations. Note that the development of such schemas and representations occurs automatically and naturally. They are simply a by-product of the way PDP systems operate. As far as the PDP system is concerned, all that has happened is that some units have become more heavily weighted or more strongly connected than others. The schema or representation is not abstracted over experiences and then stored somewhere; it is simply the likelihood of a pattern of activation given appropriate input.[3] In such a conception, the schema or representation is dynamic and somewhat fluid. We will shortly see that memories can operate in a very similar way.

Fluency and automaticity also emerge naturally from the operation of the James–Hebb rule of PDP systems. "Fluency" refers to the fact that prior experiences automatically make processing of subsequent experiences easier (Jacoby et al., 1992). The James–Hebb rule of PDP systems states that units that fire together once are more likely to do so on subsequent occasions. That is, their connection strength increases. It is exactly the same conception. PDP thereby provides a theoretical underpinning for fluency. Whatever has been experienced is more fluent and therefore easier to process the next time it appears because of increased connection weights between the units. "Automaticity" refers to the fact that, with practice, complex series of behaviors can run off with relative ease. The behavior is automatically activated and tends to run off as soon as relevant cues become available. It is hard to stop the behavior once it is initiated. And it is extremely difficult to alter an automatic behavior (Schneider & Shiffrin, 1977; Shiffrin & Schneider, 1977—also see Chapters 6 & 15). Once again, the James–Hebb rule is implicated. The amount of practice required to create automaticity would affect the level of the connection weights. Moreover, many units would be involved. Because of the very powerful connections, activation of any of the units involved would very likely result in activation of all of the others. This accounts for activation by relevant cues. Strong connection weights would make it very difficult to stop a behavior once it has begun, and make it even harder to alter any aspect of it. The remarkably complex behaviors that can become automatic are simply a function of the number of units trained. Thus, automaticity also emerges naturally from PDP functioning. Further, PDP can account for both types of automaticity identified by Bargh et al. (2012). As far as a PDP system is concerned, it does not matter whether the practice is focused and conscious (postconscious automaticity) or implicit and unconscious (preconscious automaticity). All that matters is that connection weights be increased through practice.

Stimulus-and-response generalizations are other properties that emerge from PDP systems (see McClelland et al., 1986, chap. 1). To the extent that a new pattern is similar to a previously learned one, it will activate a similar set of units. The result of this activation is to extend responding appropriate to one pattern to other, similar patterns. A generalization gradient is therefore also a natural consequence of PDP. That is, the more similar to one another two things are, the more similar will be the response to both of them. As their similarities lessen, so will the similarity of responding to them. This is due to the fact that as similarity lessens, so does commonality or overlap of processing units. This means that people will react similarly to similar things in proportion to their similarity. This is usually an adaptive way to respond to the stimuli the world presents to us. Stimulus generalization flows directly out of course coding and the James–Hebb rule. No complex interpretations or translations of stimuli from one form to another are required. There is no need for a special set of processors that compares input to some standard. It is another byproduct of PDP functioning.

Human cognition constantly and automatically corrects for the errors that are endemic to our interactions with our environment. We seem to effortlessly fill in blanks and correct mistakes. Think of all of the errors of speech we hear daily, all of the incomplete sentences we have to make sense of. Although these tasks do not constitute a problem for the human information processing system, computer programmers have been struggling to find a way to handle them for decades. We still cannot carry on an extended verbal conversation with a computer despite its superior speed and computational capabilities.

Filling in of missing values and correcting for minor mistakes flows naturally from the James-Hebb rule. When any units are activated, this will automatically increase the likelihood that other units they are strongly connected to (i.e., that they have strong connection weights with) will also be activated. These other units often represent the missing information. So, if we hear an unfinished sentence or one with a word incorrectly placed, we finish it or place the word in its correct location. If I write or say, "The rain in Spain falls mainly on the plan (sic)," we know the correct word is *plain*. We may even believe that that is what we read or heard. If we catch a glimpse of someone familiar to us, we fill in what we did not see and correctly identify her.

This is true not only for words and person recognition. It is a fact of all perception. Almost a century ago, Gestalt psychologists (e.g., Koffka, 1922) recognized our tendency to complete incomplete objects and to fill in blanks to as to create meaningful wholes. For example, observe the following stimuli presented in Figure 20.1.

You almost cannot help but fill them in and see them as a square and a circle. If I show you CAƬ, you see the pattern following the A as a T because it completes the word CAT. But if I show you LOVƂ, you are likely to see the same pattern as an E because then it completes the familiar word LOVE. These rules have consistently been utilized by creative vanity plate owners. For example, one of our graduate students had a license plate that read: Phd2b. (For more on the commonalities of Gestalt psychology and PDP, see Holyoak & Spellman, 1993.)

Our tendency to fill in is not always advantageous to us. We can misidentify someone who resembles a person we are familiar with as that person. We have a hard time noticing typos despite our most diligent efforts. Proofreading is difficult because we fill in correct words and letters. We cannot stop the James–Hebb rule from operating. It is out of our control and (not so parenthetically) unconscious. This is an area where computers are far superior to us. (Thank God for spell check.)

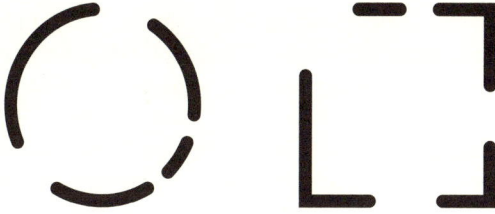

FIGURE 20.1. Filling in incomplete figures.

Yet another emergent property is what has been termed "content-addressable memory" (Hinton et al., 1986, chap. 3). Content-addressable memory is related to the filling in of missing values. People can recall events from partial descriptions and even from associatively related events. They can do this even if some parts of the partial description are wrong. For example, if I ask a baseball fan, "Who broke Babe Ruth's record of 719 home runs?," she will have a relatively easy time telling me that it was Henry Aaron and that he finished his career with 755 home runs. This will happen even though Babe Ruth only hit 714 home runs and every baseball fan knows that. (Of course, she might correct me, but she will still get the answer right.) This property is extremely difficult to implement on a computer because items are stored in specific locations known as addresses. Just one minor mistake, as we all know to our sorrow, and a computer will fail to retrieve what we are looking for.

In a PDP system, a memory, in fact a representation of any kind, does not have a physical existence anywhere in the system (Hinton et al., 1986, chap. 3). Rather than being stored, memories are actually re-created every time they are called up. (The same holds true for schemas and representations.) Memories can appear to be recalled because of permanent changes in connection weights, as specified by the James–Hebb rule. If one aspect of a memory is activated, the rest is likely to be as well. This explains content-addressable memory. It also explains the notorious unreliability of memory. Rather than existing as permanent engrams, they are constructed just like any other sort of representation. In fact, as far as a PDP system is concerned, there is no difference between a schema, a representation, and a memory. All are constructed through changes in connection weights as specified by the James–Hebb rule. Memories are not copies of events, like videos. Each time we recall something, we reconstruct it. Whatever cues are available at the time participate in this reconstruction by activating extra units. So do representations having units in common with those of the memory. These factors can modify and even distort the memory. There is no sharp distinction between an accurate, genuine memory and a plausible recon-struction. At least since the time of Bartlett (1932), we have known that memory is plastic in this way. Subsequent studies have confirmed this (Carlston & Smith, 1996; Neisser, 1981; van Gelder, 1991). (See Loftus, 2017, and Schacter, 2001, for reviews of this work.) The problem with eyewitness testimony is a perfect example of this plasticity (see Malpass & Koehnken, 1996, and Howe & Knott, 2015, for reviews). All of this flows naturally from PDP tenets and all of it is unconscious. Here PDP can account for implicit memory much as it does for implicit learning. It is about connection weights, constraint satisfaction, and context.[4]

THE DYNAMICS OF PDP: CONSTRAINT SATISFACTION AND THE SETTLING OF THE SYSTEM

Each unit in a PDP system can be part of a vast number of possible rep-resentations. Further, the units are highly and intricately interconnected. In fact, it is theoretically possible that every single unit in the system will be affected by any event to some degree. The entire PDP system can be conceptualized as a single huge meta-representation in which all previ-ously experienced and innate patterns are superposed onto one another. This would make a PDP system one big uninterpretable mush ball (see Smith, 1996).

If this were all there were to a PDP system, it would never be able to resolve its input into anything coherent or meaningful. Fortunately, differences in unit connection weights, both positive and negative, save it from this fate. Certain units are very unlikely to activate in tandem because they inhibit one another. Other units are almost certain to co-activate because their connection weights are highly positive. And there is everything in between. Mutually inhibitory and excitatory connec-tions limit the possible patterns of activation. In the parlance of PDP, they constrain the possible conclusions a PDP system can reach or the solutions it can arrive at. They are therefore termed *"constraints"* (see Westen & Gabbard, 2002). External stimulation and internal states of the system provide further constraints by causing the activation of some and inhibiting the activation of other units. These constraints further delimit possible PDP solutions. Each unit in the system may be con-ceptualized as a minipremise that, if true, increases the likelihood of other minipremises being true. At the same time, if the minipremise is true, the likelihood of still other minipremises being true is diminished. Minipremises that are likely to covary have positive connection weights; those likely to be false if the original minipremise is true have nega-tive connection weights. An example may make this clearer. If it is day (premise 1), the probability of seeing the sun (premise 2) is increased, whereas the likelihood of seeing the moon (premise 3) is decreased. A PDP system traffics in much smaller premises than this but that is the idea.

Let us set the PDP system in motion to see how this can work. Assume that an external stimulus has impinged upon someone's visual sense receptors and has activated some PDP input units. Activation of these units will then change the probability that other units (input, hidden, and output) will be activated. These units, in turn, will affect other units and so on throughout the system. Other environmental events, recent history, and contemporaneous internal states will add to this mix by also activating and inhibiting units. The probability of each of these units becoming activated or inhibited will be a function of their various connection weights.

Let us be more concrete. Say the object impinging upon the person's visual receptors consists largely of straight lines. PDP units representing straightness will then become activated. Other units related to the property of straightness in that person's experience (e.g., stationary) now are more likely to become activated. If something is composed of unmoving straight lines, it is unlikely to be curved or moving. Units related to curvature and movement therefore become inhibited. I (JW) am in my office, at my desk typing. I am concerned about how my co-author and the book audience will react to this example. Units related to these factors are also activated; those negatively related to my location, activity, and mood are inhibited. These effects, in turn, cause excitation and inhibition of yet other units. Finally, I tentatively reveal that I perceive a file cabinet to my left (which has straight lines and is stationary).

In this example, there were only a few constraints. In the actual operation of a PDP system, there is an enormously large number of them. The PDP system must sort it all out by iteratively seeking to satisfy all of the constraints it encounters (Rumelhart & McClelland, 1986, chap. 4). This takes some time but finally (typically in a second or less), a coherent pattern of activation emerges. The system is said to "*settle*" into a solution.

The particular solution the system settles into can be thought of as the intersection of the units that remains active when all of the excitatory and inhibitory activity has run its course (see Hinton et al., 1986, chap. 3). The overall pattern of stably active units captures what the "settled" system is representing. This can be a perception, a memory, a wish, a behavior, and so on (Rumelhart et al., 1986, chap. 2). In order to reach this kind of steady state of activation in 1 second or less, which is the time period required for most human operations, the system can only cycle about 100 times (the 100-step rule). This means that many of the constraints the system encounters must be satisfied simultaneously (Rumelhart et al., 1986).

Constraints in the human environment do not complement one another neatly and perfectly so as to allow for a single unambiguous solution. The system must therefore equilibrate to a solution that satisfies as many constraints as possible as completely as possible. It must try to achieve the best match possible at a particular point in time (McClelland et al., 1986, chap. 1). The better the match, the more stable the equilibrium reached by the system when it settles (Norman, 1986, chap. 26). But the match is never perfect. The best match is therefore the one that violates the microinferences represented by the constraints less than alternative matches do (Hinton et al., 1986, chap 3). It is a kind of compromise.

IMPLICATIONS OF PDP FOR UNCONSCIOUS PROCESSING

The fact that there is no one neat solution to the settling of a PDP system (no perfect match) has implications for unconscious processes not usually addressed (at least explicitly) by PDP theorists. In general, it seems that multiple solutions are attempted before the system settles on any one of them. We have no conscious access to any of these prior rejected solutions, but that does not mean that they did not exist or played no role in processing or in behavior. For example, Hinton et al. (1986, chap. 3) offered a PDP explanation for our capacity to choose the correct meaning of polysemous words. They suggested that the graphemic string we see (e.g., *bank*) will affect the input sememe (meaning) units required to activate both meanings. The constraints of a sentence in which the string is embedded, however (syntactic features), and/or the perceiver's location and recent history (he may be by a cash machine or in a boat on a river) will strongly activate units related to one of those meanings. Activation of that meaning will then suppress or inhibit activation of the other meaning (see Kawamoto & Anderson, 1984). This means that both meanings became available but that one of them was eventually suppressed. The perceiver does not recall that both solutions were briefly available or that one was suppressed because it all happens so quickly and all of it happens unconsciously. All she is left with is the solution the system ultimately settled upon.

If we could intervene and look at the system before the final suppression, we should see that both solutions are active. And that may be just what Marcel (1983a, 1983b) did. By presenting polysemous words subliminally, the constraints that usually lead to choosing just one of their meanings may not have been active (see Chapter 7). In terms of the Hinton et al. example, neither meaning may have been activated strongly enough to suppress the other. Both therefore were equally influential. PDP thereby provides a sensible scaffolding for Marcel's (1983b) shoot-first-and-ask-questions-later model of processing (see Chapter 8). A similar process may account for Spence's (1964; Spence & Bressler, 1962; Spence & Holland, 1962) findings (see Chapter 6). The sememe units related to the word *cheese* may have been activated by subliminal presentations of that word or by its presence in a word list. This made associated words easier to recall until the critical word itself emerged and constrained that recall. Thus, PDP may offer an understanding of the restricting effects of awareness.

As long as we are speculating, the tip-of-the tongue phenomenon (TOT) may be amenable to a similar explanation. In TOT (Brown, 1991, 2012), we remember associates of the word or name we are trying to recall but not the word itself. Possibly we have activated the sememe units ("I know he's a playwright"; "He was married to a movie star") and some of the grapheme units ("There's an *M* in his name"), but the system has not yet settled on a solution. We can feel the system striving to satisfy these constraints. We have everything but final closure: Arthur Miller, a playwright once married to the movie star Marilyn Monroe.

The lack of perfect matches in the settling of a PDP system suggests other implications rarely addressed by PDP theorists. These may be more far-reaching and systemic than those offered above. Constraints may not simply fail to fit perfectly; they can, in principle, be orthogonal, contradictory, and even oppositional. This means that conflict is an inherent part of PDP. PDP will try to satisfy as many constraints as possible, blending them together as best as the system can (Cleeremans, 2014; Maia & Cleeremans, 2005). Sometimes this will work just fine and sometimes no solution will fit very well. This means compromise is also central to PDP functioning. Such compromises may be minor, but it is also possible that major compromises may be required if any solution is to be found. If some constraints are simply ignored or seriously bent to fit the compromise, then distortion of the instigating event can result. For instance, we know from the trauma literature (e.g., Resick, Monson, & Chard, 2017) that one possible consequence of suffering a traumatic event may be the formation of certain pervasive and automatic negative beliefs about ourselves (e.g., "It was my fault for being raped"; "I must have invited it"; "I deserve to be punished"; and many other iterations of similar automatic thoughts). This phenomenon can also be explained in terms of conflicting constraints. As Resick, et al. (2017) point out, in such a traumatic situation, our mind may struggle to reconcile a belief in a just world—one where good things happen to good people—and a healthy sense of self—How can I see myself as good if something terrible happened to me? In other words, the traumatized mind feels locked between two options: seeing the world as one where random horrible things can happen to good people or seeing oneself as bad and deserving of whatever trauma and suffering were inflicted on one. In the latter compromise, at least the world can still be seen as having some predictability. We sacrifice ourselves in order to gain a sense of control and avoid seeing the world as randomly horrific, with no rhyme or reason. (Of course, these are not the only two options for making sense of a trauma, but they are commonly found in individuals who develop PTSD after a traumatic event.) And, finally, no matter what, a stable equilibrium is never really reached by the system because we do not live in a static world. The system is constantly in flux and only relatively stable for brief periods. This means that the system must be able to tolerate a chronic ambiguity. All of these events occur unconsciously. We are unaware of conflicting constraints, relative goodness of compromise, or the instability and ambiguity of equilibrium.

If all of the above is true, important implications follow. These have not been emphasized because most of the work in PDP has, so far, concerned perception, memory, and language. Mild distortions and compromises in such processes are theoretically meaningful but practically trivial. In real-world functioning, however, people have goals, concerns, affects, moods, and motives. They also have relationships with other people. The situations they encounter are complex, often ambiguous, and personally meaningful. In PDP terms, all of these should function as constraints that influence the solution the system settles into. Smith (1996) made a similar point but did not follow it with a discussion of the implications.

First, as Westen and Gabbard (2002) realized, the mind is not only cognitively and perceptually self-regulating, it is also affectively self-regulating. This means that the solutions a PDP system settles into are as constrained by conscious and unconscious internal psychological states as they are by the physical stimulation impinging from outside. This opens up New Look (see Chapter 5) research to new interpretations. Perceptual defense and vigilance can be understood as efforts to satisfy the affective constraints aroused by the stimulation in concert with the physical constraints of the stimulus. For those who are defensive, units related to affect inhibit those related to perception. These individuals therefore required longer presentations to make out threatening stimuli. Vigilant individuals, in contrast, have positive connection weights between affective and perceptual units. They therefore quickly recognized threatening stimuli. Issues of response bias fall by the wayside in this analysis. Positive and negative connection weights are response biases by definition. The phenomenon, far from being mysterious, is easily handled by PDP precepts.

PDP can also be considered a psychodynamic model of the mind. It has conflict and compromise built in, and it is never static. Moreover, all of its operations occur unconsciously. It is as much an unconscious dynamic model of the mind as were Herbart's (1824, 1834/1850) or Freud's (1900, 1915, 1923). Westen and Gabbard (2002) explicitly made the connection between PDP and psychoanalysis. If we assume unconscious affective and motivational constraints, if we further assume that such constraints are at least as powerful as perceptual and environmental constraints, many psychoanalytic tenets can flow naturally from PDP principles. These include defense, symptomatology, transference, and the ameliorative effects of psychotherapy. Defense and symptomatology are simply compromises between affective and environmental constraints. We have already determined that constraints may not allow for good fits and that the compromise the system settles into need not be optimally adaptive.

Symptoms and defenses fall under this heading. Transference simply refers to units that were originally connected and strengthened, via the James–Hebb rule, during early interpersonal interactions. These units still form an important part of all PDP systems activated in interpersonal interactions. Andersen (1999) has conducted research on transference that connects responses to early interpersonal cues with current interpersonal relations. Psychotherapy (be it psychodynamic or otherwise) involves changing connection weights (instantiated as associative connections discovered in the treatment) so that the solutions the systems settle into will be more adaptive and satisfying.

EVALUATION OF PDP MODELS

We have been writing of the dynamics of PDP systems, as do PDP theorists, as though they had volitional aspects (e.g., "It tries to reach the best match"). But the process of settling into a solution is anything but volitional. It is simply a by-product of the interactions of qualitatively and quantitatively different connections. Some connections are positive (excitatory) and some are negative (inhibitory). Some are more excitatory or inhibitory than others. And there are an awful lot of these connections. The arithmetic solution to this mélange of connection weights provides the wherewithal for settling the system. There is no executive or homunculus directing the process. There is no need for psychoanalytic conceptions like psychic energy or hypothetical entities like id, ego, and superego. Psychic energy can be subsumed under connection weight, and Freud's mental agencies can simply be thought of as shorthand description for internal, environmental, and societal constraints. PDP models do not need conceptions like Herbart's (1824, 1850) competing ideas or Janet's (1920; Kihlstrom, 1984; Perry & Laurence, 1984) automatisms (see Chapters 2 and 3). They do not need the stored representations and schemas posited by traditional cognitive psychology (e.g., Goldstein, 2011) or by the representation theory of Fodor and Pylshyn (2015). Instead, the settling of the PDP system is simply another emergent property of the PDP units and the James–Hebb rule. The system operates automatically and unconsciously.

The kinds of PDP properties I have described led to many positive, even effusive reactions to the PDP enterprise. PDP models have been hailed as a new cognitive revolution (Clark, 1993; Ramsey, Stitch, & Garon, 1991; Schneider, 1987). The two volumes edited by Rumelhart, McClelland, et al. (1986) have taken on almost mystical overtones and have been referred to as "the PDP bible" (Smith, 1996).

To be fair, not everyone is thrilled with PDP thinking. Fodor and Pylyshyn (1988) as well as Pinker and Prince (1988) have offered trenchant critiques. Additionally, PDP has not yet come close to successfully modeling genuinely complex and meaningful psychological phenomena. There are few experiments that actually test its predictions. The work thus far consists largely of computer simulations of relatively simple processes and metaphorical use of PDP tenets to account for complex phenomena (as we have done here). Nonetheless, reference to and use of PDP models grew rapidly. If it realizes even a portion of the potential being predicted, it will be a truly remarkable achievement. And, for our purposes, it shows how unconscious processes have become so uncontroversial that there is no longer a need to justify positing them. They are now part of the accepted canon in these models. Formerly contentious research like the New Look and subliminal priming fit easily into current conceptions like PDP. Even controversial, psychoanalytic tenets may not be far behind (see Westen & Gabbard, 2002).

MASSIVE MODULARITY VERSUS PDP: WHAT TO DO?

We seem to have two incompatible models of the brain/mind in massive modularity and PDP. Massive modularity is awash in rule-driven functioning. Each module has a set of evolutionarily based rules that control and constrain its operation. The functioning of each module is carried out relatively locally, with possibly some central area where the various independently operating modules can meet and confer. PDP, on the other hand, is practically rule-free. The model is entirely based on the operation of units (made up of groups of neurons) and the situation that activates those units. PDP operations are all, or virtually all, empirically based. Functioning is based on which units happen to be activated. And the particular units that are activated literally depend upon experience. Constraints are not rule-driven or due to separate units processing information independently of one another. Constraints are based on patterns of activation, which are a product of experience or environmental conditions. Processing in PDP is distributed throughout the mind/brain rather than locally as in massive modularity. The only thing the two models seem to have in common is that, in both, processing occurs in parallel rather than serially. How do we choose between them? Must we choose? Is there an alternative? Is there a way to reconcile them? We don't have to. No. Kind of. We think so.

ISSUES WITH MASSIVE MODULARITY

If we look at the literature, we see that each model has weaknesses, often pointed out by the alternative model (cf. McClelland & Patterson, 2002; Pinker & Mehler, 1988; Pinker & Ulman, 2002). Let's start with criticisms of massive modularity. The brain/mind shows evidence of context effects (Rogers & McClelland, 2014; Rumelhart, 1977). This is one of the central tenets of PDP but hard to explain by a model (massive modularity) that says that modules operate independently of one another. Next, what are deemed modules often share anatomical parts with other modules. M. L. Anderson (2010, 2014) has pointed out that the degree of localization and specialization required by massive modularity may not exist (also see Poldrack, 2006). Rather, many structures in the brain/mind are activated by varied tasks and experiences. What we see are overlapping rather than isolable structures. Prinz (2006) may have provided the most trenchant critique of this aspect of massive modularity. He goes after the factor most cited as corroboration for massive modularity, the specificity of brain damage and neuroimaging studies. He cites evidence indicating that the results of these studies are often inconsistent. Reports are usually based on single-person findings that have fortuitously come to the attention of the researcher. It is not easy and sometimes not ethical to find large groups of people with the same deficit. This means conclusions are based on the brain structure of very few individuals and replication is nigh on impossible. These individual findings (they can be considered case studies) are then generalized to the entire human race. Another problem is that the researcher assumes localization and then searches for it. Whatever he finds that is wrong or damaged in the brain is then implicated as uniquely causing the deficit. But well-known deficits, argues Prinz, are often associated with lesions in very different parts of the brain. Additionally, lesions in the same area of the brain can have different effects in different individuals. Finally, similar brain areas are active during many different tasks so that a lesion in one specific area often produces multiple deficits. This should not be the case in a specialized, modular brain. Prinz also concluded that neuroimaging studies often turn up large-scale networks rather than the small, localized regions called for by massive modularity. For example, researchers do not agree on the exact location of Broca's area, which is supposed to underlie language production (Poeppel, 1996). Pulvermuller (1999) found that every lobe of the brain seems to be involved in some aspect of language production. Further, these networks are also often spatially distributed rather than localized. It seems that neural networks (it is hard to call them "modules" anymore if these criticisms are accurate) are not as local, specialized, domain-specific, encapsulated, inaccessible, and innate as massive modularity would have it.

There are also logical problems with massive modularity (Fodor, 2000). How can a massively modular brain/mind assign a problem to the correct module? It is also hard to understand how a massively modular brain/mind could solve novel, abstract, or general problems. A fixed architecture with rigid rules of functioning simply would not be flexible enough. Perhaps the general workspace is where both assignment and intermodular problem solving takes place, but then that workspace cannot itself be modular.

ISSUES WITH PDP

PDP has also been trenchantly critiqued. Many of these critiques can be found in a book edited by Pinker and Mehler (1988). Even though the book is 30 years old, the criticisms still hold up. More recently, M. L. Anderson (2010) provided some more current critiques. PDP offers a very plastic view of mind/brain functioning. Taken to its logical conclusion, this would indicate that everyone would evidence a different organization of the brain/mind attributable to differences in their experiences. There should be cultural differences in brain organization as well if PDP tenets are to be believed. Instead, we find cross-cultural and interpersonal regularities across brains. Additionally, if units have the kind of flexibility attributed to them by PDP, people would have an almost infinite capacity to adjust and change. This is clearly not the case. Finally, just on a concrete level, if neural units are as flexible as PDP asserts, then circuits underlying different functions ought to be relatively localized, as expected by massive modularity but for a different reason. Maintaining long-distance connections would use up more energy than would short-distance connections. Since all neurons are basically the same, we should expect networks to be short-distance affairs so as to save said energy. But networks are distributed, a quality acknowledged in the very name of the model: parallel *distributed* processing. Finally, the appeal of PDP is in its simplicity (conceptually) and the way many brain/mind functions can be derived from its tenets. But the model has yet to deliver on truly complex behavior, whereas massive modularity has tackled big issues.

NOW WHAT?

Although both massive modularity and PDP can be powerfully critiqued, each has something to offer. Putting those things together may get us to a more viable model of brain/mind functioning. We believe such an integration has been offered in the form of neural reuse. Several neural reuse models exist. The main ones for our purposes are the <u>neuronal recycling hypothesis</u> (Dehaene & Cohen, 2007), the <u>neural exploitation hypothesis</u> (Gallese, 2003a, 2003b, 2007; Gallese & Lakoff, 2005), and the <u>massive redeployment hypothesis</u> (M. L. Anderson, 2010, 2014). The latter is the most comprehensive, in our opinion, so we embed the others in it while pointing out significant differences among them.

We next review neural reuse and indicate how it addresses the weaknesses of massive modularity and connectionism. Then we will attempt to employ some of its tenets to address those weaknesses and create a new model that we think captures what is important in each and that can hold up. We think this can underlie the findings we have presented about unconscious processes and generate important clinical implications. It is particularly relevant to what has come to be called embodied cognition (Lakoff, 2012, 2014), which is currently generating a lot of research and theory and which is rife with clinical implications—see Chapter 17.

NOTES

1. See the McGurk effect (McGurk & MacDonald, 1976), a perceptual phenomenon in which the perception of a sound changes based on the visual stimulus it is paired with.
2. This is a neurophysiological expression of the old doctrine of associationism. Systematic exposition of this view goes back at least to Locke (1690/1975) and Hume (1738/1975).

3. Such patterns need not be limited to concrete representations or schemas like restaurants or conferences. In principle, they could include abstract concepts like truth and beauty. These kinds of abstract conceptions could have developed exactly as concrete representations did, namely through repeated experiences that have something central in common.

4. The often acrimonious debate over so-called repressed memories may owe some of its contradictory findings to a failure to understand content-addressable memory in a PDP manner. Memories are neither invariably true nor invariably false; they are constructions. They can be constructed out of whole cloth, given the right inputs (e.g., Loftus, 1997). They can also represent genuine events with minimal distortions (e.g., Davies & Frawley, 1994).

CHAPTER 21

From Exaptation to Neural Reuse

Neural reuse models rely, in part, on the evolutionary principle of exaptation, introduced into the literature by Gould and Vrba (1982). *Exaptation* refers to co-opting a structure or characteristic to perform a function it did not originally evolve to do. This can come about in one of two ways. One is that a characteristic or structure evolved for one reason but came, over evolutionary time, to serve another. A well-known example is feathers. It is believed that they first evolved for temperature regulation. Later, they were adapted (exapted) for flight. The second type of exaptation is when a characteristic or structure that exists independently of natural selection (just happens to be there, so to speak) is co-opted for an adaptation enhancing use. An example of this kind of exaptation was first identified by Darwin (1859/2002; cf. Gould & Vrba, 1982). Mammalian skulls have sutures or fibrous joints at birth. This allows for some elasticity of the skull, which, as Darwin put it, is "a beautiful adaptation for aiding parturition." But, as Darwin also realized, sutures are also present in the skulls of birds and reptiles as they emerge from their eggs. There is no need for skull flexibility in these animals. So, as Darwin continued, "we may infer that this structure has arisen from the laws of growth, and has been taken advantage of in the parturition of the higher animals" (p. 197). Thus, unfused sutures in newborn mammals, although very useful structures, are not an adaptation because they were not built by selection pressures to function as they do in mammals. They existed fortuitously and as long as they are taken advantage of by evolution, they too are exaptations. This is a useful concept because it allows for a kind of evolutionary shortcut. Rather than evolve a whole new structure, an existing structure is recruited for the needed function (see

M. L. Anderson, 2010, 2014). It also avoids the term *pre-adaptation* that was in use (Bock, 1959; Mayr, 1960) and which suggests a kind of teleology to evolutionary changes (Gould & Vrba, 1982). Now let us turn this to the brain/mind.

M. L. ANDERSON'S MASSIVE REDEPLOYMENT HYPOTHESIS

We believe that M. L. Anderson's massive redeployment hypothesis (2010, 2014) provides the most comprehensive framework for neural reuse models. The core principle of this model is that neural circuits established for one purpose, through evolution, are often exapted by the same evolution or by normal development and put to other uses. But they also retain their original functions. Hence, neural circuits serve multiple roles (hence neural reuse) including their original purpose. These multiple-use circuits are relatively low level rather than the modules dedicated to high-level functioning posited by massive modularity. The low-level dedicated circuits posited by neural reuse are used and then reused for various purposes in different cognitive and task domains. This leads to a differentiation between what are called "workings" and "uses."

Workings and Uses

The terms workings and uses was introduced by Bergeron (2008). Anderson's neural reuse theory makes considerable use of these conceptions. The *working* of a brain/mind structure or network is what it does. It is the low-level operation (computation) it performs. Workings are set and immutable, based on evolutionary history, and have a fixed anatomical location. A use refers to what the structure (working) can be used for. A *use* refers to the high-level operation to which the circuit makes a contribution, of which it is a part. A use can be spread out throughout the brain/mind depending upon which workings contribute to it. Many workings can be and are combined to create a new use over evolutionary or developmental time.

Contrasting the Massive Redeployment Hypothesis with Massive Modularity and Connectionism

The aforementioned conceptions of exaptation, workings, and uses and the neural reuse they support lead to several predictions. First, high-level operations should be largely comprised of combinations of low-level neural circuitry rather than independently evolved modules. Next, we would predict that a typical brain region would support (be exapted for) many brain/mind functions, across many task categories. The individual workings would perform a similar calculation or information-processing operation in each of the different functions of which they are a part. What would differentiate these higher-level functions from one another would be the combination of workings that make up each (use). This means that *patterns of neural co-activation distinguish between functions (uses) more than localized brain regions (workings) do.* Next, the older a brain function (the earlier it appeared in evolutionary time), the more localized its components (workings) should be. Relatedly, the more recent a function, the more spread out across the brain (more distributed rather than localized) its components should be. So, more recent functions (uses) should be characterized by more and more widely scattered brain areas than are evolutionarily older functions. This is because the later a function developed in evolutionary time, the more likely it is that there would be existing neural circuits that could be exapted for that function. And there is no a priori reason to suppose that the workings exapted into a use reside next to one another. They could be anywhere in the brain. Related to this, there ought to be a correlation between the phylogenetic age of a brain area (working) and the frequency with which it appears in different cognitive functions (uses). This is because the older that part of the brain, the more opportunities it would have and therefore the more likely it would be to become part of later developing brain/mind functions.

Neural reuse differs from both massive modularity and connectionism, occupying a middle position between them. In neural reuse, the units of the brain/mind are workings, not modules. Unless a working is somehow redefined as a module (or mini-module), this is antithetical to massive modularity. Even if we change the definition of module to the low-level functions characterized by workings (and get closer to what Fodor had in mind), modules in a massively modular brain/mind ought to be local and not distributed. Finally, in the massively modular brain/mind, sharing of neuronal networks should not be the norm, if it exists at all.

In PDP, there are no workings, no set operations of groups of neurons, as this would impinge on the flexibility that makes connectionism so radical and interesting. Instead, neurons are connected because they happen to fire together often enough to result in a meaningful connection weight. And if all neurons are essentially the same and their organization is a product of experience, as connectionism avers, it would make economic sense for the neurons of a function to be relatively tightly grouped rather than distributed. This would save the energy cost of connecting the units across great brain distances.

There are also differences between neural reuse and the other models in their understanding of the flexibility of the brain/mind. Neural reuse agrees with connectionism that the brain/mind is a network but posits more a priori organization to that network than does connectionism. The fact that the operations of the workings do not change means that there are limits to the uses they can be put to and to the operation of said uses. So the system is not as plastic as is a connectionist mind/brain. Neural reuse agrees with massive modularity that there is an a priori organization to the mind/brain. But the functioning of the neural reuse mind/brain is more flexible than is hypothesized by massive modularity because its a priori units are lower level and because of the many ways that they can be reused and combined.

EMPIRICAL SUPPORT FOR NEURAL REUSE

Prinz's (2006) critique of modularity (summarized earlier) questioned the veracity of localization by citing evidence showing that functions are distributed throughout the brain and that areas often cited as performing a unique function actually perform many. These same data can be cited in support of neural reuse. M. L. Anderson, Kinnison, and Pessoa (2013) provide more recent data that support this argument. In addition, M. L. Anderson (2008) looked at co-activation patterns in the brain (which brain regions were likely to act together under which task conditions) and found that different tasks were characterized by different patterns of co-activation among the regions of the brain. Further, there is not an obvious connection between tasks that seemed to impinge on one another. For example, there is cognitive interference between language and motor control (Glenberg & Kaschak, 2002) and between memory and audition (Baddeley & Hitch, 1974), suggesting that these apparently unrelated functions have some neural components in common such that when a working or set of workings is activated in one of them, it is harder to do the other because that working is already "occupied." But it is not always interference. Glenberg et al. (2007) reported that manipulating objects can aid in reading comprehension, suggesting some underlying neuronal connection between these two apparently independent operations. These data support neural reuse over massive modularity. M. L. Anderson (2010, 2014) also reports data that indicate that the more recently evolved a function, the more its neuronal underpinnings are scattered throughout the brain. This goes against both massive modularity and connectionism but is right in line with neural reuse. There are also data that seem to specifically support neural reuse over connectionism. As we discussed earlier, there is cross-cultural invariance in the neurophysiological locations of many acquired practices. This should vary from person to person and from culture to culture if connectionism is correct, but it does not.

Probably the most impressive evidence favoring neural reuse is contained in the Neuro-Image based Co-Activation Matrix (NICAM) database (*www.agcognition.org/projects.html*). This is a project organized and maintained by Anderson and Chaovalitwongse that compiles fMRI studies and applies data mining and graph theory to investigate functional cooperation between brain regions (M. L. Anderson, Brumbaugh, & Suben, 2010). As of 2010, this database contained 2,603 studies from 824 journal articles (M. L. Anderson, 2010). The analytic strategy is to subtract whole-brain activity generated by an experimental task from whole-brain activity assessed during a control task. In this way, whatever the two tasks have in common gets subtracted out. What is left (the result) represents the brain region(s) that uniquely underlie(s) the experimental task. The results of these calculations indicate that regions of the brain tend to be reused across tasks. Thus, there is powerful, replicated, evidence that neural reuse occurs.

Neural reuse seems a viable model. And massive redeployment seems a useful way of conceptualizing it. There are some missing pieces, however, that we believe can be filled in by other neural reuse models, specifically the neuronal recycling model of Dehaene (Dehaene & Cohen, 2007) and the neural exploitation hypothesis of Gallese and Lakoff (Gallese, 2007; Gallese & Lakoff, 2005). The former fills in the role of development and experience; the latter focuses on metaphor and on embodied cognition (although massive redeployment also predicts and explains embodied cognition). We first outline those models and then try to determine whether and how they fit with massive modularity and connectionism.

DEHAENE'S NEURONAL RECYCLING HYPOTHESIS

The massive redeployment hypothesis focuses on evolutionary exaptation. M. L. Anderson (2010) did not deny that neural reuse occurs as part of development, contributes to learning, and may underlie functions that could not have been a part of our phylogenetic history (like reading, writing, music, and math), but this was not his main interest. He is primarily interested in evolutionary exaptation (M. L. Anderson, 2010, 2014). But there is a model of neural reuse that deals with functions that develop over our lifetimes rather than over evolutionary time. This neuronal recycling hypothesis (Dehaene & Cohen, 2007) focuses on processes that allow people to acquire capacities that could not have been the direct result of evolution. Reading, for example, is a cultural invention that cannot be a product of evolution. Abilities like reading (and writing) emerged too recently for evolution to have generated neural circuits specialized for them. These cultural abilities have to be learned by each and every one of us. Therefore, the brain structures that support them must be assigned and/or shaped during individual development. There is no way for a massive modularity model to account for this. A connectionist model would just aver that this is another example of the overall plasticity of the brain/mind. But the evidence indicates that the same brain circuits are associated with reading interindividually and cross-culturally (Dehaene & Cohen, 2007). Connectionism would have a hard time with this uniformity, as we discussed above.

Neuronal recycling argues that learned functions like reading and writing develop by utilizing and reconfiguring already existing brain circuitry. That is, these cognitive functions find circuits (workings) that can be co-opted for their use. So, this model argues for exaptation that occurs outside of and much more quickly than evolution. Since workings are the product of evolution and are therefore innate, there are constraints on what can be learned and how it can be learned. In a nutshell, cultural inventions make use of evolutionarily older brain circuits to support new skills but necessarily inherit many of their constraints. This has epistemological implications. Our knowledge and ability to obtain knowledge depend upon the tractability (or lack thereof) of these reused circuits.

The neuronal recycling brain/mind is more plastic than is that of massive modularity since it is a neural reuse model. Its plasticity is a result of an ability to exapt over the life span as well as over evolutionary time so it is also more plastic than massive redeployment. But it is not as plastic as connectionism since exaptations require the use of and are constrained by evolutionarily based structures (workings).

METAPHORS AND EMBODIED COGNITION: THE NEURONAL EXPLOITATION MODEL

The final (and probably most controversial) neural reuse model we discuss is the neuronal exploitation model of Gallese and Lakoff (Gallese, 2007; Gallese & Lakoff, 2005). What is relevant about this model for our purposes is that it emphasizes and provides an explanation for embodied cognition, which we reviewed in Chapter 18. M. L. Anderson's (2010, 2014) massive redeployment hypothesis also discusses and predicts embodied cognition, but the neuronal exploitation model is centered on it and on metaphor. To describe this model, we have to journey from Lakoff's early work on metaphor through his later work on metaphor and embodied cognition through the discovery of what were termed "mirror neurons" by Gallese and others. This work began with conceptual metaphor theory, developed into neural metaphor theory, and, finally, into the neural exploitation hypothesis. Embodied cognition as a form of neural reuse underlies the latter two models; mirror neurons are central to the neural exploitation hypothesis.

Decades ago, Lakoff (Lakoff & Johnson, 1980a) began to systematically study metaphor and presciently realized its importance to understanding cognition in general (Lakoff, 2012, 2014; Lakoff & Johnson, 1999, review much of the development and results of this work). (Also see Chapter 18.) Before this seminal work, cognition was seen as involving the manipulation of arbitrary symbols or computations to represent real-world experience (e.g., Fodor, 1975; Fodor & Pylyshyn, 1988) and sometimes still is (e.g., Fodor & Pylyshyn, 2015). An example of such arbitrary mapping is an alphabet. There is no inherent reason that the letter *D* should have the look and sound that it does. Similarly, there is no necessary connection between the word *dog* and the animal it represents. But Lakoff and Johnson thought that the connection between realms of experience, which we call metaphor, was different. They wondered about the connection between intimacy and closeness, why a relationship is often conceptualized as a container, and how it is that purposes are often seen as destinations. They concluded that there are experiential connections between real-world experiences and these kinds of low-level conceptual metaphors. They pointed out that intimacy requires being physically close, relationships often involve (especially early in life) living in a common space, and to achieve a purpose, one often has to travel to a specific location. They then argued that these experience-based primitive metaphors combine to form complex metaphors like *Life is a journey*. Thus, the structure and logic of one domain of thinking guides or structures another domain of thinking. Metaphor is not arbitrary symbol making. It is a translation from one domain to another in a way that makes concrete, experiential sense.

This led to another, related question, namely how are metaphors mapped? How is the experience of one domain (physical experience, like closeness) mapped onto another domain (internal/subjective experience, like intimacy)? Is this mapping based on arbitrary symbolic representations, as was believed for basic cognition? That is, are the carriers of thought nonphysically based, abstract, logical, linguistic, or computational such that the relation between signifier and signified is arbitrary, like an alphabet (see Fodor, 1975; Fodor & Pylyshyn, 1988, 2015)? Are they built analogically from experience but still require a kind of translation from one form or representation to another (e.g., Bargh & Morsella, 2008; Boroditsky & Ramscar, 2002; Matlock, Ramscar, & Boroditsky,

2005; Williams et al., 2009)? Or are some of the same neural circuits used for both? And if the latter, what are these units? To use the terminology we have been employing, what workings have been exapted to the uses of higher-level cognition?

The answer, if this conceptualization is correct, is that our thoughts are largely tied to sensory and motor circuits (these are the workings). In other words, higher-order cognitive processes are tied to our perceptions and actions. They are not disembodied arbitrary symbols but are dependent upon bodily functions and so are literally embodied. And "embodied" is the term that came to represent this idea in the literature (see Chapter 18). It did not take long before this kind of thinking was extended from metaphors to all higher-level cognition.[1]

The exaptation of sensory and motor workings, central to the idea of embodied cognition, makes evolutionary sense. Before animals capable of reflection and of talking to one another could exist, their predecessors had to be able to sense the environment and react to it. They would not have survived otherwise. This means that sensory and motor circuits had to develop first. In fact, Brooks (1991) argues that most of animal evolution has been devoted to the development of these attributes. It is reasonable, from a neural reuse point of view, to suppose that it was mostly these sensorimotor circuits that were exapted to serve higher-level functions. If this is so, then animals evolved from sensing and moving to thinking, planning, and communicating through language (see Kiverstein, 2010).

In addition to logic, there are a great deal of data that support the exaptation of sensory and motor neurons to higher-level cognitive functioning. In fact, the whole literature on embodied cognition strongly supports this hypothesis. Early on, Damasio and his colleagues showed that when participants were asked to think about verbs, motor circuits in the brain were activated, whereas when they were asked to think about nouns, neural circuits dedicated to visual processing fired (Damasio & Tranel, 1993; Damasio, Everitt, & Bishop, 1996; Martin, Haxby, Lalonde, Wiggs, & Ungerleider, 1995; Martin, Wiggs, Ungerleider, & Haxby, 1996; Martin, Ungerleider, & Haxby, 2000). Thus, stimulating one domain of thinking (parts of speech) involved activating structures seemingly involved in another (sensory–visual and motor processing). Ekman, Levenson, and Friesen (1983) reported that anger results in raised skin temperature, elevated blood pressure, and interference with visual perception and fine motor control. Lakoff (1987) related this finding to emotional metaphors like boiling mad, blind with rage, etc., thereby demonstrating that emotional metaphors are related to the physiology of emotions. (Also see Kövecses, 2000, 2002.) Damasio et al. (1996) then found that the emotional bodily experiences reported by

Ekman et al. can be connected to somatosensory neural circuits. This suggests that emotions may actually be constituted by the bodily effects reported by Ekman et al. The metaphors examined by Lakoff and by Kövecses make sense as a reflection of these bodily states.[2]

There are now too many studies supporting an association between bodily and mental states to cite. It is, for all practical purposes, a truism and explains the current interest in and support of embodied cognition. (We reviewed this area, to some degree, in Chapter 18.) Lakoff (2014) cites and summarizes dozens of supportive studies. Here we mention a few that we believe relate to psychotherapy. In all, metaphors and behaviors evidence shared circuitry. Singer et al. (2004) reported that psychological and physical pain have neural circuits in common. The circuits that fired when a person was in physical pain were the same as those that fired when observing pain in a loved one. They fired to a lesser degree when observing the pain of a stranger. Zhong and Liljenquist (2006) had participants recall either a moral or an immoral act and then asked them to choose between a gift of a pencil or of antiseptic wipes. Those asked to recall an immoral act were more likely to choose the wipes. Perhaps more interesting, because of the parallels in the New Testament (Pontius Pilate) and Shakespeare (Lady Macbeth), participants who were given an opportunity to wash their hands were less likely to accede to a request for help. They had washed their hands of guilt/responsibility. In a study reviewed in Chapter 18, Williams and Bargh (2008a) reported that participants who held a warm cup of coffee were more likely to rate a stranger as warm and offer him a job than were those who held a cold beverage. These kinds of findings hold for abstract expressions as well. Glenberg and Kaschak (2002) asked respondents to move their hands to a button, located either close to or away from their bodies, if a sentence was sensible. This was easier to do when the content of the sentence was coordinate with the directional movement. This result was obtained even when the sentence described transfer of information rather than actual movement. *John told Jane the story* was just as effective as *John left his house.* Thus, language and movement are coordinate. Finally, two studies demonstrated that the relationship between metaphor and behavior goes both ways. Zhong and Leonardelli (2008) found that participants asked to remember being socially accepted judged a room to be warmer than those asked to remember being snubbed. Lee and Schwarz (2011) showed both sides of this relationship in one study. They found that fishy smells induced suspicion and that suspicious participants were better able to discriminate a fish oil smell from other smelly oils.

These data seem to show that sensorimotor embodiment plays a role in abstract concepts. Conceptual metaphor theory understood this as a translation of the concrete (sensing and moving) into the abstract (metaphor). In this model, there had to be some sort of step, some sort of transformation, to be able to move from one domain to the other, from the physical to the abstract. With the development of the neural theory of metaphor, it was no longer necessary to translate the physical into the mental. In this kind of model (and other neural reuse models), neural circuitry for both the concrete (physical) and the abstract (mental) are, to a large degree, one and the same. As a result, the mystery of translation evaporates. The division between concrete and abstract is not ontological in this conception. Instead, it is based on whether the object of study is inside or outside of the organism. Physical objects, their properties and actions in the world, are outside the person and are therefore seen as concrete. Emotions, metaphors, needs, ideas, and complex cognitions are seen as abstract because they are inside the person. But both are processed the same way. From the point of view of brain processes, there is no difference between inside and outside, between abstract and concrete. There is no difference in how these different experiences are processed. All are embodied in the brain. This neural theory of metaphor (Lakoff, 2014) is a neater, more parsimonious theory than one requiring the extra step of translation from one domain to another.

Mirror Neurons

How do we get from sensing and moving to thinking and planning? Lakoff and his associates (see Lakoff, 2014) have argued that sensorimotor workings were exapted for this purpose. This could not have happened all at once. It must have taken place gradually over evolutionary time. There should be intermediate steps, if this is true, and there should be examples of such intermediate steps in lower animals. One model that instantiates these intermediate steps (and here is where it becomes controversial) involves what have come to be called "mirror neurons."

In the late 20th century, scientists at the University of Parma in Italy (di Pellegrino, Fadiga, Fogassi, Gallese, & Rizzolatti, 1992; Ferrari, Gallese, Rizzolatti, & Fogassi, 2003; Gallese, Fadiga, Fogassi, & Rizzolatti, 1996; Rizzolatti, Fadiga, Gallese, & Fogassi, 1996) reported that certain neurons in the brains of macaque monkeys fired both when the monkeys engaged in an activity and when the monkeys observed other monkeys or people engaged in the same activity. Thus, the same neurons fired when observing an action as when executing it. These neurons were said to "mirror" the behavior of the other, as though the observing monkey was itself acting. Hence the name "mirror neurons." In our terminology, this is a rudimentary form of embodied cognition. These investigators later reported that they had found mirror neurons in humans (Gallese, 2003a, 2003b, 2006; Gallese, Keysers, & Rizzolatti, 2004; Rizzolatti, Fogassi, & Gallese, 2001). (Also see Keysers, Kaas, & Gazzola, 2015; Mukamel, Ekstrom, Kaplan, Iacobini, & Fried, 2010; and Wicker et al., 2003, for reports of mirror neurons discovered in different parts of the human brain.)

The Parma group understood their findings to indicate a neurally direct (no mediation by other structures, no translation into another form) mechanism for understanding action in others. That is, through this embodied simulation, the brain/mind models the actions of another, thereby "understanding" it in a direct, physical way. In monkeys, this may be as far as it has gone. But Gallese and others (Gallese, 2007; Gallese & Goldman, 1998; Gallese & Lakoff, 2005), have argued that mirror neurons, in the form of specialized sensory–motor and premotor neurons, have been exapted to wider and more sophisticated uses in humans.

Gallese pointed out that most of our understanding of social interactions is immediate and unconscious just like the behavior reading of monkeys. This argues for continuity between the behavior reading of monkeys and the social understanding evidenced in humans. Gallese further argued that there is no reason to believe that understanding the intentions of others utilizes a cognitive strategy totally unrelated to predicting the consequences of their observed behaviors. In his view, both involve embodied simulation. Embodied simulation can therefore provide direct access to the meaning of actions and, perhaps more importantly, the intentions of those engaged in those actions. Lakoff and Gallese (Gallese, 2007; Gallese & Lakoff, 2005) called this the neural exploitation hypothesis.

Gallese (2007) cited data to back up this model. Broca's region, long thought to be devoted to speech, turns out to also underlie face and mouth movement (Bookheimer, 2002; Nishitani, Schurmann, Amunts, & Hari, 2005; Rizzolatti & Craighero, 2004). Similarly, Gentilucci, 2003; Gentilucci, Benuzzi, Gangitano, & Grimaldi, 2001; Gentilucci, Santunione, Roy, & Stefanini, 2004) reported a close relationship between speech production and both the execution and observation of arm and hand gestures. All of this suggests that speech and the physical gestures that accompany it are coded as a single signal. (Also see Glenberg & Kaschak, 2002, cited above.)

Goldin-Meadow (1999) presented evidence that supported this conclusion. She found that speech and speech-related hand gestures are produced by the same neural circuits. Speech and nonverbal communication are therefore parts of the same system.[3] So when Freud said, "He that has eyes to see and ears to hear may convince himself that no mortal can keep a secret. If his lips are silent, he chatters with his fingertips; betrayal oozes out of him at every pore" (Freud, 1905, p. 77), he may have been voicing a neurological as well as a clinical truth. Even earlier, Darwin (1872/1998) said the same thing, a bit less poetically: "Movements of expression . . . reveal the thoughts and intentions of others more truly than do words, which may be falsified" (p. 359). Nonverbal communication is just as much communication as is verbal communication because they come from the same source. This has enormous clinical implications, as it instructs us to look at and take very seriously our patients' gestures and other nonverbal signs. They really may be as meaningful as clinical lore has suggested. Further, the therapeutic connection can go both ways. Therapists usually think of translating actions and gestures into words to further their therapeutic goals. But it may also be possible to work with bodily gestures directly to achieve some therapeutic and learning ends. Brooks and Goldin–Meadow (2016) reported exactly this. They taught children to move their hands in specified ways and found that it enhanced their mathematical problem solving. Similarly, Glenberg, Brown, and Levin (2007) reported that manipulating objects can improve reading comprehension.

Scientists and philosophers reacted powerfully to the discovery and possible implications of mirror neurons. The distinguished neuroscientist Ramachandran (2000) gave an invited inaugural address for the leading organization for brain research (Society for Neuroscience), celebrating the "Decade of the Brain." He entitled it "Mirror Neurons and Imitation Learning as the Driving Force Behind 'The Great Leap Forward' in Human Evolution." In this talk, he asserted that "mirror neurons will do for psychology what DNA did for biology: they will provide a unifying framework and help explain a host of mental abilities that have hitherto remained mysterious and inaccessible to experiments." Not everyone is on board the mirror neuron train, however. There are many who disagree vehemently with the idea that mirror neurons underlie higher mental processes or even that they are consequential.

Hickok (2009, 2014) authored a highly cited paper, critical of the aforementioned view of mirror neurons, and then penned a book whose title *The Myth of Mirror Neurons* tells you all you need to know about his position. Methods, assumptions, and conclusions are all reviewed in detail; Hickok concludes that mirror neurons have been oversold at best and may be nothing special at worst. His arguments have been disputed by advocates of mirror neurons, of course. They cite data that suggest that, contrary to Hickok's review, there are mirror neurons in humans (e.g., Keysers et al., 2010; Rizzolatti & Sinigaglia, 2010; Wicker et al., 2003) and that focal damage to them results in poorer understanding of action (Binder et al., 2017). The reader interested in sorting it out is referred to two excellent sources wherein both positions are presented. One was a special issue of *Perspectives on Psychological Science* that had what was essentially a debate between advocates and opponents of mirror neurons (Gallese, Gernsbacher, Heyes, Hickok, & Iaconoi, 2011; Glenberg, 2011a, 2011b). Another, more recent debate was conducted in the *American Journal of Psychology* (Glenberg, 2015; Hickok, 2015; Rizzolatti & Sinigaglia, 2015a, 2015b).

As best we understand it, the central critique of mirror neurons boils down to one basic argument: It is not true or even possible that mirror neurons can divine intentions. Another system besides mirror neurons is needed to process and determine intentions. Hickok (2009, 2014) is probably the foremost proponent of this view.[4] And he is not alone. Csibra (2007) says that interpretation of action must come from a higher-level system, which must precede any contribution that mirror neurons make. Kosgonogov (2012) similarly argues that the mirror neuron system can only come into play after another brain structure works out the goal of the observed action. Churchland (2011) also argues that intentions must be coded at a level above that of individual neurons. Jacob (2009) points out that just because one has a motor representation of someone else's action (which is what mirror neurons basically do) does not mean that this also represents the other person's mind. He sees this as a category mistake.

Mirror neuron advocates seem to be of two minds about this criticism (see Hickok, 2015). Thus, Rizzolatti et al. (2001) and Rizzolatti and Craighero (2004) assert that mirror neurons are "the basis for action understanding," whereas Rizzolatti and Sinigaglia (2015) say that "to speak of the mirror mechanism as the basis of action understanding is mere nonsense" (p. 529). But this contradiction may be more apparent than real. Whereas early papers by the Parma group and other advocates of mirror neurons focus on the indispensability of mirror neurons, later papers offer a more nuanced view. The current position seems to be that mirror neurons are part of a larger system (Glenberg, 2015; Rizzolatti & Sinigaglia, 2015a, 2015b; also see Eagle, Gallese, and Migone (2009). We think that the controversy can be addressed by agreeing that a distributed system underlies action understanding and higher mental processes and that sensory and motor workings form a part of that system. Hickok (2015) himself states that he is "quite sympathetic to the idea that sensory and motor systems play a substantial role in . . . 'higher cognition'" (p. 549). Goldman (2012) avowedly proposes a neural reuse model of higher cognition that focuses on affect and sensation rather than on motor neurons and writes that Gallese and Sinigaglia (2011) have come to agree with him. (Gallese is a member of the original Parma group.)

Whether or not mirror neurons pan out to be a revolution in neuroscience (e.g., Ramachandran, 2000) or a false road (e.g., Hickok, 2009, 2014) does not critically affect our thesis that neural reuse underlies brain/mind functioning (cf. Eagle et al., 2009; Goldman, 2012). It just tells us that one model of neural reuse (the neural exploitation hypothesis) may or may not be completely correct in its central reliance on mirror neurons. But whether mirror neurons are "the" exapted workings or not, the essence of the neural exploitation hypothesis is that the neural circuitry that controls how we move our body is also part of higher mental functioning. It is avowedly a neural reuse model (cf. Goldman, 2012) with sensory and motor (and maybe affective) circuits co-opted or exapted to higher-order cognitive uses. This is in keeping with all other neural reuse models. It differs in that the neural exploitation hypothesis focuses more strongly on sensory and motor circuits. Anderson (2010) avers that other workings have been exapted to higher processes as well. The neural exploitation model further holds that mirror neurons are at the center of it all, which, as we have shown, is debatable. But even if the criticisms of mirror neurons are true (mirror neurons are not the essential basis of higher-order functioning) or if mirror neurons only constitute a part of the system underlying higher cognition, the exaptation of sensorimotor neurons underlies an important part of higher cognitive processes and has enormous clinical implications. What these criticisms suggest is that we are not yet ready to implicate a particular kind of neuron as underlying higher mental processes and being "the" exapted working.

So we stand by neural reuse as the best model currently available. And we think future research will either support the centrality of mirror neurons to the combination of workings underlying complex cognition or not. Our bet is that it will be shown to have an important role among several important workings, but, again, our thesis does not rise or fall with the eventual fate of the mirror neuron model of action understanding.

SUMMARY AND CLINICAL IMPLICATIONS OF NEURAL REUSE

Neural reuse occupies a middle position between massive modularity and connectionism (see Gomilaa & Calvoba, 2010). Workings can be organized in multiple ways, but they operate in the same way, do the same thing, in every organization of neural circuits (use) of which they are a part. This means that the brain/mind is more organized and set than in connectionism but not as preordained as in massive modularity. Thus, there is more plasticity than in massive modularity but not as much as in connectionism. To put it in terms of the neural reuse model, the brain/mind has innate functional biases, as represented by its evolutionary-based workings. Additionally, the person can develop workings (within limits), especially early in life. These then also serve to bias functioning. When experience and environmental contingencies are consistent with these innate biases, plasticity and reuse can work together adaptively. But when experiences or environmental contingencies are inconsistent with these evolutionary-based biases, then these processes come into conflict. This can lead to problems in adaptation. This relates to Seligman's (1970) view of preparedness and contrapreparedness, articulated decades ago. Seligman argued that certain associations are more easily learned than others because of the evolutionary history of the organism. At the time, this notion was considered radical because it indicated that ease of learning depended upon what was being learned and not on universal laws of learning. Seligman (1971) related this to phobias shortly afterward, and, more recently, Öhman and Mineka (2001) did the same. By this reasoning, phobias are not random examples of traumatic conditioning or fortuitous learning. We are predisposed to some (e.g., spiders and snakes) more than to others (e.g., horses and birds—see Weinberger et al., 2011). Öhman and Mineka posited a "fear module," in accord with massive modularity. But we would aver that neural reuse makes more sense since people differ so much in terms of their level of fear and what they are fearful of. There is more plasticity to phobia and to its treatment than massive modularity would seem to allow. A bias, due to workings, makes more sense than an encapsulated module that somehow varies enormously across individuals. Likewise, it does not make sense in a massive modularity model for exposure to affect such fears. But it does (Emmelkamp, 2004; Weinberger, 1995, 2014). Moreover, even exposure that is out of awareness has some effects (Siegel & Weinberger, 2012; Weinberger et al., 2011), thereby implicating unconscious processes in phobias and their treatment.

The biases inherent in the workings central to the model of neural reuse can also lead to limits in treating psychological problems. Although psychotherapy could be effective in this model (and it is effective; see Weinberger, 2014), it would be predicted to work best by altering configurations of workings rather than by directly changing uses or altering the component workings themselves, especially in adults where most workings are fixed. This does not mean that change is impossible, as it seems to be in massive modularity. As M. L. Anderson (2010, p. 298) put it: "Plasticity always remains a possibility, whether in response to extraordinary task demands or to physical injury." We would like to believe that psychotherapy could also take advantage of this plasticity.

But the possibility and extent of change would be more limited than many therapists would like due to the impermeability of already existing workings. Workings rarely change but it may be possible (with difficulty) to change their organization within a whole. Changing high-level personality processes (uses) would therefore be extraordinarily difficult. To be more concrete, to speak at the level of therapy, psychotherapy should work best when it attempts to modify coping strategies than when it attempts to change personality characteristics or basic ways of relating to the world (see Heatherton & Nichols, 1994; Heatherton & Weinberger, 1994; Jurist, 2018; Weinberger, 1994).

We would also expect that, following successful therapy, there would be two coping mechanisms. One would be the original, developed through evolution and over the patient's lifetime; the other would be new, developed over the course of psychotherapy. They would overlap because their workings would overlap. Whether the old maladaptive learning or the new more adaptive coping would be active in a situation would depend upon which organization was triggered. And this could be expected to depend upon context, which would favor one organization over the other. So, this model would predict (as would connectionism) that context would be critical to whether adaptive behavior appears or not. Related to this, we would expect that psychotherapeutic change would not always dominate and might not last since the old organization of workings would not be eliminated and could reappear over time and under certain conditions. In this way, relapse flows naturally from neural reuse theory.

The work on metaphor also suggests some important implications for psychotherapy. Listening to our patients' associations and paying attention to their nonverbal communications takes on new meaning in the context of neural reuse theory. Associations reveal the way our patients organize the world and themselves. Nonverbal behavior can help tell us what the patient is thinking and feeling since the same workings underlie both. And nonverbal behavior is hard to censor (cf. Darwin, 1872/1998; Freud, 1905). Psychodynamic theory refers extensively to derivatives and to primary process, which are associatively connected to patients' issues and are frequently thought to underlie them. Often these are bodily based. Nonverbal, bodily communication is also of primary importance in psychodynamic therapy. This takes on important new meaning once we accept the concept of embodied cognition and affect. Cognitive therapy also makes extensive use of metaphor (Stott, Mansell, Salkovskis, Lavender, & Cartwright–Hatton, 2010). This can now be seen as a way of dealing directly with the embodied workings that may underlie a patient's issues. Symptoms are no longer just symptoms. They are embodied representations of the problem. For example,

Lindeman and Abramson (2008) link internal symptoms of depression to bodily states. Thus, the feeling that one is helpless to affect one's outcomes is turned into the metaphor of an inability to overcome physical inertia, often reported by depressed patients. This metaphor of physical incapacity becomes simulated cognitively, which then results in both internal and physiological lethargy. The metaphor becomes physical and psychic reality.

An interesting and unique prediction this model would make is based on the idea that the same workings can underlie very different types of behaviors. A lot of apparently qualitatively different functions may actually have a lot in common. That is, a lot of functions are connected because they share workings. This suggests that addressing those common workings could affect functioning. Perhaps we can indirectly affect one function by intervening in another. Working with metaphor is one way. The therapist can work with a metaphor on the assumption that he is addressing the underlying workings at the same time. Essentially, the therapist would interpret the metaphor, trying to get at the underlying bodily state so as to understand what needs to be changed. Perhaps this is what underlies the effectiveness of mentalization, as reported by Fonagy (Allen & Fonagy, 2014; Bateman & Fonagy, 2015; Fonagy & Allison, 2014; Luyten & Fonagy, 2015). After all, mentalization is a form of mind reading. It requires that you put yourself in the mental state of another. Although it seems a higher-order skill and requires training, Fonagy also reports that borderline patients are good at it in a perverse sort of way. This suggests that at least certain aspects of it are automatic and unconscious. And Fonagy does differentiate between automatic versus controlled mentalization (Bateman & Fonagy, 2015; Fonagy & Allison, 2014). Gallese (2007) goes so far as to aver that most mind reading and most social interaction do not involve reflection, are automatic, and are unconscious. Mentalization may function this way as well, at least in part.

Even more radical, the therapist may seek to directly change physical behavior in the belief that this will also change a psychological state. This is not a simple or intuitively obvious task. One would need to know what workings underlie which psychological states. For example, as cited above, Brooks and Goldin–Meadow (2016) showed that having children move their hands in specified ways enhanced their mathematical problem solving. Similarly, Glenberg et al. (2007) reported that having children manipulate objects improved reading comprehension. Perhaps there are other movements or connections that are linked to different kinds of functioning. Then we could intervene at this level in order to affect the psychological state that we are really interested in altering. We encounter this kind of reasoning in music or art therapy. More recently evolved therapeutic approaches for the treatment of trauma also rely heavily on the body as a vehicle for change (e.g., Ogden's, 2015, sensorimotor psychotherapy or Levine's, 1997, somatic experiencing). Perhaps this kind of direct action on workings is what underlies the reported effectiveness (Bradley, Greene, Russ, Dutra, & Westen, 2005) of eye movement desensitization and reprocessing (EMDR) therapy. The apparently odd interventions of having patients move their eyes in specified ways and (sometimes) tapping their knees is said to be part of why this treatment works. There is no obvious reason for engaging in such acts to positively affect well-being unless the problems people are having and the actions they undertake in these forms of therapy are connected. If this is correct, it would behoove researchers to identify the workings that underlie different psychopathologies so as to more directly address them. Most thinking in this area has focused on sensory and motor reactions, but if Anderson is right, this is only part of the picture and workings are not limited to these functions.

INTEGRATING MASSIVE MODULARITY, CONNECTIONISM, AND NEURAL REUSE

We have reviewed three major models of the brain/mind: massive modularity, connectionism, and neural reuse. They seem to contradict each other. Each has strengths and weaknesses, so there is no clear way to choose between them. Must we choose one and jettison the others? Or is there a way to maximize the strengths, minimize the weaknesses, and keep them all? We believe there is and that neural reuse is the model that can do it.

The strength of PDP is its ability to model a great deal of psychological functioning through very simple principles, namely, frequency of units firing together and a resultant connection weight. PDP is careful not to identify a unit with a single neuron. PDP theorists seem to be saying that a unit consists of a group of neurons that all tend to fire together (as a unit). So the only change that would be needed would be to call workings the unit. The PDP model would lose some of its flexibility in this way but would maintain most of what makes the model so appealing. Moreover, not all workings are present at birth, as M. L. Anderson (2010) and especially Dehaene and Cohen (2007) make clear. They can be created through experience, particularly early life experience. The PDP model would also no longer be vulnerable to the criticism that it is infinitely plastic and therefore capable of doing anything, which is clearly not the case for the brain/mind. Massive modularity would have to give up the idea of localization and encapsulation as absolute entities.

It would have to accept overlapping modules composed of different organizations of the same workings. This would address the distributed nature of processing and the overlap between parts of the brain underlying different functions. In this conceptualization, the workings would constitute a kind of mini-module, more in line with what Fodor had in mind originally (encapsulated, localized, etc.). This is not a stretch for massive modularity. In fact, Carruthers (2010) has argued that this kind of overlap is actually not antithetical to massive modularity but fits in well with it.

There is an interesting collaboration that supports integrating both PDP and massive modularity into a neural reuse framework. One version of connectionism is termed Leabra (local, error-driven and associative, biologically realistic algorithm; Aisa, Mingus, & O'Reilly, 2008; O'Reilly, 1998; O'Reilly & Munkata, 2000). The Leabra team collaborated with the ACT–R team, which is more identified with massive modularity. What both teams discovered to their surprise was that their similarities outweighed their differences, despite coming from two very different orientations. In fact, they integrated their views into what they termed the SAL (synthesis of ACT–R and Leabra) architecture of the mind (Jilk, Labiere, O'Reilly, & Anderson, 2008). This led J. R. Anderson to conclude that Leabra and ACT–R could both employ neural reuse as an organizing principle. Thus, there are precedents and modeling that support the idea of integrating massive modularity and connectionism.

IMPLICATIONS OF THE INTEGRATED MODEL

All of the models are avowedly biological in their thinking. Being biological, all look to evolution for explanations of the functioning and structure of the brain/mind. Although massive modularity is most strongly identified with evolutionary psychology, all of the models make use of evolutionary precepts. They can all agree that the brain/mind evolved so as to maximize survival and procreation in a particular environment, probably that of the Pleistocene era. Parallel processing is also common to all of the models. Doing many things at once allows the brain/mind to operate in the sophisticated way that it does despite its slow pace of operation. All of the models also have epistemological implications. They vary in the degree to which they have an empirical versus innate emphasis, but all agree that how we gain knowledge and what we are able to know is constrained by the structure of the brain/mind. What gives us the flexibility we do have as well as our capacity for learning and change, besides parallel processing, is the vast number of neurons in our central nervous system, which allows for the combinatorial possibilities that both PDP and neural reuse emphasize. Although massive modularity offers less flexibility, the aforementioned huge number of neurons means that there can be a very large number of modules. So there is flexibility in this model as well.

These commonalities have important implications for unconscious processes and for psychotherapy. The emphasis on evolution supports the massive modularity assertion that our species is best adapted for a Pleistocene existence. This means that we are not necessarily adapted for our modern, fast-paced, and technological society. What we want and feel we need, as well as our way of looking at the world, are not necessarily coordinated with our best interests or the demands and constraints of our current environment. Obvious examples are our love of sugar, fats, and salt. This was adaptive when these resources were scarce but are now often maladaptive since we can (and do) create products with exaggerated amounts of what we crave (see Lieberman, 2014).[5] Less obvious but just as important is our difficulty with the stresses and strains of the modern world. We are simply not built for it. For example, the simple ingroup/outgroup functioning that is natural to us, worked in an environment that was geographically local and familially based. But this mode of functioning does not work well in a global environment where ingroup/outgroup has come to be based on race, religion, nationality, or political beliefs. (For a wonderful short tome on the potential connection between living in the modern world and mental illness, see Sebastian Junger's [2016] book *Tribe*.)

The idea that a great deal of our functioning is unconscious is consistent with this evolutionary view. After all, we retain much of what our evolutionary ancestors brought to bear, and most of that was unconscious. What really brings unconscious processes to the fore, however, is parallel processing, which is central to all of the models. If many processes occur simultaneously, it would not be possible for them all to achieve awareness. As a result, the unconscious is built into this conception. Additionally, many of the old arguments against unconscious processes, reviewed earlier in this book, evaporate. Since many processes occur simultaneously, there does not have to be priority of one over the other temporally. For example, the priority of structure over meaning is no longer an issue. The current controversy over the priority of affect over cognition is another example. Although this has not yet been definitively resolved, we suspect that it too may evaporate.

Another by-product of parallel processing is conflict. If many processes are occurring at once, it is reasonable to expect that not all would be in alignment. Some would complement one another, some would be orthogonal to others, and some would be antithetical (see Weinberger & McClelland, 1990). And yet, all would be occurring simultaneously. So conflict is built into any complex system that operates via parallel processing. That is, conflict is normative and ubiquitous. Resistance, a form of conflict, should therefore also be normative and ubiquitous. Moreover, much of this would have to be unconscious. The person would not be aware of much of this conflict. And, even if aware, he might not be able to do much about it since different, relatively noninteracting, systems could be involved. Further, pointing out irrational behavior or faulty information processing may not be effective in and of itself for the same reason. Any encapsulation or use of workings that are not compatible with more adaptive behavior would help create or strengthen this difficulty. Finally, since we were built for an environment vastly different from the one we find ourselves in, this can be expected to occur often. This is most obvious in phobias and reactions to trauma but would be true of any difficulty or irrational behavior. Related to conflict is compromise. The world does not offer us experiences that perfectly match and repeat. It does not offer us exactly what our minds are prepared for or desire. Thus, the brain/mind must settle for as close an approximation as is possible. And this too is unconscious.

Learning in this model is variable and largely unconscious. Any innate a priori way of approaching information and environmental contingencies would suggest a very limited capacity to learn and/or to change. You can't do much with inherited proclivities. Additionally, the model suggests that the nature of learning, when it is possible at all (the different versions of the model differ in the extent to which it is possible), would mostly be what has come to be called implicit learning (reviewed earlier in this book). That is, experience would cause certain units to fire together and/or create new workings and/or change the configurations of workings within larger neural networks. Such learning would be almost, if not entirely, unconscious. Moreover, it would be strongly affected by context as different sets of units or workings are created or strengthened in different situations. And since the environment is not fixed, such learning would be messy or fuzzy. That is, boundary conditions of what is learned would not be clearly defined. Multiple solutions would be calculated until contextual constraints cause the person to settle on one (a form of compromise). This kind of learning leads to generalizations and the creation of schemas that capture the central commonalities of recurring experiences but can and do also tolerate differences in detail and nuance. Sometimes this works, as in having a schema of a restaurant or classroom, and sometimes it can go awry, as in having a stereotype for a race or religion. Further, in line with the principle of compromise, this learning and these schemas would be approximations rather than accurate representations of experience since experience never exactly repeats. Schemas, plans, and such would therefore also be compromises and have fuzzy boundaries. Such compromises may be minor, but it is also possible that major compromises may be required if any solution is to be found. If some constraints (contextual factors) are ignored or seriously bent to fit the compromise, then distortion of an experience can result. It is important to note that the constraints that underlie these compromises are not limited to physical factors but include emotional and motivational states as well (cf. Westen & Gabbard, 2002). And, finally, no matter what, a stable equilibrium is never really reached by the system because we live in a dynamic, ever-changing world. The system is constantly in flux and can only achieve relative stability for brief periods of time. So the system is dynamic. One consequence of this is that the system must be able to tolerate chronic ambiguity. All of these events occur unconsciously. We are unaware of conflicting constraints, relative goodness of compromise, or the instability and ambiguity of equilibrium.

The seemingly trivial truism that we think with our brains leads to the radical idea that thought is embodied (Lakoff, 2014). We need to pay attention to the body and to metaphors that invoke physical events to explain mental and emotional processes. And, again, all of this is unconscious.

Finally, once developed through learning, networks would be difficult to alter, as they would tend to go off automatically and unconsciously. So this model emphasizes early learning over later learning, conflict, strong context effects, compromise, generalizations, and the creation of schemas. None of this would exactly mirror experience. Some could distort it in important ways. And virtually all of it would be unconscious.

To summarize, this model predicts some innate modes of responding, which would be relatively impervious to experience. There would also be learned modes of responding that are sensitive to context, that can represent accurate or distorted views of reality, that get generalized both appropriately and inappropriately, that are easier to form early than later in life, and that are difficult to change once formed. Most, if not all, of this would be unconscious. And all of it would be embodied. We would concur with Clark (2013) that the brain/mind can be thought of as an implicit prediction engine. We would add that the predictions would not be perfect reflections of the regularities of experience but the best fit across all of them (i.e., compromises), given the extant constraints.

All of this suggests that psychotherapy, as an agent of change, would not be an easy affair. Additionally, it might need to be relatively long term and deal with change across contexts. It would not be easy to change long-standing ways of functioning that are partly based on innate and early-developing workings that have generalized across many contexts. Why should it be any easier or quicker to change an idiosyncratic and chronic maladaptive way of behaving that results in depression or anxiety than it would be to change a societally based chronic maladaptive way of behaving that results in bias and discrimination? Both would have some basis in innate workings and both would also be based on early creation of workings. Both should take a long time and a lot of work to change. Both would have to address the different contexts in which the targeted behaviors appear. Additionally, psychotherapy might have to traffic in compromises. On the more optimistic side, it might also be the case that attention to workings that underlie both low-level physical and high-level mental operations, perhaps through the study of metaphor and nonverbal communication, might provide a way for psychotherapy to be more effective. We discuss the psychotherapeutic implications of these models in more detail in the next chapter.

What is not built into computational models in any systematic way is consciousness. Modern models of the brain/mind easily encompass unconscious processes; conscious processes and rationality, not so much. One possibility that covers consciousness is the global workspace. Here is an area where modules and/or neural networks, composed of different configurations of workings, can meet. Here is where they can communicate with one another. And here is where consciousness can reside. But here, the models do not agree. Some do not posit such a central executive or common medium. This is an area that will have to remain open for the present.

NOTES

1. This conception fits nicely with the classical Gestalt psychology notion of *isomorphism*, which states that our experiences are organized exactly as are our perceptions. That is, our brain mapping of each is topographically identical (Köhler, 1976).

2. This also supports the classical view of James (1890) that the bodily conditions associated with emotions are the emotions.

3. If this is true, it can explain why we move our hands when we talk, even when the person we are talking to cannot see those movements. They are part of the same neurological system.

4. Hickok makes a case for the superior temporal sulcus (STS) and sees it as more essential than the motor system implicated by mirror neuron advocates.

5. Ethologists take advantage of built-in innate releasing mechanisms to study the behavior of animals. Two classic examples are the attack behavior of the male stickleback and the egg-retrieving behavior of the graylag goose. Male sticklebacks react aggressively to the red belly of another male stickleback

during mating season. Tinbergen (1951) was able to get male sticklebacks to attack a crude model of another male stickleback whose only defining feature was that its underside was painted red. Lorenz (1991) showed that the graylag goose will attempt to bring egg-like objects with exaggerated features (too large) into their nests as though they were displaced eggs. They even preferred these "supernormal stimuli" to actual goose eggs. Geese are unlikely to find such objects in their natural environment. But we humans are likely to find supernormal stimuli like sugary cereals in ours and prefer them to fruit (see Lieberman, 2014). My (JW) sons display this behavior every morning and, to tell the truth, so do I. For a more recent but more pop book on this topic, see Alcock (2013). For a book more focused on evolutionarily based human adaptations and their consequences in our modern society, see Lieberman (2014).

CHAPTER 22

A Model of the Unconscious

Theory and Implications for Psychotherapy

We have come a long way in this book. What we would like to do now is discuss the fruits of this journey. We are fully aware that the conclusions we draw are liable to change as more data are collected and more theoretical innovations are offered. But we think they represent an accurate view of the current state of knowledge about the unconscious.

THE UNCONSCIOUS EXISTS AND IT IS IMPORTANT

We now know that unconscious processes are genuine. Considering how long it took for their existence to be acknowledged, this is not a trivial accomplishment. We also learned that they are important. In fact, unconscious processing is the default mode of functioning—the primary process. Additionally, it tends to *be broad, expansive, and uncritical. Unconscious processes come to the fore when the person adopts a passive, noncritical attitude*, whereas focus and efforts to figure out what is going on favor consciousness. Ironic processes, as described by Wegner (1989, 1994), demonstrated this empirically, and it is almost a given in most therapeutic models.

At the same time, *unconscious processes often show stereotypy, rigidity, and resistance to change.* The early work on automaticity, as well as a lot of research on what has been termed "spontaneous recovery" (in psychotherapy we call it "relapse"), make this aspect of unconscious processes clear. In contrast, *conscious processes manifest the flexibility that unconscious processes lack.* Finally, there *are no pure conscious or unconscious processes and no absolute differentiation between them.* All mental operations are a mixture, with some showing more of the characteristics of conscious and some showing more of the characteristics of unconscious processes. All of the features of unconscious processes that we described above are relative rather than absolute.

UNCONSCIOUS PROCESSES CAN BE EXAMINED SYSTEMATICALLY

Once the existence and import of unconscious processes were established, and once there were some hypotheses concerning the nature of these processes, systematic work on their operation began in earnest. We reviewed this research in the areas of heuristics, implicit memory, implicit learning, implicit motivation, automaticity, attribution theory, affective primacy, and embodied cognition. What did it tell us?

First and foremost, the work in all of these areas demonstrates that much of unconscious functioning is *normative.* By this we mean that unconscious processes are not necessarily set in motion by conflict or pathology nor are they manifestations of conflict and psychopathology. They are simply part of how the mind/brain is designed and operates to help us negotiate our lives. *Unconscious processes are a normal, integral part of how we function in the world and with each other.* That this functioning is not always optimal is not central to the way unconscious processes operate.

Next, we know a bit about how unconscious processes are organized. They do not operate in a rational fashion. But they are not irrational for motivational reasons; they are that way because they are *organized associatively* rather than logically and/or hierarchically. That is why we referred to them as <u>arational</u> and cautioned against conceptualizing them as irrational. The ego, if we want to use that term to refer to these normative processes, is a great deal more important and central to our functioning than Freud and even the ego psychologists believed. This underestimation of the ubiquity of normative unconscious processing is not unique to psychoanalytic theories. Normative unconscious processes have been shown to be more important and more central to our functioning than any school of psychology taught or believed.

Conscious processing must therefore be less essential than most theorists have heretofore argued (i.e., it is not the primary process). Instead of conscious processes predominating, all mental processes are at least partly unconscious, with various (often small) degrees of conscious processing. So unconscious processing is not simply part of our normal functioning, it underlies most of it. If we believe in Gazzaniga's interpreter or Kurzban and Aktipis's social cognitive interface, there is virtually no conscious processing at all.

And what is unconscious processing concerned with? It focuses on what is *salient* to the person. It learns through experience but in an uncritical, literally empirical fashion. Whatever is salient and happens to have covaried with an experience becomes associated with that experience and learned (within limits). This associative learning affects our understanding of and response to the experience. The more ambiguous the situation, the more likely unconscious learning processes are to come to an idiosyncratic understanding of it. Each time we have that experience, the associative network it is connected with (what has been learned) also gets triggered. This understanding then gets "locked in," all without our realizing it. Our understanding of and reactions to our experiences can therefore be right, somewhat off, biased, and even spectacularly wrong. Which of these happens depends upon the associative networks connected to those experiences, which, in turn, depend upon whatever was salient and therefore connected to the experience at the time. When the implicit association between a behavior and the reasons we engage in it are not explicitly available, Gazzaniga's interpreter or Kurzban and Aktipis SCI kicks in and we make something up (i.e., we rationalize).

The aforementioned unconscious processes function dynamically. Many processes are going on at the same time (in parallel). If we hone in on one for illustrative purposes, we would see the following. Many stimuli, both internal and external, are impinging upon us. We notice and respond to whichever of these is most salient to us. Often this is affect but sometimes not. We immediately categorize whatever is salient as good or bad, to be approached or avoided. And then we form empirically based ways of understanding our experiences (implicit learning). All of this is grounded in our physical functioning (embodied).

Importantly, unconscious functioning is never an all-or-nothing affair. It can have some of the characteristics outlined above but lack others. Which characteristics a particular process exhibits depends upon many factors that we have yet to understand and identify. But the bottom line is that all of our functioning is a mix of affect and cognition, of implicit and explicit, and of the four properties of automaticity. Functioning is more likely to evince unconscious properties when we are tired, passive, distracted, or stressed. It is more likely to manifest properties associated with consciousness when we are focused and attentive. Finally, we have not found a brain locus for unconscious processes. We tentatively settled on a model proposed by Reber that argues that unconscious processes are distributed throughout the brain and represent its overall functioning. Explicit processes, on the other hand, may be more localizable in the brain.

NEURAL REUSE: A COMPUTATIONAL NEUROSCIENCE MODEL OF UNCONSCIOUS PROCESSES

Once we described a bit about how unconscious processes operate, we tried to identify a model that could incorporate the data from the various areas of empirical inquiry we reviewed. We arrived at one based on computational neuroscience. We reviewed three such models: massive modularity, parallel distributed processing (PDP), and neural reuse. Although they seem antithetical, we argued that these models can and should be integrated. We offered a modified neural reuse model as the best fit for the findings we reported. Instead of the large function modules posited by massive modularity, this model proposes the more delimited workings posited by neural reuse. Instead of the almost infinitely malleable small units proposed by PDP, this model posits somewhat larger units (workings), designed for a particular purpose by evolution, that can be coopted or exapted for other uses. Additionally, it is also possible in this model, to some degree, to construct new workings based on experience. With these changes, massive modularity and PDP were integrated into the aforementioned modified neural reuse model.

What all of these models have in common and what is retained by our integrated version is that processing must occur in parallel. Thus, one of the conclusions we have come to flows from this type of model: the brain/mind operates in parallel. This means that much of our functioning takes place and must take place unconsciously. Moreover, unconscious processes are now seen as primary to our functioning. These conclusions must follow if we perform many operations simultaneously (in parallel). Because this is how the brain/mind works, such processes are normal, not pathological. So the existence of ubiquitous, normative unconscious processes, which fits with the empirical data, is now a necessity.

In this model, functioning is a result of preexisting workings, workings exapted for new purposes but also still serving their original purpose, and workings developed through experience. So, functioning is based on preexisting modes of operation, on new ways of combining those operations, and/or on the vagaries of experience that create new operations. Although this model allows for some flexibility in our functioning, it also posits some limits. We cannot transcend our workings. We are stuck with many of them. Even when we combine them in new ways, they still retain their original function, and there is only so much leeway to create new ones. Thus, the model is more flexible than is massive modularity but not as plastic as is PDP. The concept of workings also supports the idea that much of our cognition, much of our mind, is literally (physically) based on (connected to) workings that originally evolved for physical (e.g., sensory and motor) purposes. This aspect of the model parsimoniously explains the now ubiquitous findings that physical stimulation leads to parallel psychological consequences. It also explains the power of metaphor. Thus, the model can account for, in fact requires, embodied cognition.

The conclusion that mental functioning is not rationally or logically organized also flows from this model. The brain is organized associatively, and therefore so is the mind. Cognition is based on preexisting associative organization in the brain supplemented to some degree by whatever changes in this organization the environment can cause. Associative structure is not rational or logical. So the finding that we normatively function arationally flows from the model as well. Again, unconscious processes are not necessarily, nor even usually, pathological. They simply reflect the way we are built. And we are built to organize our experiences associatively.

This model also predicts that whatever learning there is, is (within the limits described below) radically empirical. This follows from the associative structure of the mind/brain and the manner in which those associative connections change with experience. Learning in this model is defined as changes in the nature and strength of associative connections in the brain/mind. Environmental and internal experiences cause certain units to fire together. As such experiences are repeated, the connection between the activated units strengthens. This is exactly what the research in implicit learning has shown. So the model accounts for implicit learning. It also explains automaticity as such connections become ingrained in the mind/brain. Preconscious and postconscious automaticity are not now qualitatively different processes. They just differ in terms of some aspects of their organization. The model also predicts some limits to learning as many workings are innate and cannot be changed to any appreciable degree. Again, the process is normal and arational rather than motivated or pathological.

The model has *compromise* between imperfectly fitting constraints built into it. The same properties of the model also lead to the phenomena of generalizations, schemas, core relational themes, context effects, and "fuzzy boundaries" between concepts. All emerge from the way the mind/brain in this model reacts to experiences and learns from them. As the person's experiences grow, certain commonalities between situations get abstracted out. The connections they have in common become strengthened across different situations. This results in generalizations and in schemas. The conditions that differentiate disparate experiences are not lost, however. They result in discrimination and context effects as some units are strengthened and others not depending upon unique aspects of an experience. Finally, since no two situations can be exactly identical, what is abstracted out as general and what is differentiated as unique or contextual are approximations. So concepts and context effects would have what are often called fuzzy boundaries. These could also be considered compromises as the system settles on the best solution available to it. So, from one aspect of the system, the manner in which it changes with experience, many psychological phenomena emerge naturally.

Conflict is also part of this model. Since many processes occur at once (parallel processing), not all will be in sync. Some simultaneous processes would be coordinate, some would be orthogonal or irrelevant, and some would be in opposition to one another. So conflict is inevitable (as the massive modularity aspect of the model avers). How would it be resolved? Through settling on the best solution, as the PDP aspect of this model would argue. Such a solution can never be ideal. Thus, compromise is built into the model as a natural outgrowth of the way it functions. And since some of the factors that would have to be integrated into any solution would include emotional and motivational processes, this integration would inevitably be messy. Additionally, the solution would have to at least partially involve idiosyncratic learning (radically empirical implicit learning). How does the system decide which constraints are paramount, which are secondary, and which are unimportant? The units that are most strongly activated would be paramount in the solution. Those less activated would be less relevant to the solution. Psychologically, the most strongly activated units are experienced as most *salient* (as we defined it earlier) in the experience. Thus, *salience would be operationalized as strongest connection.* This could be a result of prior experience or of preexisting workings that evolved to be strongest. These could be, and often are, emotions and motivations but they could also be other kinds of evolutionarily based workings or they could be idiosyncratic experiences that occurred frequently enough to become salient. Put it all together and the result would be truly messy, and normatively so. Finally, since many of the workings involved in a solution evolved for an evolutionary period that no longer exists, it gets even messier and could easily shift into a normatively maladaptive solution.

All of this means *we have an evolved, associatively organized, embodied brain/mind that operates in parallel.* The units of the brain/mind are workings that both evolved and developed with experience. Each working is designed to perform a specific function, and the assortment of workings can be combined in multiple ways. Some workings and combinations of workings would be more salient than others and hence more likely to underlie any solution the system comes to. The result is *normatively unconscious, arational functioning that has some preset modes of functioning and that learns, within limits, in a radically empirical fashion. The dynamics of this system have conflict and compromise built into them. Generalizations, schemas, core relational themes, context effects, and fuzzy boundaries biased by the saliency of certain workings and sets of workings are emergent properties of these dynamics.* Finally, any concern over localization of function evaporates. Functions are distributed. Further, a great deal of functioning, like learning, is due to general properties of the model rather than localized in specific areas of the brain. Thus Reber's hypothesis seems supported by this model.

WHAT'S MISSING?

This model may not yet clearly account for a dynamic unconscious. It is either missing and needs to be developed or it is an emergent property of the model we have outlined. Thus, the ideas of conflict and compromise, the never totally satisfactory settling of the system, the fact that among the aspects of experience that have to be considered in this settling are emotional and motivational factors as well as idiosyncratically learned responses, may mean that a dynamic unconscious can flow from the model as is. Or not. Time, further study, and more theorizing will have to address this question. And what of consciousness? Its place and mode of operation are not well described in this model. It could exist as an aspect of the general workspace posited by some adherents of massive modularity. It could be an emergent quality of the model we have sketched. Or it could be epiphenomenal or even illusory as Gazzaniga, Kurzban, Libet, and Wegner have argued.

It is ironic that the study of unconscious processes began with consciousness as a given and unconsciousness as questionable, whereas now unconsciousness is a given and consciousness is mysterious and questionable. Such are the vagaries of intellectual progress. So we make a prediction to come full circle with the quote by Bergson that we presented near the beginning of this book. Bergson predicted study and understanding of unconscious processes: "To explore the unconscious, to work in the subterranean of the mind with especially adequate methods, this will be the main task of psychology in the opening [20th] century. I do not doubt that fine discoveries will follow, as important perhaps as have been in the preceding centuries those of physical and natural sciences" (Bergson, 1901, quoted in Ellenberger, 1970, p. 321). We are confident that the 21st century will be noted for its leaps forward in understanding the mind. Developments in this century will powerfully further our understanding of unconscious processes and provide us with a workable model of the mind and explain consciousness. We hope this book represents a small step forward in that enterprise.

THE UNCONSCIOUS IN CLINICAL WORK

When we compare the effectiveness of different psychotherapies (Weinberger, 1995, 2014), we find they all work equally well (or badly). Current therapy models have no explanations for this phenomenon. Different schools offer contradictory views of what is ameliorative, yet the outcomes they yield seem to be no different from one another. They predict lasting change, yet change does not last. Relapse is the norm rather than the exception. And when there are speculations about why therapy works, when it does work, the models underlying the various treatments take little if any account of current work on the brain/mind or on unconscious processes. As we stated in our opening chapter, this suggests that currently existing treatment modalities may be outmoded (cf. Weinberger, 1995, 2014).

Beck's cognitive therapy, for example, still harkens back to his writings of the 1970s. The model, even in its current form, does not really take recent findings on unconscious processes into account. Cognitive therapies do not attribute enough importance to the normative aspects of unconscious functioning. For example, Socratic dialogue is probably not effective because of the rational sense it offers to patients, which then challenges and replaces their illogical thinking. Instead, it may be effective because it allows for alternative learning that can compete with older, more established learning, in the context of a therapeutic relationship (which provides an affective component to the new learning). Additionally, monitoring automatic thoughts and challenging them is not a simple process. As we saw, ironic processes can cause such monitoring to backfire. Finally, it may take a long time for new learning to solidify so that the short-term therapy currently favored may have to be either lengthened considerably or supplemented periodically.

Psychodynamic work is also based on decades-old models. Additionally, much of the literature refers to clinical material but shows relatively little regard for empirical understandings of how the brain/mind operates. And although psychodynamic models do pay attention to the importance of affect in organizing experience, these models, like their cognitive counterparts, do not take the normative nature of unconscious processes into account. Further, there is no systematic rationale to explain why insight, or emotional experiences, or the therapeutic relationship should result in change (assuming that they do). There is certainly no systematic viable theory of unconscious processes. There seems to be some insight in recent relational models that there is no hard-and-fast separation between conscious and unconscious processes and some understanding that the way people come to understand these experiences is strongly affected by emotional and relational factors. But referring to this as "unformulated" is not clarifying.

Although person-centered therapy does not emphasize unconscious processes (Mearns & Thorne, 2000; Schaffer, 1978), they seem to be an important part of the model. (We saw this kind of thing early in the history of psychology as well; see Chapter 3.) The person is said to possess an inborn motive to develop or self-actualize of which she is not aware. As Rogers (1980) writes, "Our organisms as a whole have a wisdom and purposiveness which goes well beyond our conscious thought" (p. 106; also see Maslow, 1943). There is also a motive for positive self-regard; it is not clear whether this motive is unconscious, conscious, or a mix of both. There is also a sense, such as we reviewed in our chapter on implicit motivation (Chapter 13), that when these motives are aligned or congruent, the person functions better. When they are misaligned or incongruent, the person functions badly and experiences negative emotions (Rogers, 1959, 1961). These concepts tend to be vaguely described and difficult to operationalize, however. One reason, as in the other therapies reviewed, is that the model is decades old and does not incorporate recent understandings of unconscious processes. Another problem is that despite the presence of these unconscious factors, Rogers (1959, 1961) seems to have eschewed systematic investigation of unconscious processes (cf. Mearns & Thorne, 2000), instead focusing on conscious experience. We would like to believe that this was, at least in part, due to the lack of understanding (and appreciation) of unconscious processing during the time that he wrote (over a half century ago). To be fair, humanistic thought and Rogers' concept of unconditional positive regard were ahead of their time in signifying the importance of relational factors in healing. To speculate, based on our current understanding of unconscious processes, the alignment of motives, the relational bond between therapist and patient, and the embodied nature of thought (all emphasized in person-centered therapy) may be powerful factors in psychotherapy and should be investigated.

IMPLICATIONS OF THE DATA ON UNCONSCIOUS PROCESSES

Throughout this book, we have derived therapeutic implications from our reviews of empirical work on unconscious processes and of brain/

mind models. Here, we attempt to summarize some of the conclusions we came to concerning unconscious processes, review the implications we drew from these conclusions, and place these implications in a theoretical context.

First, the mind/brain is organized associatively. This means that we should strive to understand our patients associatively rather than rationally. For instance, using Socratic questions and challenging unhealthy beliefs to treat a patient with an eating disorder, determining how the search for positive self-regard led to a distortion of eating behaviors, or even gaining insight into, say, issues of control or a wish to disappear through restrictive eating, only scratches the surface. We have to also use an embodiment lens to understand how the sensation of eating/feeling full is connected to affective states and implicitly learned messages for each patient individually. For instance, restrictive eating may be used as a means of "disappearing" because not being seen may mean safety for someone who has been sexually assaulted. In this case, appealing to a patient's sense of self-preservation ("you have to eat to stay alive") may directly conflict with what self-preservation means to her. Interventions of the exposure-response prevention type may not be effective because they simply will not be utilized by the patient. And mirroring the person's feelings and understandings of her eating disorder may not address the habitual nature and meaning of the eating disorder behaviors or other possible motives underlying the disorder. Thus, it may also be worthwhile to explore how this patient's behaviors are not simply a way to obtain self-regard or make sense of the world. The behaviors may also reflect other implicit motivations (e.g., power vs. intimacy). For example, if the patient's primary motivation is intimacy, but an interpersonal trauma has occurred, this will likely result in significant difficulty in forging and utilizing a safe and secure bond with the therapist. In other words, the emphasis on rational versus irrational emphasized by both psychodynamic and cognitive therapy may be misplaced. It is more important to understand how our patients understand the world associatively. Some of these understandings will reflect reality accurately; some will not. But the underlying reasons will be arational, not rational or irrational. Likewise, the emphasis on a single motive of self-regard in conflict with a need to self-actualize and/or an emphasis on making sense of the world may not cover all that is going on. There are other implicit motives that may need to be addressed.

Next, most, if not all, mental processes involve both conscious and unconscious aspects. This is basic and normal. If we do not accept this fact, we risk confounding unconscious processes with psychopathology and conscious processes with health. Janet made this mistake over a century ago and others have repeated it since; we should not fall into this trap.[1] Third, unconscious processes are real and, for the most part, are the default most prominent part of our functioning. They are the primary process.

If the above is true, then our experiences are represented as networks of associations. Further, research has shown that whatever is salient in an experience is given pride of place in the associative network representing that experience and treated as though it caused the experience. When such implicit learning is repeated, the associative network strengthens. The understanding of and reactions to the experience generated by the network can then become entrenched or automatized and become self-perpetuating (and it does not take much). This is particularly true of learning that occurred early in life. This hardening of automatized behavior occurs whether the learning was once conscious and became unconscious (postconscious automaticity) or whether the learning was entirely unconscious (preconscious automaticity). For example, we all carry unconscious mental models of attachment that we are not cognizant of throughout our lives. This normative unconscious process may prove maladaptive when the internalized patterns do not represent true causal relationships or are based on past connections that no longer hold. We may internalize anxieties or maladaptive social strategies through such learning. This kind of learning may also underlie phobias, aversions, fetishes, and the like.

Affective experiences are often (but not always) more salient than nonaffective experiences and therefore frequently become central to our representations. What is more, negative affect is usually more salient than is positive affect. This is a normal consequence of our evolutionary past. I am happy, life is good, move on. But when I am sad or anxious or angry, that signals a threat to my well-being (existence) and must be attended to. The process is not inherently pathological, but its application to particular life circumstances may be. An important clinical task, then, may be to investigate when and how (and why) such normative processes cross over into pathology, such as depression, trauma, and anxiety.

Affect may not only serve an attention-capturing function (salience) but may also be used to categorize experiences. It is normative to tend to group together stimuli that elicit the same emotional response. Moreover, emotional arousal may increase the likelihood of doing so. If the person is subject to inconsistent, adverse, and therefore emotionally arousing experiences, this can lead to the clinical phenomenon of "splitting" wherein a patient vacillates between all good and all bad characterizations of others. Additionally, we know that when someone survives traumatic experiences, salient sensory perceptions can become strongly associated with the negative affect and physiological responses triggered by the trauma. He may then have a strong negative reaction, for example, to a song that was playing in the background when he got into a car accident. Sometimes he may not even realize why this song causes him so much distress because this process is largely unconscious.

Associative learning and organization centered on salient stimuli means we are especially sensitive to stimuli that support our preexisting beliefs and biases. This may explain the apparent automatic seeking out of stimuli that confirm preexisting beliefs and biases that seems to be characteristic of many disorders, notably depression and anxiety.[2] Since this process takes place automatically, we are not aware of these dynamics. Research on obsessions and addictive disorders demonstrates that simple exposure to triggers (even below the threshold of conscious perception) may be sufficient to cause an automatic behavioral reaction that bypasses conscious thought. We know from the addiction literature, for example, that a negative affective reaction is a powerful predictor of relapse—I feel bad, therefore I quickly and automatically crave a drink. What is more, awareness that this chain of internal events just took place does not mean my craving will diminish.

And then there is the resistance patients routinely show to our clinical interpretations of their behaviors. Even though our patients often do not know what drives their behavior, they tend to believe (and insist) that they do know. And they offer explanations of their issues that may or may not be reflective of the true reasons behind them. These explanations may represent their best guess about causality (attribution theory), be based on a need to provide a coherent narrative (the interpreter), or on an unconscious desire for smooth and beneficial interactions (social cognitive interface—SCI). As a result, we cannot take our patients' understanding of what is going on with them at face value. Therapists are not immune to such confabulations either. They are just as liable to make these kinds of mistakes as are their patients. The therapist must therefore be aware of potential biases and take care to justify her interpretations and explanations for patient behaviors.

Biases are not random. There are built-in systematic biases concerning how people understand their experiences. The keys to these attributional biases are salience and self-image. Because the situations we find ourselves in are more salient to us than our personalities, we are more likely to view our own behavior as environmentally caused. Because the overt behaviors of others are more salient to us than are situational constraints, we tend to attribute their behaviors to dispositional factors. I am angry because you made me angry, but you are angry because you are an angry person. So, in psychotherapy, patients will tend to see their own behavior as dependent on situational constraints whereas the behaviors of others are due to their personality characteristics. Additionally, if a person holds a generally positive view of herself, she will tend to attribute success to internal factors and failures to external factors in contradistinction to the usual bias of understanding one's own behaviors as situationally caused. By the same token, individuals who tend to hold stable negative self-images are likely to attribute failures to dispositional factors and success to chance.

Therapists are just as potentially susceptible to these kinds of biases as are their patients. They are more likely to attribute their patients' behaviors to their enduring personality characteristics than to the situation. Their own behavior, however, is likely to be seen as situational. For example, when the patient rejects the therapist's character-based interpretation, the therapist might see this as resistance. Treatment outcome is no different; therapists tend to attribute patient-initiated termination to either patient improvement or environmental factors rather than to patient dissatisfaction. Self-image also operates as most therapists tend to understand their patients in line with their own personal and theoretical predilections.

Studies in the area of embodied cognition demonstrate that thoughts are, to a large degree, encoded physically. Moreover, these bodily experiences structure our personal narratives in ways that are not consciously accessible. We feel warm physically so we feel more positively toward another. We push something away physically, and we are more likely to reject an idea or person. Having such experiences vicariously can result in similar effects. We do not even necessarily need a full-blown physical experience; a simple physiological reaction to a stimulus is sufficient to bring up a psychic one. And we're often not aware of any of it. It is largely unconscious. This all suggests that intervening on a physical level can affect psychological phenomena just as intervening on a psychological level can affect both psychological and physical phenomena.

Another factor that is important to psychotherapy is the relationship between unconscious and conscious processes. An important example is that what we believe we are motivated to do and what we implicitly strive for may be (and often are) two separate things (also see above discussion of person-centered therapy and Chapter 13 on implicit motivation). This has significant implications for a person's functioning as well as for the person's mental and physical health. For instance, one may be implicitly motivated to seek closeness and intimacy, but if he is pursuing a job that focuses on achievement, he may feel like something is missing. Such misalignment of motives leads to psychological discomfort, even pain. Conversely, alignment of implicit and explicit motives leads to an increased sense of well-being.

One of us (VS), for instance, works extensively with military veterans, for whom the concept of closeness and intimacy can be loaded and complex. On the one hand, military personnel are trained to leave no one behind and, indeed, often develop intensely loyal and close bonds and a sense of camaraderie. However, by its nature, the military relies on a strict structure and hierarchy in which power is clearly delineated through a ranking system. In that sense, someone with predominantly implicit intimacy motivation may struggle in navigating the hierarchy and even struggle to accomplish certain missions that may threaten relationships. As a result, she may also be more prone to experiencing moral injury and posttraumatic stress resulting from relational trauma. However, such an individual may also be more likely to engage in treatment and gain more from it through a positive therapeutic alliance (which has an implicit hierarchy built into it).

A THEORETICAL MODEL

Finally, we turned to computational neuroscience for a model that could underlie the above phenomena. That is, we employed computational neuroscience to create our clinical meta-theory. We proposed a modified neural reuse model as a good fit for the empirical data we reviewed. We presented the model and the clinical implications we derived from it in detail in Chapter 21. Its main points are as follows.

Like all modern computational neuroscience models, ours posits a largely unconscious, parallel processing, and associatively organized mind/brain. More specifically, our modified neural reuse model focused on what we termed workings and exaptation of those workings to new uses. Workings are tightly organized, low-level neural networks with a specific function and location in the brain. They do what they do and nothing else. They are immutable. Workings can be evolutionarily based, a result of development, or created through learning. A use is a relatively high-level operation that is composed of some combination of workings. Exaptation refers to coopting a working so that it can be used to help perform a function (have a use) it was not originally designed for. These factors enabled us to incorporate, indeed required that we incorporate, implicit learning and memory, automaticity, embodied cognition, and salience. Regardless of whether a working is exapted through evolution, coopted by developmental needs, or created through learning, *early workings bias later experiences*. Later in life, if the environment is congruent with these biases, neural reuse and plasticity can work together, creating an adaptive equilibrium within the system. However, if biases and the environment are incongruent, this may create significant conflict and problems in adaptation. This is consistent with Seligman's notion that, within a species, some things are learned more easily than others.

Clinically, neural reuse is applicable in explaining many pathological phenomena. For instance, many phobias are partly evolutionary predispositions and partly learning—but learning that takes place easily due to that evolutionary predisposition.

Additionally, the model predicts conflict and compromise as inevitable and ubiquitous. Finally, it predicts that therapy can work but would be limited in its effectiveness. It could lead to the learning of new coping mechanisms but not to personality change. Moreover, the old learning would not be replaced by the new. Rather, they would exist side by side so to speak, with one predominating in some situations and the other more likely in others. As a result, relapse would be expected, and long-term effectiveness would probably require long-term or repeated treatments. Thus, this modified neural reuse model can incorporate much of the research data on therapeutic effectiveness that we reviewed.

PRACTICAL IMPLICATIONS FOR TREATMENT

How do we operationalize the model of treatment we are proposing? This problem too has been considered in several places in this book. Here we try to summarize the conclusions we arrived at. First, we suggest providing some psychoeducation to our patients. Most (but not all) contemporary therapy models recommend this as well, but focus on different types of *psychoeducation*. We suggest it is essential to tell our patients about the associative structure of the mind. We would discuss the unconscious nature of much of our functioning, how much of our thinking and feeling relies upon physical properties and functions (is embodied), how we often have opposing needs and wants, and how all of this is normal and usually adaptive but can go wrong under certain conditions. Moreover, we would explain that some of our predilections are more suited to an evolutionary past that no longer exists and can therefore lead to maladaptive outcomes. All of this could serve to reassure our patients that they are not fundamentally off. Rather, certain normative processes have led to some currently maladaptive behaviors. We would also recommend being honest about the possibilities and limits of psychotherapy. Change is difficult and can take a while, relapse can occur and may require further therapy down the road, and we cannot produce miracles. Nevertheless, we often are able to help someone improve the quality of her life. In general, psychotherapy is effective.

One area we would particularly recommend discussing with patients, along with psychoeducation about the treatment itself, is the human propensity for systematic bias. A similar notion of "truthfulness" has recently been emphasized as a crucial component of therapy beyond the therapeutic alliance (Jurist, 2018). Providing our patients with psychoeducation about how biases operate normatively may serve to alleviate feelings of confusion, self-criticism, guilt, and shame, which can otherwise adversely affect the therapeutic process. Additionally, it is incumbent upon the therapist to investigate the possibility that she is seeing normative attributional bias in her patient before interpreting pathology or resistance. The patient should conduct a similar self-search. Does he behave similarly across situations? What seems to be situational to him may, in fact, be dispositional. Additionally, the therapist should pay close attention to her patient's self-image so as to better understand how she structures and interprets the world. Similar self-attention on the part of the therapist concerning her own predilections would also be beneficial.

We also would recommend some strategies beyond psychoeducation. Several clinical strategies flow from embodiment, for example. Embodiment calls for and explains why *metaphors* can be such an effective aspect of psychotherapy. Metaphors reflect the physical part of our experiences in ways that simple descriptive language cannot. Clinicians should pay attention to the metaphors used by patients in treatment as well as help them work toward creating new, more adaptive ones. We would aver that patients in successful treatments develop healthy core metaphorical themes. Metaphors in such treatments can be used to represent internal embodied experiences (e.g., depression as a physical burden, which can be lifted) and to connect such experiences with cognition and language so as to facilitate expression and restructuring. The therapeutic relationship, which we know to be a critical aspect of successful psychotherapy, may owe part of its effectiveness to eliciting embodied feelings of working together (in sync), warmth, (building) trust, and safety (solid). So a therapist should be aware of and try to maximize such feelings in the therapeutic setting. It may be that the therapeutic relationship is also enhanced by how able the therapist is to show understanding of the patient's narrative, conveyed through the use of metaphors—creating the extremely important feeling of being "gotten."

Neural reuse supports the importance of listening to the metaphors our patients offer as clues to what is going on at the physical/psychological interface. It also should lead the therapist to pay attention to nonverbal behavior as metaphorically communicating our patients' inner workings. Finally, *embodiment*, as related to neural reuse, suggests that we can intervene physically as well as psychologically by providing relevant physical experiences that can have psychological consequences. Since many functions have some underlying neural circuitry (workings) in common, we may be able to affect one type of functioning by altering an aspect of another. Targeting physical behavior, then, may result in psychological change. Thus, neural reuse may be able to explain the growing popularity of various treatment modalities that involve more holistic interventions than conventional talk therapy, such as body psychotherapy, art and dance therapy, and eye movement desensitization and reprocessing. One strong recommendation we have for future research is to try to identify relevant workings so that we may better target the ones that matter instead of the hit-and-miss (often faddy) identification of bodily interventions that is currently most common.

All of this may impact how we understand our patients' clinical presentation, how we help them make sense of their problems, and how we approach treating these problems. Affective salience explains why simply challenging negative cognitions may not be sufficient to lead to improvement. These cognitions are affectively charged and feel true to the patient. So even though a particular cluster of thoughts is challenged, the negative affective state associated with them is likely to continue to impact how events are perceived and interpretations of them made. In fact, the mere process of challenging said cognitions may engender negative affect and thus become counterproductive. After all, why would I want to challenge beliefs and perceptions that I associate with being self-protective? A more effective approach may be to work toward generating a context of positive affective states and an internal sense of safety (e.g., through the therapeutic relationship) before therapeutic work can focus on addressing negative cognitions.

Finally, what we have learned of automaticity provides us with a powerful intervention. That is, the automaticity that helps make maladaptive behaviors so recalcitrant may also hold the key to changing them. Making the unconscious conscious or unmasking automatic thoughts may only represent a first step toward healing and engaging in more adaptive behavioral patterns. This can tell us what has gone wrong and what needs to be changed. What may need to happen next is that new, adaptive functioning needs to be identified. And then, these, now conscious, modes of behavior and/or thinking and/or feeling must be made unconscious (automatic) through (possibly laborious) practice. So *making the conscious unconscious could be a powerful therapeutic technique.*

That is not the end, however. The older maladaptive knowledge is unlikely to be eradicated. The new, more adaptive learning does not replace it. Rather, this new learning is built on top of it, so to speak. Moreover, the old learning will be more likely to be enacted in the contexts in which it was learned, just as the new learning will be more likely to be enacted in the contexts in which it was learned. The old learning will also tend to rear its ugly head during periods of heightened stress when the system is overtaxed so that old habits come to the fore. When this happens, resisting its impact will require considerable effort and even added psychotherapy. We must consistently engage in the new behaviors, monitoring the impact of older patterns of thought and action and reinforcing new learning brought about through psychotherapy. So a major goal of therapy is first to bring maladaptive unconscious automatic processes to awareness. We next need to identify solutions. And finally, we must make these better coping behaviors/thoughts/feelings automatic and unconscious.

In this scenario, it is not impossible to alter maladaptive behaviors, affective reactions, and habits of thought, but it is not easy either. As a result, successful therapy is likely to take time, effortful repetition, and continuous monitoring. And with all of that, relapse can be expected much of the time because the new learning brought about through psychotherapy does not eliminate the old maladaptive learning but rather overlaps with it and is subject to context effects. Thus, it may take long-term or many repetitions of therapy, followed by many relapses before effects become long lasting, if this occurs at all. That is, effective therapy is long-term therapy and/or interventions that are repeated periodically.

We have offered a tentative beginning of a model of psychotherapy based on current understanding of unconscious processes and of the functioning of the mind/brain. It may have great or little value; time will tell. Let us call this model _normative implicit psychotherapy (NIP)_. NIP sees therapy as effective but limited but does not yet know how effective it can be or what those limitations are. Yet, it offers an optimistic view of healing, as it takes into consideration how to harness what we know about the brain/mind works within its limitations, but also recognizes its unique normative unconscious strengths. It is our hope that future integration of knowledge in all of the fields we strove to examine in this book will lead us to more effective and efficient treatments in the (near) future. And we hope this knowledge will be regularly reviewed so as to keep the theories and practice of psychotherapy current. After all, we all want to become better therapists and help our patients in the best ways possible.

NOTES

1. Relational psychoanalytic theorists often laud Janet for emphasizing dissociation over repression. They do not equate dissociation with pathology as did Janet, however (see e.g., Bromberg, 1998, 2006, 2011).

2. It also can help account for the robustness of stereotypes and intransient political beliefs.

Glossary

Affective primacy: Affectively charged information is processed separately from as well as more readily and more quickly than is cognitive information.

Arational: Process that is neither rational, irrational, logical, nor motivated but simply represents the way the mind/brain operates normatively. Most of unconscious processing is arational. AI is arational, and so are computational models of the mind/brain.

Attribution theory: People continuously monitor themselves and their environment, inferring causes of their own behaviors, of the behaviors of others, and of the events taking place around them. These causal attributions are processed (and sometimes distorted) in accordance with preexisting causal beliefs.

Automaticity: Once mental processes have been sufficiently rehearsed (whether consciously–postconsciously or unconsciously–preconsciously), they begin operating autonomously, often circumventing intentionality and awareness. An automatic process must contain at least one of the following features: unconscious, efficient, unintentional, or uncontrollable.

Computational models: Describe mental knowledge structures and how they operate (cognitive architecture). They are attempts to empirically address questions of epistemology. The goal is to understand cognition (defined broadly so as to include motivation and emotion) dynamically, that is, in a process-oriented fashion. The original computational models were modeled after computers. Current ones are modeled after the brain.

Connectionism: A computational model of the mind/brain in which there are innumerable, mappable connections between units (small networks of neurons or aspects of cognition) widely distributed throughout the brain/mind. These units interact such that many mental/neurological processes take place simultaneously (in parallel). This, in turn, allows for complex cognitive and neurological functioning. The most prominent connectionist model is parallel distributed processing (PDP).

Controlled processing: Conscious, more effortful, but also more flexible, counterpart to automatic processing. Control processes allow us to digest and respond to new information in novel ways.

Dipsychism: The idea that there are two minds operating in parallel, one of which is conscious and the other of which is unconscious.

Dual-processing models: Two information-processing systems that operate in parallel. One is more impressionistic, automatic, and unconscious. The other is more reflective, controlled, and conscious. The former operates as the default; the latter requires effort and can override the former.

Embodied cognition: The idea that our thought parallels and is based on the physical body, largely sensory and motor functioning. The theoretical proposition is that cognitive states are embedded in the body—that is, embodied. In other words, higher-level mental processes are grounded to some degree (have parallels) in the body's sensory and motor systems.

Exaptation: Coopting a structure or characteristic to perform a function it did not originally evolve to do. This can come about in one of two ways. One is that a characteristic or structure evolved for one reason but came, over evolutionary time, to serve another (e.g., feathers). The second type of exaptation is when a characteristic or structure that exists independently of natural selection (it just happens to be there, so to speak) is coopted for an adaptation-enhancing use (e.g., fibrous joints in the skull at birth).

Explicit memory: A person's conscious, verbalizable recollection of some event.

Fodor module: Computational model of modules wherein the modules perform specific and limited functions. Fodor characterizes modules as having nine properties.

Heuristic: An unconscious cognitive strategy for making a judgment or solving a problem that does not involve logic or effort. It could be described as a strategic shortcut for solving a problem or reaching a conclusion that bypasses effortful, logical reasoning. It functions as a cognitive rule of thumb, allowing for quick and effortless judgments and decision making.

Implicit learning: Learning that takes place outside of awareness, such that the person does not realize what he has learned; it consists of acquiring knowledge of relations between experiences without intention, without realizing that one is doing so, and without being able to verbalize what one has learned.

Implicit memory: It is present when a person performs an action, voices an attitude, or in some other way appears to have been influenced by a prior event even though she denies any memory of that event. That is, there is a measurable effect of past experiences that the person does not consciously recall.

Implicit motive: Unconscious psychosocial motivators of behavior, usually assessed through narratives.

James–Hebb rule: Through past association, units become more likely to become active together in the future. The more often their activation has been associated, the greater the likelihood of their coactivation on subsequent occasions. Whatever they represent will thereby become activated as well. The system has "learned" something in the sense that a new connection has been made. The strength of the connection is analogous to the degree of the learning. The greater the connection strength, the better the learning.

Massive modularity: The brain/mind is mostly, if not entirely, modular. This includes sophisticated central processes.

Massive redeployment hypothesis: Developed by M. L. Anderson (2010, 2014), this hypothesis provides the most comprehensive framework for neural reuse models. It argues that neural circuits established for one purpose, through evolution, are often exapted (see term above in Glossary) by the same evolution or by normal development and put to other uses. Hence, neural circuits serve multiple roles (neural reuse), including their original purpose as well as new ones determined by evolution.

Mere exposure effect: Repeated presentations of novel stimuli increases people's liking of them.

Module: A set of highly interconnected neurons with relatively few connections to other sets of neurons (i.e., a relatively circumscribed set of neurons).

Neural exploitation hypothesis: The idea, proposed by Gallese (2007) and Gallese and Lakoff (2005), that embodied simulation (mentally simulating the actions of others) can provide direct access to the meaning of those actions as well as the intentions of those engaged in those actions.

Neural reuse: Low-level dedicated neural circuits that developed for one function but are then also used for other psychological processes.

Neuronal recycling hypothesis: Proposed by Dehaene and Cohen (2007), it focuses on processes that allow people to acquire capacities that could not have been the direct result of evolution. It argues that learned functions like reading and writing, for example, develop by utilizing and reconfiguring already existing brain circuitry.

Normative implicit psychotherapy (NIP): The model of therapy this book develops, as detailed in the final chapter. It centers around normative unconscious processes.

Normative unconscious processes: Unconscious processes that are not conflictual or motivated as is the dynamic unconscious posited by psychoanalytic theories; rather, they are universal and operate independently of repressed material, defenses, or deprivation experiences.

Parallel distributed processing (PDP): This theory postulates that the brain consists of an extremely large number of highly interconnected and generalized, small-unit processing elements, distributed throughout the brain. A myriad of such processes occur simultaneously throughout the information-processing system (the brain/mind).

Polypsychism: The mind consists of a cluster of subpersonalities, subject to a central executive personality that contains everyday consciousness.

Postconscious automaticity: A result of repeated rehearsal and, at least initially, some conscious thought or intention. These processes require prior or concurrent intentionality and conscious repetition in order to become automatic.

Preconscious automaticity: Not consciously learned or rehearsed until becoming automatic. They are learned outside of awareness. They result from sensory or perceptual input, which then implicitly and effortlessly impacts conscious higher mental processes.

Priming: The influence of a recent exposure (say of a word) on subsequent performance (like choosing a word from a list).

Scaffolding: Language and thought become formed through physical interactions during the first few years of life.

Self-attributed motive: Conscious psychosocial motivator of behavior, usually assessed through self-report.

Subliminal priming: Priming (see above for definition) wherein the initial exposure (the prime) is presented subliminally (i.e., outside of awareness).

Unit in a PDP system: Groups of neurons that inevitably fire together.

Use: What a working can be used for. A relatively high-level operation that is composed of some combination of workings. It refers to the high-level operation to which the circuit (working) makes a contribution, of which it is a part. A use can be spread out throughout the brain/mind depending upon which workings contribute to it. Many workings can be and typically are combined to create a new use over evolutionary or developmental time.

Workings: Tightly organized, low-level neural networks with a specific function and location in the brain. They do what they do and nothing else. They are immutable. Workings can be evolutionarily based, a result of development, or created through learning. What a brain/mind structure or network does (i.e., the low-level operation—computation—it performs). A working is set and immutable and has a fixed anatomical location.

References

Abend, S. (1990). Unconscious fantasies, structural theory, and compromise formation. *Journal of the American Psychoanalytic Association, 38*(1), 61–73.

Adair, J. G. (1978). The combined probabilities of 345 studies: Only half the story? *Behavioral and Brain Sciences, 3,* 386–387.

Adams, J. (1957). Laboratory studies of behavior without awareness. *Psychological Bulletin, 54,* 383–405.

Ainsworth, M. D. S., Blehar, M. C., Waters, E., & Wall, S. (1978). *Patterns of attachment: A psychological study of the Strange Situation.* Oxford, UK: Erlbaum.

Aisa, B., Mingus, B., & O'Reilly, R. (2008). The emergent neural modeling system. *Neural Networks, 21,* 1146–1152.

Ajzen, I., & Fishbein, M. (1970). The prediction of behavior from attitudinal and normative variables. *Journal of Experimental Social Psychology, 6,* 466–487.

Alcock, J. (2013). *Animal behavior: An evolutionary approach.* Sunderland, MA: Sinauer.

Allen, J. G., & Fonagy, P. (2014). Mentalizing in psychotherapy. In R. E. Hales, S. C. Yudofsky, & L. W. Roberts (Eds.), *The American Psychiatric Publishing textbook of psychiatry* (6th ed., pp. 1095–1118). Arlington, VA: American Psychiatric Publishing.

Allen, R., & Reber, A. S. (1980). Very long term memory for tacit knowledge. *Cognition, 8,* 175–185.

Allers, R., & Teler, J. (1960). On the utilization of unnoticed impressions in associations. *Psychological Issues, 2,* 121–154. (Original work published 1924)

Alpers, G. W., & Gerdes, A. B. (2007). Here is looking at you: Emotional faces predominate in binocular rivalry. *Emotion, 7,* 495–506.

Alpers, G. W., & Pauli, P. (2006). Emotional pictures predominate in binocular rivalry. *Cognition and Emotion, 20,* 596–607.

Alpers, G. W., Ruhleder, M., Walz, N., Muhlberger, A., & Pauli, P. (2005). Binocular rivalry between emotional and neutral stimuli: A validation using fear conditioning and EEG. *International Journal of Psychophysiology, 57,* 25–32.

Ambady, N., & Rosenthal, R. (1992). Thin slices of expressive behavior as predictors of interpersonal consequences: A meta-analysis. *Psychological Bulletin, 111,* 256–274.

Ambady, N., & Rosenthal, R. (1993). Half a minute: Predicting teacher evaluations from thin slices of nonverbal behavior and physical attractiveness. *Journal of Personality and Social Psychology, 64,* 431–441.

American Psychiatric Association. (2013). *Diagnostic and statistical manual of mental Disorders* (5th ed.). Arlington, VA: Author.

Andersen, S. M., & Przybylinski, E. (2012). Experiments on transference in interpersonal relations: Implications for treatment. *Psychotherapy, 49,* 370–383.

Anderson, E., Siegel, E., White, D., & Barrett, L. F. (2012). Out of sight but not out of mind: Unseen affective faces influence evaluations and social impressions. *Emotion, 12,* 1210–1221.

Anderson, J. R. (2007). *How can the human mind occur in the physical universe?* Oxford, UK: Oxford University Press.

Anderson, M. L. (2008). Circuit sharing and the implementation of intelligent systems. *Connection Science, 20,* 239–251.

Anderson, M. L. (2010). Neural reuse: A fundamental organizational principle of the brain. *Behavioral and Brain Sciences, 33,* 245–313.

Anderson, M. L. (2014). *After phrenology: Neural reuse and the interactive brain.* Cambridge, MA: MIT Press.

Anderson, M. L., Brumbaugh, J., & Suben, A. (2010). Investigating functional cooperation in the human brain using simple graph-theoretic methods. In W. Chaovalitwongse, P. Pardola, & P. Xanthopoulos (Eds.), *Computational neuroscience* (Vol. 38, pp. 31–42). New York: Springer.

Anderson, M. L., Kinnison J., & Pessoa L. (2013). Describing functional diversity of brain regions and brain networks. *NeuroImage, 73,* 50–58.

Angell, J. R. (1907). The province of functional psychology. *Psychological Review, 14,* 61–91.

Antoniadis, E. A., Winslow, J. T., Davis, M., & Amaral, D. G. (2007). Role of the primate amygdala in fear-potentiated startle: Effects of chronic lesions in the rhesus monkey. *Journal of Neuroscience, 27,* 7386–7396.

Araujo, S. F. (2012). Why did Wundt abandon his early theory of the unconscious?: Towards a new interpretation of Wundt's psychological project. *History of Psychology, 15,* 33–49.

Arey, L. (1960). The indirect representation of sexual stimuli by schizophrenic and normal subjects. *Journal of Abnormal and Social Psychology, 61*(3), 424–441.

Ariam, S., & Siller J. (1982). Effects of subliminal oneness stimuli in Hebrew on academic performance of Israeli high school students: Further evidence on the adaptation-enhancing effects of symbiotic fantasies on another culture using another language. *Journal of Abnormal Psychology, 91,* 343–349.

Arlow, J. (1953). Masturbation and symptom formation. *Journal of the American Psychoanalytic Association, 1,* 45–58.

Arlow, J. (1961). Ego psychology and the study of mythology. *Journal of the American Psychoanalytic Association, 9,* 371–393.

Arlow, J. (1963). Conflict, regression and symptom formation. *International Journal of Psych-analysis, 44,* 12–22.

Arlow, J. (1969). Unconscious fantasy and disturbances of conscious experience. *Psychoanalytic Quarterly, 38,* 1–27.

Arlow, J. (1987). The dynamics of interpretation. *Psychoanalytic Quarterly, 56,* 68–87.

Arlow, J., & Brenner, C. (1964). *Psychoanalytic concepts and the structural theory.* New York: International Universities Press.

Aron, L. (1996). *A meeting of minds: Mutuality in psychoanalysis.* Hillsdale, NJ: Analytic Press.

Aron, L., & Starr, K. (2013). *A psychotherapy for the people: Toward a progressive psychoanalysis.* New York: Routledge.

Asch, S. E. (1946). Forming impressions of personality. *Journal of Abnormal and Social Psychology, 41,* 258–290.

Atas, A., Faivre, N., Timmermans, B., Cleeremans, A., & Kouider, S. (2014). Nonconscious learning from crowded sequences. *Psychological Science, 25,* 113–119.

Atkinson, J. W., & Walker, E. L. (1956). The affiliation motive and perceptual sensitivity to faces. *Journal of Abnormal and Social Psychology, 53,* 38–41.

Atwood, G. E., & Stolorow, R. D. (1984). *Structures of subjectivity: Explorations in psychoanalytic phenomenology.* Hillsdale, NJ: Analytic Press.

Augustinack, J. C., ven der Kouwe, A. J. W., Salat, D. H., Benner, T. Stevens, A. A., Annese, J., et al. (2014). H. M.'s contributions to neuroscience: A review and autopsy studies. *Hippocampus, 24,* 1267–1286.

Augustine, Saint, Bishop of Hippo. (2009). *The city of God* (M. Dods, Trans.). Peabody, MA: Hendrickson.

Bachant, J. L., Lynch, A. A., & Richards, A. D. (1995). The evolution of drive in contemporary psychoanalysis: A reply to Gill. *Psychoanalytic Psychology, 12*(4), 565–573.

Baddeley, A. D. (1995). Working memory. In M. S. Gazzaniga (Ed.), *The cognitive neurosciences* (pp. 755–764). Cambridge, MA: MIT Press.

Baddeley, A. D., & Hitch, G. J. (1974). Working memory. In G. A. Bower (Ed.), *Recent advances in learning and motivation* (Vol. 8, pp. 47–90). New York: Academic Press.

Baddeley, A. D., & Hitch, G. J. (2000). Development of working memory: Should the Pascual-Leone and the Baddeley and Hitch models be merged? *Journal of Experimental Child Psychology, 77,* 128–137.

Bak, R. C. (1954). The schizophrenic defense against aggression. *International Journal of Psychoanalysis, 35,* 129–134.

Baker, L. E. (1938). The pupillary response conditioned to subliminal auditory stimuli. *Psychological Monographs, 50,* 1–32.

Balay, J., & Shevrin, H. (1989). SPA is subliminal, but is it psychodynamically activating? *American Psychologist, 44,* 1423–1426.

Banaji, M. R., & Greenwald, A. G. (2013). *Blindspot: Hidden biases of good people.* New York: Delacorte Press.

Bandura, A. (1969). *Principles of behavior modification.* New York: Holt, Rinehart & Winston.

Bannerman, R. L., Milders, M., De Gelder, B., & Sahraie, A. (2008). Influence of emotional facial expressions on binocular rivalry. *Ophthalmic and Physiological Optics, 28*(4), 317–326.

Bar-Anan, Y., Wilson, T. D., & Hassin, R. R. (2010). Inaccurate self-knowledge formation as a result of automatic behavior. *Journal of Experimental Social Psychology, 46,* 884–894.

Bargh, J. A. (1989) Conditional automaticity: Varieties of automatic influence on social perception and cognition. In J. Uleman & J. Bargh (Eds.), *Unintended thought* (pp. 3–51). New York: Guilford Press.

Bargh, J. A. (1992). The ecology of automaticity: Toward establishing the conditions needed to produce automatic processing effects. *American Journal of Psychology, 105,* 181–199.

Bargh, J. A. (1994). The Four Horsemen of automaticity: Awareness, efficiency, intention, and control in social cognition. In R. S. Wyer, Jr., & T. K. Srull (Eds.), *Handbook of social cognition* (2nd ed., pp. 1–40). Hillsdale, NJ: Erlbaum.

Bargh, J. A. (1996) Automaticity in social psychology. In E. T. Higgins & A. W. Kruglanski (Eds.), *Social psychology: Handbook of basic principles* (pp. 169–183). New York: Guilford Press.

Bargh, J. A. (1997). The automaticity of everyday life. In R. S. Wyer, Jr. (Ed.), *Advances in social cognition* (Vol. 10, pp. 1–61). Mahwah, NJ: Erlbaum.

Bargh, J. A. (2006). What have we been priming all these years?: On the development, mechanisms, and ecology of nonconscious social behavior. *European Journal of Social Psychology, 36,* 147–168.

Bargh, J. A. (2011). Unconscious thought theory and its discontents: A critique of the critiques. *Social Cognition, 29,* 629–647.

Bargh, J. A. (2016). The devil made me do it. In A. Miller (Ed.), *The social psychology of good and evil* (pp 69–91). New York: Guilford Press.

Bargh, J. A. (2017). *Before you know it.* New York: Simon & Schuster.

Bargh, J. A., & Chartrand, T. (1999). The unbearable automaticity of being. *American Psychologist, 54*(7), 462–479.

Bargh, J. A., Chen, M., & Burrows, L. (1996). Automaticity of social behavior: Direct effect of trait construct and stereotype activation on action. *Journal of Personality and Social Psychology, 71,* 230–244.

Bargh, J. A., & Ferguson, M. (2000). Beyond behaviorism: On the automaticity of higher mental processes. *Psychological Bulletin, 126,* 925–945.

Bargh, J. A., & Morsella, E. (2008). The unconscious mind. *Perspectives on Psychological Science: A Journal of the Association for Psychological Science, 3,* 73–79.

Bargh, J. A., & Morsella, E. (2010). Unconscious behavioral guidance systems. In C. Agnew, D. Carlston, W. Graziano, & J. Kelly (Eds.), *Then a miracle occurs: Focusing on behavior in social psychological theory and research* (pp. 89–118). New York: Oxford University Press.

Bargh, J. A., Schwader, K., Hailey S., Dyer, R., & Boothby, E. (2012). Automaticity in social-cognitive processes. *Trends in Cognitive Science, 16*(12), 593–605.

Bartlett, F. C. (1932). *Remembering: A study in experimental and social psychology.* Cambridge, UK: Cambridge University Press.

Bateman, A., & Fonagy, P. (2015). Borderline personality disorder and mood disorders: Mentalizing as a framework for integrated treatment. *Journal of Clinical Psychology, 71*(8), 792–804.

Batterink, L. J., Reber, P. J., Neville, H. J., & Paller, K. A. (2015). Implicit and explicit contributions to statistical learning. *Journal of Memory and Language, 83,* 62–78.

Bauer, R. M. (1984). Autonomic recognition of names and faces in prosopagnosia: A neuropsychological application of the Guilty Knowledge Test. *Neuropsychologia, 22,* 457–469.

Baumann, N., Kaschel, R., & Kuhl, J. (2005). Striving for unwanted goals: Stress-dependent discrepancies between explicit and implicit achievement motives reduce subjective well-being and increase psychosomatic symptoms. *Journal of Personality and Social Psychology, 89,* 781–799.

Baumeister, R., Bratslavsky, E., Finkenauer, C., & Vohs, K. (2001). Bad is stronger than good. *Review of General Psychology, 5,* 323–370.

Baumrind, D. (1964). Some thoughts on ethics in research: After reading Milgram's "Behavioural study of obedience." *American Psychologist, 19,* 421–423.

Beck, A. T. (1972). *Depression: Causes and treatment.* Philadelphia: University of Pennsylvania Press.

Beck, A. T. (1976). *Cognitive therapy and the emotional disorders.* New York: International Universities Press.

Beck, A. T., Rush, A., Shaw, B., & Emery, G. (1979). *Cognitive therapy of depression.* New York: Guilford Press.

Benjamin, A. A. (2010). Representational explanations of "process" dissociations in recognition: The DRYAD theory of aging and memory judgments. *Psychological Review, 117,* 1055–1079.

Benjamin, J. (1995). Recognition and destruction: An outline of intersubjectivity. In *Like subjects, love objects: Essays on recognition and sexual difference.* New Haven, CT: Yale University Press.

Benoit, R. G., & Schacter, D. L. (2015). Specifying the core network supporting episodic simulation and episodic memory by activation likelihood estimation. *Neuropsychologia, 75,* 450–457.

Beres, D. (1962). The unconscious fantasy. *Psychoanalytic Quarterly, 31,* 309–328.

Bergeron, V. (2008). *Cognitive architecture and the brain.* Unpublished doctoral dissertation, Department of Philosophy, University of British Columbia.

Bergmann, G. (1978). *The metaphysics of logical positivism*. Santa Barbara, CA: Praeger. (Original work published 1950)

Bernston, G. G., Boysen, S. T., & Cacioppo, J. T. (1993). Neurobehaviorlal organization and the cardinal principle of evaluative bivalence. *Annals of the New York Academy of Sciences, 702,* 75–102.

Berry, C. J., Shanks, D. R., & Henson, R. N. A. (2008). A single-system account of the relationship between priming, recognition, and fluency. *Journal of Experimental Psychology: Learning, Memory, and Cognition, 34,* 97–111.

Berry, C. J., Shanks, D. R., & Henson, R. N. A. (2012). Models of recognition, repetition priming, and fluency: Exploring a new framework. *Psychological Review, 119,* 40–79.

Berry, C. J., Shanks, D. R., Li, S., Rains, L. S., & Henson, R. N. A. (2010). Can "pure" implicit memory be isolated?: A test of a single-system model of recognition and repetition priming. *Canadian Journal of Experimental Psychology, 64,* 241–255.

Berry, C. J., Shanks, D. R., Speekenbrink, M., & Henson, R. N. A. (2012). Models of recognition, repetition priming, and fluency: Exploring a new framework. *Psychological Review, 119,* 40–79.

Berry, D. C., & Broadbent, D. E. (1988). Interactive tasks and the implicit-explicit distinction. *British Journal of Psychology, 79,* 251–272.

Berry, D. C., & Dienes, Z. (1993). *Implicit learning: Theoretical and empirical issues*. Hillsdale, NJ: Erlbaum.

Bertrand, A. (1823). *Traite du somnambulisme et des differentes modifications qu'il presente* [*Treatise on somnambulism and its various modifications*]. Paris: J.G. Dentu.

Bettelheim, B. (1983). *Freud and man's soul: An important re-interpretation of Freudian theory*. New York: Vintage Books.

Biernat, M. (1989). Motives and values to achieve: Different constructs with different effects. *Journal of Personality, 57,* 69–95.

Binder, E., Dovern, A., Hesse, M., Ebke, M., Karbe, H., Saliger, J., et al. (2017). Lesion evidence for a human mirror neuron system. *Cortex, 90,* 125–137.

Birdsall, T. G. (1955). The theory of signal detectability. In H. Quastler (Ed.), *Information theory in psychology* (pp. 391–402). Glencoe, IL: Free Press.

Bisiach, E., Vallar, G., Perani, D., & Papagno, C. (1986). Unawareness of disease following lesions of the right hemisphere: Anosognosia for hemiplegia and anosognosia for hemianopia. *Neuropsychologia, 24,* 471–482.

Blatt, S. J., Wein, S. J., Chevron, E., & Quinlan, D. M. (1979). Parental representations and depression in normal young adults. *Journal of Abnormal Psychology, 88,* 388–397.

Blum, G. S. (1954). An experimental reunion of psychoanalytic theory with perceptual vigilance and defense. *Journal of Abnormal and Social Psychology, 49,* 94–98.

Blumer, H. (1969). *Symbolic interactionism: Perspective and method*. Englewood Cliffs,NJ: Prentice-Hall.

Blumstein, S. E., Milbert, W., & Shrier, R. (1983). Semantic processing in aphasia: Evidence from an auditory lexical decision task. *Brain and Language, 17,* 301–315.

Bock, W. J. (1959). Preadaptation and multiple evolutionary pathways. *Evolution, 13,* 194–211.

Boehme, J. (2016). *Aurora.* St. Louis, MO: Kraus House.

Bonnano, G. A., & Stilling, N. A. (1986). Preference, familiarity, and recognition after repeated brief exposures to random geometric shapes. *American Journal of Psychology, 99,* 403–415.

Bookheimer, S. (2002). Functional MRI of language: New approaches to understanding the cortical organization of semantic processing. *Annual Review of Neuroscience, 25,* 151–188.

Boring, E. G. (1950). *A history of experimental psychology* (2nd ed.). Englewood Cliffs, NJ: Prentice-Hall.

Bornstein, R. F. (1989). Exposure and affect: Overview and meta-analysis of research, 1968–1987. *Psychological Bulletin, 106,* 265–289.

Bornstein, R. F. (1992). Subliminal mere exposure effects. In R. F. Bornstein & T. F. Pittman (Eds.), *Perception without awareness: Cognitive, clinical, and social perspectives* (pp. 191–210). New York: Guilford Press.

Bornstein, R. F., & Becker-Matero, N. (2011). Reconnecting psychoanalysis to mainstream psychology: Metaphor as glue. *Psychoanalytic Inquiry, 31,* 172–184.

Bornstein, R. F., & D'Agostino, P. R. (1992). Stimulus recognition and the mere exposure effect. *Journal of Personality and Social Psychology, 63,* 545–552.

Bornstein, R. F., & D'Agostino, P. R. (1994). The attribution and discounting of perceptual fluency: Preliminary tests of a perceptual fluency/attributional model of the mere exposure effect. *Social Cognition, 12,* 103–128.

Bornstein, R. F., & Masling, J. M. (Eds.). (1998). *Empirical perspectives on the psychoanalytic unconscious.* Washington, DC: American Psychological Association.

Bornstein, R. F., & Pittman, T. S. (1992). *Perception without awareness: Cognitive, clinical, and social perspectives.* New York: Guilford Press.

Boroditsky, L., & Ramscar, M. (2002). The roles of body and mind in abstract thought. *Psychological Science, 13,* 185–189.

Bowers, K. S. (1984). On being unconsciously influenced and informed. In K. S. Bowers & D. Meichenbaum (Eds.), *The unconscious reconsidered* (pp. 227–272). New York: Wiley.

Bowlby, J. (1969). *Attachment and loss: Vol. 1. Attachment.* New York: Basic Books.

Boyatzis, R. E. (1972). Affiliation motivation: A review and a new perspective. In D. C. McClelland & R. S. Steele (Eds.), *Human motivation: A book of readings* (pp. 252–278). Morristown, NJ: General Learning Press.

Bradley, R., Greene, J., Russ, E., Dutra, L., & Westen, D. (2005). A multidimensional meta-analysis of psychotherapy for PTSD. *American Journal of Psychiatry, 162,* 214–227.

Braid, J. (1976). *Neuryphnology: Or, the rationale of nervous sleep, considered in relation with animal magnetism.* New York: Arno Press. (Original work published 1843)

Breitmeyer, B. (1984). *Visual masking: An integrative approach.* Oxford, UK: Clarendon Press.

Breitmeyer, B., & Öğmen, H. (2006). *Visual masking: Time slices through conscious and unconscious vision.* Oxford, UK: Oxford University Press.

Brenner, C. (1982). The concept of the superego: A reformulation. *Psychoanalytic Quarterly, 51,* 501–525.

Bricker, P. D., & Chapanis, A. (1953). Do incorrectly perceived tachistoscopically presented stimuli convey some information? *Psychological Review, 60,* 181–188.

Bridgman, P. (1938). Operational analysis. *Philosophy of Science, 5,* 114–131.

Broadbent, D. E. (1957). A mechanical model for human attention and immediate memory. *Psychological Review, 64,* 205–215.

Broadbent, D. E. (1958). *Perception and communication.* New York: Oxford University Press.

Broadbent, D. E. (1971). *Decision and stress.* London: Academic Press.

Broadbent, D. E., & Gregory, M. (1967). Psychological refractory period and the length of time required to make a decision. *Proceedings of the Royal Society, Series B, 158,* 222–231.

Broca, P. (2011). Remarks on the seat of spoken language, followed by a case of aphasia. *Neuropsychology Review, 21,* 227–229. (Original work published 1861)

Brody, N. (1972). *Personality: Research and theory.* New York: Academic Press.

Bromberg, P. (1998). *Standing in spaces: Essays on dissociation, trauma and clinical process.* New York: Routledge.

Bromberg, P. (2006). *Awakening the dreamer: Clinical journeys.* New York: Routledge.

Bromberg, P. (2011). *The shadow of the tsunami: And the growth of the relational mind.* New York: Routledge.

Bronstein, A. A., & Rodin, G. C. (1983). An experimental study of internalization fantasies in schizophrenic men. *Psychotherapy: Theory, Research and Practice, 20,* 408–416.

Brooks, D. N., & Baddeley, A. (1976). What can amnesic patients learn? *Neuropsychologia, 14,* 111–122.

Brooks, N., & Goldin-Meadow, S. (2016). Moving to learn: How guiding the hands can set the stage for learning. *Cognitive Science, 40,* 1831–1849.

Brooks, R. (1991). Intelligence without representation. *Artificial Intelligence, 47,* 139–160.

Broughton, J. (2002). *Descartes's method of doubt.* Princeton, NJ: Princeton University Press.

Brown, A. S. (1991). A review of the tip-of-the-tongue experience. *Psychological Bulletin, 109,* 204–223.

Brown, A. S. (2012). *The tip of the tongue state: Essays in cognitive psychology.* New York: Psychology Press.

Brown, B. (2015). *Daring greatly: How the courage to be vulnerable transforms the way we live, love, parent, and lead.* New York: Avery.

Brown, T. A., & Barlow, D. H. (1995). Long-term outcome in cognitive-behavioral treatment of panic disorder: Clinical predictors and alternative strategies for assessment. *Journal of Consulting and Clinical Psychology, 63,* 754–765.

Brown, W. P. (1961). *Conceptions of perceptual defense* (*British Journal of Psychology Monograph Supplements, 35*). London: Cambridge University Press.

Bruner, J. S., & Postman, L. (1947). Emotional selectivity in perception and reaction. *Journal of Personality, 16,* 69–77.

Bruner, J. S., & Postman, L. (1949). On the perception of incongruity: A paradigm. *Journal of Personality, 18,* 206–223.

Brunstein, J. C., & Maier, G. W. (2005). Implicit and self-attributed motives to achieve: Two separate but interacting needs. *Journal of Personality and Social Psychology, 89,* 205–222.

Brunstein, J. C., Schultheiss, O. C., & Grassmann, R. (1998). Personal goals and emotional well-being: The moderating role of motive dispositions. *Journal of Personality and Social Psychology, 75,* 494–508.

Bryant-Tuckett, R., & Silverman L. H. (1984). Effects of the subliminal stimulation of symbiotic fantasies on the academic performance of emotionally handicapped students. *Journal of Counseling Psychology, 31,* 295–305.

Buchner, A., & Brandt, M. (2003). Further evidence for systematic reliability differences between explicit and implicit memory tests. *Quarterly Journal of Experimental Psychology, 56A,* 193–209.

Buchner, A., & Wippich, W. (2000). On the reliability of implicit and explicit memory measures. *Cognitive Psychology, 40,* 227–259.

Buranelli, V. (1975). *The wizard from Vienna: Franz Anton Mesmer.* New York: Coward, McCann & Geoghegan.

Buss, D. M. (1999). *Evolutionary psychology: The new science of the mind.* Needham Heights, MA: Allyn & Bacon.

Butters, N., Heindel, W. C., & Salmon, D. P. (1990). Dissociation of implicit memory in dementia: Neurological implications. *Bulletin of the Psychonomic Society, 28,* 359–366.

Byrne, D. (1959). The effects of a subliminal food stimulus on verbal responses. *Journal of Applied Psychology, 43,* 249–252.

Byrne, D. (1961). Interpersonal attraction and attitude similarity. *Journal of Abnormal and Social Psychology, 62,* 713–715.

Cacioppo, J. T., & Bernston, G. G. (1994). Relationship between attitudes and evaluative space: A critical review, with emphasis on the separability of positive and negative substrates. *Psychological Bulletin, 115,* 401–423.

Cahill, L., Uncapher, M., Kilpatrick, L., Alkire, M. T., & Turner, J. (2004). Sex-related hemispheric lateralization of amygdala function in emotionally influenced memory: An fMRI investigation. *Learning and Memory, 11,* 261–266.

Caliskan, A., Bryson, J. J., & Narayanan, A. (2017). Semantics derived automatically from language corpora contain human-like biases. *Science, 356,* 183–186.

Calvo, M. G., Avero, P., & Nummenmaa, L. (2011). Primacy of emotional vs. semantic scene recognition in peripheral vision. *Cognition and Emotion, 25,* 1358–1375.

Calvo, M. G., & Nummenmaa, L. (2008). Detection of emotional faces: Salient physical features guide effective visual search. *Journal of Experimental Psychology: General, 137*, 471–494.

Campbell, K., & Sedikides, C. (1999). Self-threat magnifies the self-serving bias: A meta-analytic integration. *Review of General Psychology, 3*, 23–43.

Caramazza, A. (1996). The brain's dictionary. *Nature, 380*, 485–486.

Carey, B. (2008, December 4). H. M., an unforgettable amnesiac, dies at 82. *New York Times*. Retrieved from *www.nytimes.com/2008/12/05/us/05hm.html*.

Carlston, D. E., & Smith, E. R. (1996). Principles of mental representation. In E. T. Higgins & A. W. Kruglanski (Eds.), *Social psychology: Handbook of basic principles* (pp. 184–210). New York: Guilford Press.

Carpenter, B., Wiener, M., & Carpenter, J. T. (1956). Predictability of perceptual defense behavior. *Journal of Abnormal and Social Psychology, 52*(3), 380–383.

Carruthers, P. (2006). *The architecture of the mind: Massive modularity and the flexibility of thought*. New York: Oxford University Press.

Carruthers, P. (2009). How we know our own minds: The relationship between mindreading and metacognition. *Behavioral and Brain Sciences, 32*, 121–138.

Carruthers, P. (2010). Introspection: Divided and partly eliminated. *Philosophy and Phenomenological Research, 80*(1), 76–111.

Casey, B. J., Tottenham, N., Liston, C., & Durston, S. (2005). Imaging the developing brain: What have we learned about cognitive development? *Trends in Cognitive Science, 9*, 104–110.

Cave, C. B. (1997). Very long-lasting priming in picture naming. *Psychological Science, 8*, 322–325.

Cermak, L. S., Talbot, R., Chandler, K., & Wolbarst, L. R. (1985). The perceptual priming phenomenon in amnesia. *Neuropsychologia, 23*, 615–622.

Cesario, J., Plaks, J. E., & Higgins, E. T. (2006). Automatic social behavior as motivation preparation to interact. *Journal of Personality and Social Psychology, 90*, 893–910.

Chalmers, D. J. (1996). *The conscious mind: In search of a fundamental theory*. New York: Oxford University Press.

Chan, K. Q., Tong, E. M., Tan, D. H., & Koh, A. H. Q. (2013). What do love and jealousy taste like? *Emotion, 13*, 1142–1149.

Chapman, C. R., & Feather, B. W. (1972). Modification of perception by classical conditioning procedures. *Journal of Experimental Psychology, 93*, 338–342.

Chen, M., & Bargh, J. (1997). Nonconscious behavioral confirmation process: The self-fulfilling consequences of automatic stereotype activation. *Journal of Experimental Social Psychology, 33*, 541–560.

Cherry, E. C. (1953). Some experiments on the recognition of speech, with one and with two ears. *Journal of the Acoustical Society of America, 25*, 975–979.

Cherry, E. C., & Taylor, W. K. (1954). Some further experiments upon the recognition of speech, with one and with two ears. *Journal of the Acoustical Society of America, 26*, 554–559.

Chomsky, N. (1957). *Syntactic structures*. The Hague, the Netherlands: Mouton.

Chun, M. M., & Phelps, E. A. (1999). Memory deficits for implicit contextual information in amnesic subjects with hippocampal damage. *Nature Neuroscience, 2*, 844–847.

Churchland, P. S. (2011). *Braintrust: What neuroscience tells us about morality*. Princeton, NJ: Princeton University Press.

Claparède, E. (1995). Recognition and selfhood. *Consciousness and Cognition, 4*, 371–378. (Original work published 1911)

Clark, A. (1993). *Associative engines: Connectionism, concepts, and representational change*. Cambridge, MA: MIT Press.

Clark, A. (2013). Whatever next?: Predictive brains, situated agents, and the future of cognitive science. *Behavioral and Brain Sciences, 36*, 181–204.

Clarke, M. (2004). *Reconstructing reason and representation*. Cambridge, MA: MIT Press.

Cleeremans, A. (2014). Connecting conscious and unconscious processing. *Cognitive Science, 38*, 1286–1315.

Cleeremans, A., & Dienes, Z. (2008). Computational models of implicit learning. In R. Sun (Ed.), *The Cambridge handbook of computational modeling* (pp. 396–421). Cambridge, UK: Cambridge University Press.

Cleeremans, A., & McClelland, J. L. (1991). Learning the structure of event sequences. *Journal of Experimental Psychology: General, 120*, 235–253.

Cohen, W. J., & Squire, L. R. (1981). Retrograde amnesia and remote memory impairment. *Neuropsychologia, 19*, 337–356.

Collins, A. M., & Loftus, E. F. (1975). A spreading-activation theory of semantic processing. *Psychological Review, 82*, 407–428.

Coltheart, M. (1987). The semantic error: Types and theories. In M. Coltheart, K. Patterson, & J. C. Marshall (Eds.), *Deep dyslexia* (2nd ed., pp. 146–159). New York: Routledge.

Comte, A. (1988). *Introduction to positive philosophy* (F. Ferre, Trans.). Indianapolis, IN: Hackett. (Original work published 1830)

Conroy, M. A., Hopkins, R. O., & Squire, L. R. (2005). On the contribution of perceptual fluency and priming to recognition memory. *Cognitive, Affective, and Behavioral Neuroscience, 5*, 14–20.

Cooley, C. H. (1902). *Human nature and the social order*. New York: Scribner.

Corteen. R. S., & Dunn, D. (1974). Shock-associated words in a nonattended message: A test for momentary awareness. *Journal of Experimental Psychology, 102*, 1143–1144.

Corteen, R. S., & Wood, B. (1972). Autonomic responses to shock-associated words in an unattended channel. *Journal of Experimental Psychology, 94*, 308–313.

Cortina, M., & Liotti, G. (2007). New approaches to understanding unconscious processes: Implicit and explicit memory systems. *International Forum of Psychoanalysis, 16*, 204–212.

Coslett, H. B., Rothi, L. G., Valenstein, E., & Heilman, K. M. (1986). Dissociations of writing and praxis: Two cases in point. *Brain and Language, 28*, 357–369.

Cox, L. (1974). *Depressive symptoms as affected by aggressive stimuli subliminally and supraliminally presented.* Unpublished doctoral dissertation, Fordham University, New York.

Cozolino, L. (2014). *The neuroscience of human relationships.* New York: Norton.

Craik, F. I. M., & Jennings, J. M. (1992). Human memory. In F. I. M. Craik & T. A. Salghouse (Eds.), *The handbook of aging and cognition* (pp. 51–110). Hillsdale, NJ: Erlbaum.

Craske, M. C., Liao, B., Brown, L., & Vervliet, B. (2012). Role of inhibition in exposure therapy. *Journal of Experimental Psychopathology, 3,* 322–345.

Craske, M. G., Treanor, M., Conway, C. C., Zbozinek, T., & Vervilet, B. (2014). Maximizing exposure therapy: An inhibitory learning approach. *Behaviour Research and Therapy, 58,* 10–23.

Crick, F. H., & Koch, C. (1990). Towards a neurobiological theory of consciousness. *Seminars in the Neurosciences, 2,* 263–275.

Csibra, G. (2007). Action mirroring and action understanding: An alternative account. In P. Haggard, Y. Rosetti, & M. Kawato (Eds.), *Sensorimotor foundations of higher cognition* (pp. 435–459). New York: Oxford University Press.

Damasio, A. R., Everitt, B., & Bishop, D. (1996). The somatic marker hypothesis and the possible functions of the prefrontal cortex [and discussion]. *Philosophical Transactions: Biological Sciences, 351*(1346), 1413–1420.

Damasio, A. R., & Tranel, D. (1993). Nouns and verbs are retrieved with differently distributed neural systems. *Proceedings of the National Academy of Sciences of the USA, 90,* 4857–4960.

Darwin, C. (1998). *The expression of the emotions in man and animals* (3rd ed.). Introduction, afterwords, and commentaries by Paul Ekman. New York: Oxford University Press. (Original work published 1872)

Darwin, C. (2002). *On the origin of species.* London: Murray. Republished Abingdon, UK: Routledge. (Original work published 1859)

Dauber, R. (1984). Subliminal psychodynamic activation in depression. *Journal of Abnormal Psychology, 93,* 9–18.

Davids, A. (1956). Personality dispositions, word frequency and word association. *Journal of Personality, 24,* 328–338.

Davies, J. M., & Frawley, M. G. (1994). *Treating the adult survivor of childhood sexual abuse: A psychoanalytic perspective.* New York: Basic Books.

Dawson, M. E., & Schell, A. M. (1982). Electrodermal responses to attended and unattended significant stimuli during dichotic listening. *Journal of Experimental Psychology: Human Perception and Performance, 8,* 315–324.

de Gelder, B., Vroomen, J., Pourtois, G., & Weiskrantz, L. (1999). Non-conscious recognition of affect in the absence of striate cortex. *NeuroReport, 10,* 3753–3759.

De Houwer, J. (2006). What are implicit measures and why are we using them?

In R. W. Wiers & A. W. Stacy (Eds.), *The handbook of implicit cognition and addiction* (pp. 11–28). Thousand Oaks, CA: SAGE.

De Houwer, J., & Moors, A. (2007). How to define and examine the implicitness of implicit measures. In B. Wittenbrink & N. Schwartz (Eds.), *Implicit measures of attitudes: Procedures and controversies* (pp. 179–194). New York: Guilford Press.

De Houwer, J., Teige-Mocigemba, S., Spruyt, A., & Moors, A. (2009). Implicit measures: A normative analysis and review. *Psychological Bulletin, 135,* 347–368.

de Roten, Y., Drapeau, M., & Michel, L. (2008). Are there positive emotions in short-term dynamic psychotherapy or is it all Freude-less? *Journal of Psychotherapy Integration, 18,* 207–221.

deCharms, R., Morrison, H. W., Reitman, W., & McClelland, D. C. (1955). Behavioral correlates of directly and indirectly measured achievement motivation. In D. C. McClelland (Ed.), *Studies in motivation* (pp. 414–423). New York: Appleton-Century-Crofts.

Dehaene, S. (2005). Evolution of human cortical circuits for reading and arithmetic: The "neuronal recycling" hypothesis. In S. Dehaene, J. R. Duhamen, M. D. Hauser, & G. Rizolatti (Eds.), *From monkey brain to human brain* (pp. 133–157). Cambridge, MA: MIT Press.

Dehaene, S. (2008). Conscious and unconscious processes: Distinct forms of evidence accumulation? In C. Engel & W. Singer (Eds.), *Better than conscious?: Decision making, the human mind, and implications for institutions* (pp. 21–49). Cambridge, MA: MIT Press.

Dehaene, S. (2009). *Reading in the brain: The science and evolution of a human invention.* New York: Penguin.

Dehaene, S. (2014). *Consciousness and the brain: Deciphering how the brain codes our thoughts.* New York: Viking.

Dehaene, S., Charles, L., King, J.-R., & Marti, S. (2014). Toward a computational theory of conscious processing. *Current Opinion in Neurobiology, 25,* 76–84.

Dehaene, S., & Cohen, L. (2007). Cultural recycling of cortical maps. *Neuron, 56,* 384–398.

Dennett, D. C. (1991). *Consciousness explained.* New York: Little, Brown & Co.

Dermot, L., Corker, K. S., Wortman, J., Connell, L., Donnellan, M. B., Lucas, R. E., et al. (2014). Replication of "Experiencing physical warmth promotes interpersonal warmth" by Williams and Bargh (2008). *Social Psychology, 45,* 216–222.

Descartes, R. (1989). *The passions of the soul* (S. H. Voss, Trans.). Indianapolis, IN: Hackett. (Original work published 1649)

Descartes, R. (2013). *Meditations on first philosophy* (I. Johnston, Trans.). Petersburg, Ontario, Canada: Broadview Press. (Original work published 1642)

Descartes, R. (2017). *Discourse on method* (I. Johnston, Trans.). Petersburg, Ontario, Canada: Broadview Press. (Original work published 1637)

D'Esposito, M., Detre, J. A., Alsop, D. C., Shin, R. K., Atlas, S., & Grossman, M. (1995). The neural basis of the central executive system of working memory. *Nature, 378,* 279–281.

Dessoir, M. (1890). *Das doppie-ich* [*The double ego*]. Liepzig, Germany: Gunther. (Cited in Ellenberger, 1970)

Deutsch, J. A., & Deutsch, D. (1963). Attention: Some theoretical considerations. *Psychological Review, 70,* 80–90.

Devine, P. (1989). Stereotypes and prejudice: Their automatic and controlled components. *Journal of Personality and Social Psychology, 56,* 5–18.

Dew, I. T. Z., & Cabeza, R. (2011). The porous boundaries between explicit and implicit memory: Behavioral and neural evidence. *Annals of the New York Academy of Science, 1224,* 174–190.

di Pellegrino, G., Fadiga, L., Fogassi, L., Gallese, V., & Rizzolatti, G. (1992). Understanding motor events: A neuropsychological study. *Experimental Brain Research, 91,* 175–80.

Dienes, Z., Broadbent, D., & Berry, D. (1991). Implicit and explicit knowledge bases in artificial grammar learning. *Journal of Experimental Psychology: Learning, Memory, and Cognition, 17,* 875–887.

Dijksterhuis, A. (2004). Think different: The merits of unconscious thought in preference development and decision making. *Journal of Personality and Social Psychology, 87,* 586–598.

Dijksterhuis, A. (2013). Exploring the relation between motivation and intuition. In J. P. Forgas, K. Fiedler, & C. Sedikides (Eds.), *Social thinking and interpersonal behavior: Sydney Symposium of Social Psychology* (pp. 101–112). New York: Psychology Press.

Dijksterhuis, A., Bos, M. W., Nordgren, L. F., & van Barren, R. B. (2006). On making the right choice: The deliberation-without-attention effect. *Science, 211,* 1005–1007.

Dijksterhuis, A., & Nordgren, L. (2006). A theory of unconscious thought. *Perspectives on Psychological Science, 1,* 95–109.

Dittrich, L. (2016). *Patient H. M.: A story of memory, madness, and family secrets.* New York: Random House.

Dixon, N. F. (1956). Symbolic associations following subliminal stimulation. *International Journal of Psycho-analysis, 37,* 159–170.

Dixon, N. F. (1958). The effect of subliminal stimulation upon autonomic and verbal behavior. *Journal of Abnormal and Social Psychology, 57,* 29–36.

Dixon, N. F. (1971). *Subliminal perception: The nature of a controversy.* New York: McGraw Hill.

Dixon, N. F. (1981). *Preconscious processing.* New York: Wiley.

Donaldson, D. I., Petersen, S. E., & Buckner, R. L. (2001). Dissociating memory retrieval processes using fMRI: Evidence that priming does not support recognition memory. *Neuron, 31,* 1047–1059.

Doré, B. P., Zerubavel, N., & Ochsner, K. N. (2015). Social cognitive neuroscience: A review of core systems. In M. Mikulincer, P. R. Shaver, E. Borgida, & J. A. Bargh (Eds.), *APA handbook of personality and social psychology: Vol. 1. Attitudes and social cognition* (pp. 693–720). Washington, DC: American Psychological Association.

Dorfman, D. D. (1967). Recognition of taboo words as a function of a priori probability. *Journal of Personality and Social Psychology, 7*, 1–10.

Draguns, J. G. (2008). Perceptgenesis: Its origins, accomplishments, and prospects. In G. J. W. Smith & I. M. Carlsson (Eds.), *Process and personality: Actualization of the personal world with process-oriented methods* (pp. 23–50). Frankfurt, Germany: Ontos Verlag.

Dulany, D. E. (1997). Consciousness in the explicit (deliberative) and implicit (evocative). In J. D. Cohen & J. W. Schooler (Eds.), *Carnegie Mellon Symposia on Cognition: Scientific approaches to consciousness* (pp. 179–212). Hillsdale, NJ: Erlbaum.

Dulany, D. E., Carlson, R. A., & Dewey, G. I. (1984). A case of syntactical learning and judgment: How conscious and how abstract? *Journal of Experimental Psychology: General, 113*, 541–555.

Dulany, D. E., Jr., & Eriksen, C. W. (1959). Accuracy of brightness discrimination as measured by concurrent verbal responses and GSRs. *Journal of Abnormal and Social Psychology, 59*, 418–423.

Dunn, J. C., & Kirsner, K. (2003). What can we infer from double dissociations? *Cortex, 39*, 1–7.

Durand, J. P. (1868). *Polyzoïsme ou pluralité animale chez l'homme*. Paris: Immprimerie Hennuyer. (Polyzoism or animal plurality in man—as cited in Ellenberger, 1970)

Dutta, A., Shah, K., Silvanto, J., & Soto, D. (2014). Neural basis of non-conscious visual working memory. *Neuroimage, 91*, 336–343.

Dykas, M. J., & Cassidy, J. (2011). Attachment and the processing of social information across the life span: Theory and evidence. *Psychological Bulletin, 137*, 19–46.

Eagle, M. (1959). The effects of subliminal stimuli of aggressive content upon conscious cognition. *Journal of Personality, 27*, 578–600.

Eagle, M. (1983). Psychoanalysis as hermeneutics. *PsyCRITIQUES, 28*, 149.

Eagle, M. N., Gallese, V., & Migone, P. (2009). Mirror neurons and mind: Commentary on Vivona. *Journal of the American Psychoanalytic Association, 57*, 559–568.

Eagly, A. H., & Chaiken, S. (1993). *The psychology of attitudes*. Orlando, FL: Harcourt-Brace-Jovanovich.

Ebbinghaus, H. (1964). *Memory: A contribution to experimental psychology*. New York: Dover. (Original work translated 1913)

Eichenbaum, H., & Cohen, N. J. (2001). *From conditioning to conscious recollection: Memory systems of the brain*. New York: Oxford University Press.

Einstein, G. O., & McDaniel, M. A. (1990). Normal aging and prospective memory. *Journal of Experimental Psychology: Learning, Memory, and Cognition, 16*, 717–726.

Ekman, P., Levenson, R., & Friesen, W. (1983). Autonomic nervous system activity distinguishes among emotions. *Science, 221*(4616), 1208–1210.

Ellenberger, H. (1970). *The discovery of the unconscious: The history and evolution of dynamic psychiatry*. New York: Basic Books.

Emmelkamp, P. (2004). *The treatment of phobic disorders: Is exposure still the treatment of choice?* New York: Wiley.

Engelbert, M., & Carruthers, P. (2010). Introspection. *Cognitive Science, 1,* 245–253.

Erdelyi, M. H. (1974). A new look at the new look: Perceptual defense and vigilance. *Psychological Review, 81,* 1–25.

Erdelyi, M. H. (1985). *Psychoanalysis: Freud's cognitive psychology.* San Francisco: Freeman.

Erdelyi, M. H. (1992). Psychodynamics and the unconscious. *American Psychologist, 47,* 784–787.

Eriksen, C. W. (1951). Perceptual defense as a function of unacceptable needs. *Journal of Abnormal and Social Psychology, 46,* 557–564.

Eriksen, C. W. (1954). The case for perceptual defense. *Psychological Review, 61,* 175–182.

Eriksen, C. W. (1956). Subception: Fact or artifact? *Psychological Review, 63,* 71–80.

Eriksen, C. W. (1957). Prediction from and interaction among multiple concurrent discriminative responses. *Journal of Experimental Psychology, 53,* 353–359.

Eriksen, C. W. (1958). Unconscious processes. In M. R. Jones (Ed.), *Nebraska Symposium on Motivation* (pp. 169–225). Lincoln: University of Nebraska Press.

Eriksen, C. W. (1959). Discrimination measured by multiple concurrent responses. *Psychological Reports, 5,* 741–750.

Eriksen, C. W. (1960). Discrimination and learning without awareness: A methodological survey and evaluation. *Psychological Review, 6,* 279–300.

Eslinger, P. J., & Damasio, A. R. (1986). Preserved motor learning in Alzheimer's disease: Implications for anatomy and behavior. *Journal of Neuroscience, 10,* 3006–3009.

Evans, R. B., & Koelsch, W. A. (1985). Psychoanalysis arrives in America. *American Psychologist, 40,* 942–948.

Exline, R. V. (1960). Effects of sex, norms, and affiliation motivation upon accuracy of perception of interpersonal preference. *Journal of Personality, 28,* 397–412.

Eysenck, H. (1963). *Uses and abuses of psychology.* Baltimore: Penguin Books.

Fairbairn, W. R. D. (1952). *Psychoanalytic studies of the personality.* Oxford, UK: Routledge & Kegan Paul.

Fallshore, M., & Schooler, J. W. (1993). Post-encoding verbalization impairs transfer on artificial grammar tasks. In *Proceedings of the 15th annual meeting of the Cognitive Science Society,* 412–416.

Faranda, F. (2014). Working with images in psychotherapy: An embodied experience of play and metaphor. *Journal of Psychotherapy Integration, 24,* 65–77.

Fazio, R. H., Sanbonmatsu, D. M., Powell, M. C., & Kardes, F. R. (1986). On the automatic activation of attitudes. *Journal of Personality and Social Psychology, 50,* 229–238.

Fechner, G. (1846). *Ueber das höchste Gut* [*Concerning the highest good*]. Frankfurt, Germany: Breitkopf & Hartel.

Fechner, G. (1873). *Einige Ideen zur Schöpfungs und Entwickelungsgeschichte der Organismen [Some ideas on the history of the creation and evolution of organisms]*. Hamburg, Germany: Verlag.

Feldman, J. A. (1985). Connectionist models and their applications: Introduction. *Cognitive Science, 9*, 1–2.

Feldman, J. A., & Ballard, D. H. (1982). Connectionist models and their properties. *Cognitive Science, 6*, 205–254.

Fenichel, O. (1945). *The psychoanalytic theory of neurosis*. New York: Norton.

Ferrari, P. F., Gallese, V., Rizzolatti, G., & Fogassi, L. (2003). Mirror neurons responding to the observation of ingestive and communicative mouth actions in the monkey ventral premotor cortex. *European Journal of Neuroscience, 17*(8), 1703–1714.

Festinger, L. (1957). *A theory of cognitive dissonance*. Stanford, CA: Stanford University Press.

Festinger, L., & Carlsmith, J. M. (1959). Cognitive consequences of forced compliance. *Journal of Abnormal and Social Psychology, 58*, 203–210.

Fichte, J. G. (1982). *The science of knowledge* (P. Heath & J. Lachs, Trans. & Eds.). Cambridge, UK: Cambridge University Press. (Original work published 1802)

Fiske, S., & Tablante, C. (2015). Stereotyping: Process and content. In M. Mikulincer, P. Shaver, E. Borgida, & J. Bargh (Eds.), *APA handbook of personality and social psychology: Vol. 1. Attitudes and social cognition* (pp. 457–507). Washington, DC: American Psychological Association.

Fitzsimons, G. M., & Bargh, J. A. (2003). Thinking of you: Nonconscious pursuit of interpersonal goals associated with relationship partners. *Journal of Personality and Social Psychology, 84*, 148–164.

Fitzsimons, G. M., & Bargh, J. A. (2004, January 29–31). *Automatic goal pursuit in close relationships*. Paper presented at the meeting of the APA Division 8, Society for Personality and Social Psychology.

Fleischman, D. A., Wilson, R. S., Gabrieli, J. D. E., Bienias, J. L., & Bennett, D. A. (2004). A longitudinal study of implicit and explicit memory of old persons. *Psychology and Aging, 19*, 617–625.

Fodor, E. M. (1990). The power motive and creativity of solutions to an engineering problem. *Journal of Research in Personality, 24*, 338–354.

Fodor, E. M. (2009). Power motivation. In M. R. Leary & R. H. Hoyle (Eds.), *Handbook of individual differences in social behavior* (pp. 426–440). New York: Guilford Press.

Fodor, E. M., & Smith, T. (1982). The power motive as an influence on group decision making. *Journal of Personality and Social Psychology, 42*, 178–185.

Fodor, J. A. (1975). *The language of thought*. Cambridge, MA: Harvard University Press.

Fodor, J. A. (1983). *Modularity of mind*. Cambridge, MA: MIT Press.

Fodor, J. A. (2000). *The mind doesn't work that way: The scope and limits of computational psychology*. Cambridge, MA: MIT Press.

Fodor, J. A., & Pylyshyn, Z. (1988). Connectionism and cognitive architecture: A critical analysis. *Cognition, 28*(1–2, 3–71).

Fodor, J. A., & Pylyshyn, Z. (2015). *Minds without meanings: An essay on the content of concepts.* Cambridge, MA: MIT Press.

Fonagy, P., & Allison, E. (2014). What is mentalization?: The concept and its foundations in developmental research. In N. Midgley & I. Vrouva (Eds.), *Minding the child: Mentalizations-based interventions with children, young people and their families* (pp. 11–34). New York: Routledge/Taylor & Francis.

Forster, P. M., & Govier, E. (1978). Discrimination without awareness. *Quarterly Journal of Experimental Psychology, 30,* 289–296.

Fowler, C. A., Wolford, G., Slade, R., & Tassinary, L. (1981). Lexical access with and without awareness. *Journal of Experimental Psychology: General, 110,* 341–362.

Fraley, C., & Shaver, P. (2000). Adult romantic attachment: Theoretical developments, emerging controversies, and unanswered questions. *Review of General Psychology, 4*(2), 132–154.

Frankel, C. (1950). Positivisim. In V. T. A. Ferm (Ed.), *A history of philosophical systems* (pp. 329–339). Freeport, NY: Books for Libraries Press.

Frensch, P. A., & Runger, D. (2003). Implicit learning. *Current Directions in Psychological Science, 12,* 13–18.

Freud, A. (1992). *The ego and the mechanisms of defense.* London: Karnac Books. (Original work published 1936)

Freud, S. (1900). *The interpretation of dreams.* Leipzig, Germany: Franz Deuticke.

Freud, S. (1904). *The psychopathology of everyday life.* New York: Macmillan.

Freud, S. (1905). *Jokes and their relation to the unconscious.* Leipzig, Germany: Franz Deuticke.

Freud, S. (1910). Five lectures on psycho-analysis. *Standard Edition, 11,* 9–55, 1957.

Freud, S. (1915). The unconscious. *Standard Edition, 14,* 159–215, 1963.

Freud, S. (1916). Introductory lectures on psycho-analysis. *Standard Edition, 22,* 1–182, 1961.

Freud, S. (1917). Mourning and melancholia. *Standard Edition, 14,* 237–258, 1963.

Freud, S. (1920). *Beyond the pleasure principle.* London: International Psychoanalytical Press.

Freud, S. (1923). The ego and the id. *Standard Edition, 19,* 1–66, 1961.

Freud, S. (1926). Inhibitions, symptoms, and anxiety. *Standard Edition, 20,* 75–175, 1959.

Freud, S. (1933). New introductory lectures on psychoanalysis. *Standard Edition, 22,* 3–184, 1959.

Freud, S. (1937). Analysis terminable and interminable. *International Journal of Psycho-analysis, 18,* 373–405.

Freud, S. (1940). Splitting of the ego in the process of defence. In *Standard Edition, 22,* 271–278, 1964.

Fribourg, A. (1981). Ego pathology in schizophrenia and fantasies of merging with the good mother. *Journal of Nervous and Mental Disease, 169,* 337–347.

Fritz, G., & Hitzig, E. (2009). Electric excitability of the cerebrum [*Uber die elektrische erregbarkeit des grosshirns*]. *Epilepsy and Behavior, 15,* 123–130. (Original work published 1870)

Fudin, R. (1986). Subliminal psychodynamic activation: Mommy and I are not yet one. *Perceptual and Motor Skills, 63,* 1159–1179.

Fuhrer, M. J., & Eriksen, C. W. (1960). The unconscious perception of the meaning of verbal stimuli. *Journal of Abnormal and Social Psychology, 61,* 432–439.

Fullerton, G. S., & Cattell, J. M. (1892). *On the perception of small differences.* Publications of the University of Pennsylvania, Philosophical Series No. 2, 1892. (Reprinted in James McKeen Cattell, *Man of science: Vol. 1. Psychological research.* Lancaster, PA. Science Press, 1947)

Gabrieli, J. D. E. (1998). Cognitive neuroscience of human memory. *Annual Review of Psychology, 49,* 87–115.

Gall, F. J. (1835). *On the functions of the brain and each of its parts* (Vol. 1, J. G. Spurzheim, co-author) (W. Lewis, Jr., Trans.). Boston: Marsh, Capen & Lyon. (Original work published 1822–1825)

Gallese, V. (2003a). The manifold nature of interpersonal relations: The quest for a common mechanism. *Philosophical Transactions of the Royal Society of London, Series B: Biological Sciences, 358,* 517–528.

Gallese, V. (2003b). The roots of empathy: The shared manifold hypothesis and the neural basis for intersubjectivity. *Psychopathology, 36,* 171–180.

Gallese, V. (2006). Intentional attunement: A neuropsychological perspective on social cognition and its disruption in autism. *Brain Research, 1079,* 15–24.

Gallese, V. (2007). Before and below "theory of mind": Embodied simulation and the neural correlates of social cognition. *Philosophical Transactions of the Royal Society of London, Series B: Biological Sciences, 362,* 359–369.

Gallese, V., Fadiga, L., Fogassi, L., & Rizzolatti, G. (1996). Action recognition in the premotor cortex. *Brain, 119*(Pt. 2), 593–609.

Gallese, V., Gernsbacher, M. A., Heyes, C., Hickok, G., & Iacoboni, M. (2011). Mirror neuron forum. *Perspectives on Psychological Science, 6,* 369–407.

Gallese, V., & Goldman, A. (1998). Mirror neurons and the simulation theory of mindreading. *Trends in Cognitive Sciences, 2,* 493–501.

Gallese, V., Keysers, C., & Rizzolatti, G. (2004). A unifying view of the basis of social cognition. *Trends in Cognitive Science, 8,* 396–403.

Gallese, V., & Lakoff, G. (2005). The brain's concepts: The role of the sensory-motor system in conceptual knowledge. *Cognitive Neuropsychology, 22,* 455–479.

Gallese, V., & Sinigaglia, C. (2011). What is so special about embodied simulation? *Trends in Cognitive Science, 15,* 512–519.

Galton, F. (1907). *Inquiries into human faculty and its development.* London: Dent & Sons.

Garcia-Marques, L., & Ferreira, M. B. (2009). The scaffolded mind: The why of embodied cognition? *European Journal of Social Psychology, 39,* 1272–1275.

Gardner, R. C. (1985). *The mind's new science: A history of the cognitive revolution.* New York: Basic Books.

Gay, P. (1988). *Freud: A life for our time.* London: Dent & Sons.

Gazzaniga, M. S. (1970). *The bisected brain.* New York: Appleton-Century-Crofts.

Gazzaniga, M. S. (1998). *The mind's past.* Berkeley: University of California Press.

Gazzaniga, M. S. (1999). The interpreter within: The glue of conscious experience. *Cerebrum: The Dana Forum on Brain Science, 1,* 68–78.

Gazzaniga, M. S. (2009). The fictional self. In D. J. H. Mathews, H. Bok, & P. V. Rabins (Eds.), *Personal identity and fractures selves: Perspectives from philosophy, ethics, and neuroscience* (pp. 174–185). Baltimore: Johns Hopkins University Press.

Gazzaniga, M. S., & LeDoux, J. E. (1978). *The integrated mind.* New York: Plenum Press.

Gazzaniga, M. S., LeDoux, J. E., & Wilson, D. H. (1977). Language, praxis, and the right hemisphere: Clues to some mechanisms of consciousness. *Neurology, 27,* 1144–1147.

Gazzaniga, M. S., & Sperry, R. W. (1967). Language after section of the cerebral commissures. *Brain, 90,* 131–148.

Geisler, C. (1986). The use of subliminal psychodynamic activation in the study of repression. *Journal of Personality and Social Psychology, 51,* 844–851.

Gentilucci, M. (2003). Grasp observation influences speech production. *European Journal of Neuroscience, 17,* 179–184.

Gentilucci, M., Benuzzi, F., Gangitano, M., & Grimaldi, S. (2001). Grasp with hand and mouth: A kinematic study on healthy subjects. *Journal of Neurophysiology, 86,* 1685–1699.

Gentilucci, M., Santunione, P., Roy, A., & Stefanini, S. (2004). Execution and observation of bringing a fruit to the mouth affect syllable pronunciation. *European Journal of Neuroscience, 19,* 190–202.

Ghinescu, R., Schachtman, T. R., Stadler, M. A., Fabiani, M., & Gratton, G. (2010). Strategic behavior without awareness?: Effects of implicit learning in the Eriksen flanker paradigm. *Memory and Cognition, 38,* 197–205.

Gigerenzer, G., & Goldstein, D. G. (1996). Mind as computer: Birth of a metaphor. *Creativity Research Journal, 9,* 131–144.

Gilbert, D., & Malone, P. (1995). The correspondence bias. *Psychological Bulletin, 117,* 21–38.

Gilead, M., Gal, O., Polak, M., & Cholow, Y. (2015). The role of nature and nurture in conceptual metaphors: The case of gustatory priming. *Social Psychology, 46,* 167–173.

Gill, M. M. (1982). *Analysis of transference: 1. Theory and technique.* New York: International Universities Press.

Gladwell, M. (2005). *Blink: The power of thinking without thinking.* New York: Little Brown.

Glauber, I. P. (1958). Freud's contributions on stuttering: Their relation to some current insights. *Journal of the American Psychoanalytic Association, 6,* 326–347.

Glenberg, A. M. (2011a). Introduction to the mirror neuron forum. *Perspectives on Psychological Science, 6,* 363–368.

Glenberg, A. M. (2011b). Positions in the mirror are closer than they appear. *Perspectives on Psychological Science, 6,* 408–410.

Glenberg, A. M. (2015). Few believe the world is flat: How embodiment is changing the scientific understanding of cognition. *Canadian Journal of Experimental Psychology, 69,* 165–171.

Glenberg, A. M., Brown, M., & Levin, J. (2007). Enhancing comprehension in small reading groups using a manipulation strategy. *Contemporary Educational Psychology, 32,* 389–399.

Glenberg, A. M., & Kaschak, M. P. (2002). Grounding language in action. *Psychonomic Bulletin and Review, 9,* 558–565.

Glisky, E. L., Schacter, D. L., & Tulving, E. (1986). Computer learning by memory-impaired patients: Acquisition and retention of complex knowledge. *Neuropsychologia, 24,* 313–328.

Gluck, M. A., & Myers, C. E. (1997). Psychobiological models of hippocampal function in learning and memory. *Annual Review of Psychology, 48,* 481–514.

Goldiamond, I. (1958). Indicators of perception: 1. Subliminal perception, subception, unconscious perception: An analysis in terms of psychophysical indicator methodology. *Psychological Bulletin, 55,* 373–411.

Goldin-Meadow, S. (1999). The role of gesture in communication and thinking. *Trends in Cognitive Science, 3,* 419–429.

Goldman, A. (2012). A moderate approach to embodied cognitive science. *Review of Philosophy and Psychology, 3,* 71–88.

Goldstein, E. B. (2011). *Cognitive psychology: Connecting mind, research, and everyday experience* (3rd. ed.). Belmont, CA: Wadsworth.

Gomila, A., & Calvo, P. (2010). Understanding brain circuits and their dynamics. *Behavioral and Brain Sciences, 33,* 274–275.

Gordon, P. C., & Holyoak, K. J. (1983). Implicit learning and generalization of the "mere exposure" effect. *Journal of Personality and Social Psychology, 45,* 492–500.

Gould, S. J., & Vrba, E. S. (1982). Exaptation—A missing term in the science of form. *Palebiology, 8,* 4–15.

Graf, P. (1990). Life span changes in implicit and explicit memory. *Bulletin of the Psychonomic Society, 28,* 353–358.

Graf, P., & Mandler, G. (1984). Activation makes words more accessible, but not necessarily more retrievable. *Journal of Verbal Learning and Verbal Behavior, 23,* 553–568.

Graf, P., & Masson, M. (1993). *Implicit memory.* Hillside, NJ: Erlbaum.

Graf, P., & Schacter, D. (1985). Implicit and explicit memory for new associations in normal and amnesic subjects. *Journal of Experimental Psychology: Learning, Memory, and Cognition, 11,* 501–518.

Graf, P., Squire, L., & Mandler, G. (1984). The information that amnesic patients do not forget. *Journal of Experimental Psychology: Learning, Memory, and Cognition, 10,* 164–178.

Greenbaum, M. (1956). Manifest anxiety and tachistoscopic recognition of facial photographs. *Perceptual and Motor Skills, 6,* 245–248.

Greenberg, J. (1991). *Oedipus and beyond: A clinical theory*. Cambridge, MA: Harvard University Press.

Greenberg, J., & Mitchell, S. A. (1983). *Object relations in psychoanalytic theory*. Cambridge, MA: Harvard University Press.

Greenspoon, J. (1955). The reinforcing effect of two spoken sounds on the frequency of two responses. *American Journal of Psychology, 68*(3), 409–416.

Greenwald, A. G. (1992). New look 3: *Unconscious* cognition reclaimed. *American Psychologist, 47*, 766–790.

Greenwald, A. G. (2017). An AI stereotype catcher. *Science, 356*, 133–134.

Greenwald, A. G., McGhee, D. E., & Schwartz, J. L. (1998). Measuring individual differences in implicit cognition: The Implicit Association Test. *Journal of Personality and Social Psychology, 74*, 1464–1480.

Greenwald, A. G., & Pettigrew, T. F. (2014). With malice toward none and charity for some: Ingroup favoritism enables discrimination. *American Psychologist, 69*, 669–684.

Groddeck, G. (1923). *The Book of the It*, Letter I and Letter II. New York: Nervous and Mental Disease Publishing.

Gross, W. L., & Greene, A. J. (2007). Analogical inference: The role of awareness in abstract learning. *Memory, 15*, 838–844.

Grünbaum, A. (1984). *The foundations of psychoanalysis: A philosophical critique*. Berkeley: University of California Press.

Guthrie, G., & Wiener, M. (1966). Subliminal perception or perception of partial cue with pictorial stimuli. *Journal of Personality and Social Psychology, 3*, 619–628.

Habermas, J. (1972). Knowledge and human interests (J. J. Shapiro, Trans.). London: Heineman.

Habib, R. (2009). Introduction to the special issue on episodic memory and the brain. *Neuropsychologia, 47*, 2155–2157.

Hadley, M. (2008). Relational theory. In J. Berzoff, L. M. Flanagan, & P. Hertz (Eds.), *Inside out and outside in: Psychodynamic clinical theory and psychopathology in contemporary multicultural contexts* (pp. 205–228). New York: Jason Aronson.

Hamlin, J. K., Wynn, K., & Bloom, P. (2007). Social evaluation by preverbal infants. *Nature, 450*, 557–560.

Hamlin, J. K., Wynn, K., & Bloom, P. (2010). Three-month-old infants show a negativity bias in social evaluation. *Developmental Science, 13*, 923–929.

Hardaway, R. (1990). Subliminal symbiotic fantasies: Facts and artifacts. *Psychological Bulletin, 107*, 177–195.

Hardy, G. R., & Legge, D. (1968). Cross-modal induction of changes in sensory thresholds. *Quarterly Journal of Experimental Psychology, 20*, 20–29.

Harrison, A. A. (1977). Mere exposure. In L. Berkowitz (Ed.), *Advances in experimental social psychology* (Vol. 10, pp. 39–83). New York: Academic Press.

Hartmann, H. (1958). *Ego psychology and the problem of adaptation* (D. Rapaport, Trans.). New York: International Universities Press. (Original work published 1939)

Hasan, M. T., Hernández-González, S., Dogbevia, G., Treviño, M., Bertocchi, I., Gruart, A., et al. (2013). Role of motor cortex NMDA receptors in learning-dependent synaptic plasticity of behaving mice. *Nature Communications, 4,* Article Number 2258, 1–9.

Hassin, R. R. (2013). Yes it can on the functional abilities of the human unconscious. *Perspectives on Psychological Science, 8,* 195–207.

Hayman, C. G., & Tulving, E. (1989). Contingent dissociation between recognition and fragmented completion: The method of triangulation. *Journal of Experimental Psychology: Learning, Memory, and Cognition, 15,* 228–240.

Heatherton, T. F., & Nichols, P. A. (1994). Conceptual issues in assessing whether personality can change. In T. Heatherton & J. Weinberger (Eds.), *Can personality change?* (pp. 3–18). Washington, DC: APA Books.

Heatherton, T. F., & Weinberger, J. (Eds.). (1994). *Can personality change?* Washington, DC: APA Books.

Hebb, D. O. (1949). *The organization of behavior: A neuropsychological theory.* New York: Wiley.

Heerey, E. A., & Velani, H. (2010). Implicit learning of social predictions. *Journal of Experimental Social Psychology, 46,* 577–581.

Hefferline, R. F., Keenan, B., & Harford, R. A. (1959). Escape and avoidance conditioning in human subjects without their observation of the response. *Science, 13,* 1338–1339.

Heidbreder, E. (1933). *Seven psychologies.* London: Century/Random House UK.

Heider, F. (1958). *The psychology of interpersonal relations.* Hillside, NJ: Erlbaum.

Heisz, J. J., Vakorin, V., Ross, B., Levine, B., & McIntosh, A. R. (2014). A trade-off between local and distributed information processing associated with remote episodic versus semantic memory. *Journal of Cognitive Neuroscience, 26,* 41–53.

Helson, H. (1964). *Adaptation-level theory: An experimental and systematic approach to behavior.* New York: Harper & Row.

Henson, R. N. (2003). Neuroimaging studies of priming. *Progress in Neurobiology, 70,* 53–81.

Herbart, J. F. (1824). *Psychologie als Wissenschaft. Neu gegründet auf Erfahrung, Metaphysik und Mathematik. Erster, synthetischer Teil [Psychology as science: Newly founded on experience, metaphysics and mathematics; First, synthetic part].* Leipzig, Germany: Voss.

Herbart, J. F. (1850). *Lehrbuch zur Psychologie [Textbook of psychology]* (2nd ed.). Reprinted in G. Hartenstein (Ed.), *Herbarts schriften zur psychologie* (Vol. 1). Leipzig, Germany: Voss. (Original work published 1834)

Herring, D. R., Jabeen, L. N., Hinojos, M., White, K. R., Taylor, J. H., & Crites, S. L., Jr. (2013). On the automatic activation of attitudes: A quarter century of evaluative priming . *Psychological Bulletin, 139,* 1062–1089.

Heynes, R. W., Veroff, J., & Atkinson, J. W. (1958). A scoring manual for the affiliation motive. In J. W. Atkinson (Ed.), *Motives in fantasy, action, and society* (pp. 205–218). Princeton, NJ: Van Nostrand.

Hickok, G. (2009). Eight problems for the mirror neuron theory of action understanding in monkeys and humans. *Journal of Cognitive Neuroscience, 21,* 1229–1243.

Hickok, G. (2014). *The myth of mirror neurons: The real neuroscience of communication and cognition.* New York: Norton.

Hickok, G. (2015). Response to Rizzolatti and Sinigaglia and to Glenberg. *American Journal of Psychology, 128,* 539–549.

Hicks, J. A., & King, L. A. (2011). Subliminal mere exposure and explicit and implicit positive affective responses. *Cognition and Emotion, 25,* 726–729.

Hilgard, E. R. (1986). *Divided consciousness: Multiple controls in human thought and action.* New York: Wiley.

Hilgard, E. R. (1992). Dissociation and theories of hypnosis. In E. Fromm & M. R. Nash (Eds.), *Contemporary hypnosis research* (pp. 69–101). New York: Guilford Press.

Hill, T., Lewicki, P., Czyzewska, M., & Boss, A. (1989). Self-perpetuating development of encoding biases in person perception. *Journal of Personality and Social Psychology, 57,* 373–387.

Hill, T., Lewicki, P., Czyzewska, M., & Schuller, G. (1990). The role of learned inferential encoding rules in the perception of faces: Effects of nonconscious self-perpetuation of a bias. *Journal of Experimental Social Psychology, 26,* 350–371.

Hinton, G. E., McClelland, J. L., & Rumelhart, D. E. (1986). Distributed representations. In D. E. Rumelhart, J. L. McClelland, & the PDP Research Group (Eds.), *Parallel distributed processing: Explorations in the microstructure of cognition* (Vol. 1, pp. 77–109). Cambridge, MA: MIT Press.

Hochberg, J. E., & Gleitman, H. (1949). Towards a reformulation of the perception–motivation dichotomy. *Journal of Personality, 18,* 180–191.

Hofer, J., Busch, H., Bond, M. H., Kartner, J., Kiessling, F., & Law, R. (2010). Is self-determined functioning a universal prerequisite for motive goal congruence?: Examining the domain of achievement in three cultures. *Journal of Personality, 78,* 747–780.

Hofer, J., & Chasiotis, A. (2003). Congruence of life goals and implicit motives as predictors of life satisfaction: Cross cultural implications of a study of Zambian male adolescents. *Motivation and Emotion, 27,* 251–272.

Hoffman, I. Z. (1998). *Ritual and spontaneity in the psychoanalytic process.* Hillsdale, NJ: Analytic Press.

Hogarth, L. (2011). The role of impulsivity in the aetiology of drug dependence: Reward sensitivity versus automaticity. *Psychopharmacology, 215,* 567–580.

Holender, D. (1986). Semantic activation without conscious identification in dichotic listening, parafoveal vision, and visual masking: A survey and appraisal. *Behavioral and Brain Sciences, 9,* 1–23.

Holyoak, K. J., & Spellman, B. A. (1993). Thinking. *Annual Review of Psychology, 44,* 265–315.

Hornstein, G. (1992). The return of the repressed: Psychology's problematic relations with psychoanalysis, 1909–1960. *American Psychologist, 47,* 254–263.

House, R. J., Woycke, J., & Fodor, E. M. (1988). Charismatic and noncharismatic leaders: Differences in behavior and effectiveness. In J. A. Conger & R. N. Kanungo (Eds.), *Charismatic leadership: The elusive factor in organizational effectiveness* (pp. 98–121). San Francisco: Jossey-Bass.

Hovland, C. I., & Weiss, W. (1951). The influence of source credibility on communication effectiveness. *Public Opinion Quarterly, 15,* 635–650.

Howard, J. H., & Ballas, J. A. (1982). Acquisition of acoustic pattern categories by exemplar observation. *Organizational Behavior and Human Performance, 30,* 157–173.

Howe, M. L., & Knott, L. M. (2015). The fallibility of memory in judicial processes: Lessons from the past and their modern consequences. *Memory, 23,* 633–656.

Howes, D. H. (1954). A statistical theory of the phenomenon of subception. *Psychological Review, 61,* 98–110.

Howes, D. H., & Solomon, R. L. (1950). A note on McGinnies' "Emotionality and perceptual defense." *Psychological Review, 57,* 229–234.

Howie, D. (1952). Perceptual defense. *Psychological Review, 59,* 308–315.

Hull, J. G., Slone, L. B., Meteyer, K. B., & Matthews, A. R. (2002). The nonconsciousness of self-consciousness. *Journal of Personality and Social Psychology, 83,* 406–424.

Hume, D. (1975). *A treatise of human nature* (L. A. Selby-Bigge, Ed., 2nd ed., revised by P. H. Nidditch). Oxford, UK: Clarendon Press. (Original work published 1738)

Hunsley, J., Aubry, T., Verstervelt, C., & Vito, D. (1999). Comparing therapist and client perspectives on reasons for psychotherapy termination. *Psychotherapy, 36,* 380–388.

Ijzerman, H., & Semin, G. R. (2009). The thermometer of social relations: Mapping social proximity on temperature. *Psychological Science, 20,* 1214–1220.

Inderbitzin, L. B., & Levy, S. T. (1990). Unconscious fantasy: A reconsideration of the concept. *Journal of the American Psychoanalytic Association, 38,* 113–130.

Ionescu, M. D., & Erdelyi, M. H. (1992). The direct recovery of subliminal stimuli. In R. F. Bornstein & T. S. Pittman (Eds.), *Perception without awareness* (pp. 143–169). New York: Guilford Press.

Isaacs, S. (1943). The nature and function of phantasy. In M. Klein, P. Heimann, S. Isaacs, & J. Riviere (Eds.), *Developments in psycho-analysis* (pp. 67–121). London: Hogarth Press.

Jackson, J. H. (1958). *Selected writings of John Hughlings Jackson* (J. Taylor, Ed.). New York: Basic Books.

Jackson, J. M. (1983). Effects of subliminal stimulation of oneness fantasies on manifest pathology in male vs. female schizophrenics. *Journal of Nervous and Mental Disease, 171,* 280–289.

Jacob, P. (2009). A philosopher's reflections on the discovery of mirror neurons. *Topics in Cognitive Science, 1,* 570–595.

Jacobson, E. (1971). *Depression: Comparative studies of normal, neurotic, and psychotic conditions.* Madison, CT: International Universities Press.

Jacoby, L. L. (1983a). Perceptual enhancement: Persistent effects of an experience. *Journal of Experimental Psychology: Learning, Memory, and Cognition, 9,* 21–38.

Jacoby, L. L. (1983b). Remembering the data: Analyzing interactive processes in reading. *Journal of Verbal Learning and Verbal Behavior, 22,* 485–508.

Jacoby, L. L., Begg, I. M., & Toth, J. P. (1997). In defense of functional independence: Violations of assumptions underlying the process-dissociation procedure? *Journal of Experimental Psychology: Learning, Memory, and Cognition, 23,* 484–495.

Jacoby, L. L., & Dallas, M. (1981). On the relationship between autobiographical memory and perceptual learning. *Journal of Experimental Psychology: General, 3,* 306–340.

Jacoby, L. L., & Kelley, C. M. (1987). Unconscious influences of memory for a prior event. *Personality and Social Psychology Bulletin, 13,* 314–336.

Jacoby, L. L., Lindsay, D. S., & Toth, J. P. (1992). Unconscious influences revealed: Attention, awareness, and control. *American Psychologist, 47,* 802–809.

Jacoby, L. L., Toth, J., Lindsay, D., & Debner, J. (1992). Lectures for a layperson: Methods for revealing unconscious processes. In R. F. Bornstein & T. S. Pittman (Eds.), *Perception without awareness: Cognitive, clinical, and social perspectives* (pp. 81–120). New York: Guilford Press.

Jacoby, L. L., & Whitehouse, K. (1989). An illusion of memory: False recognition influenced by unconscious perception. *Journal of Experimental Psychology: General, 118,* 126–135.

James, W. (1920). *The letters of William James* (Vol. 2). Boston: Atlantic Monthly Press.

James, W. (1929). *The varieties of religious experience: A study in human nature* (20th ed.). New York: Longmans, Green. (Original work published 1902)

James, W. (1950). *The principles of psychology* (Vols. 1 & 2). New York: Holt. (Original work published 1890)

Janaway, C. (2002). *Schopenhauer: A very short introduction.* New York: Oxford University Press.

Janet, P. (1920). *The major symptoms of hysteria.* New York: Macmillan.

Jernigan, T. L., & Ostergaard, A. L. (1993). Word priming and recognition memory both affected by mesial temporal lobe damage. *Neuropsychology, 7,* 14–26.

Jiang, Y. V., Swallow, K. M., & Sun, L. (2014). Egocentric coding of space for incidentally learned attention: Effects of scene context and task instructions. *Journal of Experimental Psychology: Learning, Memory, and Cognition, 40,* 233–250.

Jiang, Y. V., Won, B.-Y., & Swallow, K. M. (2014). First saccadic eye movement reveals persistent attentional guidance by implicit learning. *Journal of Experimental Psychology: Human Perception and Performance, 40,* 1161–1173.

Jilk, D., Lebiere, C., O'Reilly, R., & Anderson, J. (2008). SAL: An explicitly pluralistic cognitive architecture. *Journal of Experimental and Theoretical Artificial Intelligence, 20,* 197–218.

Johnson, M. K., Kim, J. K., & Risse, G. (1985). Do alcoholic Korsakoff's syndrome patients acquire affective reactions? *Journal of Experimental Psychology: Learning, Memory, and Cognition, 11,* 22–36.

Jones, E. (1955). *The life and work of Sigmund Freud* (Vols. 1–3). New York: Basic Books.

Jones, E., & Harris, V. (1967). The attribution of attitudes. *Journal of Experimental Social Psychology, 3,* 1–24.

Jones, E., & Nisbett, R. (1972). The actor and the observer: Divergent perceptions of the causes of behavior. In E. Jones, D. Kanouse, H. Kelley, R. Nisbett, S. Valins, & B. Weiner (Eds.), *Attribution: Perceiving the causes of behavior* (pp. 79–94). Morristown, NJ: General Learning Press.

Josephs, L. (1995). *Balancing empathy and interpretation: Relational character analysis.* Lanham, MD: Jason Aronson.

Jurchis, R., & Opre, A. (2016). Unconscious learning of cognitive structures with emotional components: Implications for cognitive behavior psychotherapies. *Cognitive Therapy and Research, 40,* 230–244.

Jung, C. G. (1928). *Two essays on analytical psychology.* London: Baillére.

Jung, C. G. (1969). *Studies in word-association.* Abingdon, UK: Taylor & Francis. (Original work published 1906)

Jung, J. (1966). Restricting effects of awareness: Serial position bias in Spence's study. *Journal of Personality and Social Psychology, 3,* 124–128.

Junger, S. (2016). *Tribe: On homecoming and belonging.* New York: Twelve.

Jurist, E. L. (2018). *Minding emotions: Cultivating mentalization in psychotherapy.* New York: Guilford Press.

Kabat-Zinn, J. (2005). *Full catastrophe living: Wisdom of your body and mind to face stress, pain, and illness: Fifteenth anniversary edition.* New York: Bantam Books.

Kahneman, D. (2011). *Thinking, fast and slow.* New York: Farrar, Straus, & Giroux.

Kahneman, D., Slovic, P., & Tversky, A. (1982). *Judgment under uncertainty: Heuristics and biases.* Cambridge, UK: Cambridge University Press.

Kahneman, D., & Tversky, A. (1979). Prospect theory: An analysis of decision under risk. *Econometrica, 47,* 263–291.

Kail, R. (1990). *The development of memory in children.* New York: Freeman/Times Books/Henry Holt & Co.

Kalin, N. H., Shelton, S. E., & Davidson, R. J. (2004). The role of the central nucleus of the amygdala in mediating fear and anxiety in the primate. *Journal of Neuroscience, 24,* 5506–5515.

Kalin, N. H., Shelton, S. E., Davidson, R. J., & Kelley, A. E. (2001). The primate amygdala mediates acute fear but not the behavioral and physiological components of anxious temperament. *Journal of Neuroscience, 21,* 2067–2074.

Kang, Y., Williams, L. E., Clark, M. S., Gray, J. R., & Bargh, J. A. (2011). Physical temperature effects on trust behavior: The role of insula. *Social Cognitive and Affective Neuroscience, 6,* 507–515.

Karabenik, S. A. (1977). Fear of success, achievement and affiliation dispositions, and the performance of men and women under individual and competitive conditions. *Journal of Personality, 45,* 117–149.

Kawamoto, A. H., & Anderson, J. A. (1984). Lexical access using a neural network. *Proceedings of the Sixth Annual Conference of the Cognitive Science Society, 204–213.*

Kelley, H. H. (1967). Attribution theory in social psychology. *Nebraska Symposium on Motivation, 15,* 192–238.

Kelly, G. (1991). *The psychology of personal constructs.* New York: Norton. (Original work published 1955)

Kelman, H. C., & Hovland, C. I. (1953). Reinstatement of the communicator in delayed measurement of opinion change. *Journal of Abnormal and Social Psychology, 48,* 327–335.

Kendall, P., Kipnis, D., & Otto-Salaj, L. (1992). When clients don't progress: Influences on and explanations for lack of therapeutic progress. *Cognitive Therapy and Research, 16,* 269–281.

Kernberg, O. F. (1975). *Borderline conditions and pathological narcissism.* Lanham, MD: Rowman & Littlefield.

Kernberg, O. F. (1976). *Object relations theory and clinical psychoanalysis.* New York: Jason Aronson.

Kernberg, O. F. (1987). The dynamic unconscious and the self. In R. Stern (Ed.), *Theories of the unconscious and theories of the self* (pp. 3–25). Hillsdale, NJ: Analytic Press.

Kernberg, O. (2004). *Contemporary controversies in psychoanalytic theory, techniques, and their applications.* New Haven, CT: Yale University Press.

Kernberg, O., Yeomans, F., Clarkin, J., & Levy, K. (2008). Transference focused psychotherapy: Overview and update. *International Journal of Psychoanalysis, 89,* 601–620.

Keysers, C., Kaas, J. H., & Gazzola, V. (2010). Somatosensation in social perception. *Nature Reviews in Neuroscience, 11,* 417–428.

Kihlstrom, J. F. (1984). Conscious, subconscious, unconscious: A cognitive perspective. In K. S. Bowers & D. Meichenbaum (Eds.), *The unconscious reconsidered* (pp. 149–211). New York: Wiley.

Kihlstrom, J. F. (1987). The cognitive unconscious. *Science, 237,* 1445–1452.

Kihlstrom, J. F. (1999). Conscious versus unconscious cognition. In R. J. Sternberg (Ed.), *The nature of cognition* (pp. 73–203). Cambridge, MA: MIT Press.

Kihlstrom, J., Dorfman, J., & Park, L. (2007). Implicit and explicit memory and learning. In M. Velmans & S. Schneider (Eds.), *The Blackwell companion to consciousness* (pp. 525–539). Oxford, UK: Blackwell.

Kihlstrom, J. F., Mulvaney, S., Tobias, B. A., & Tobis, I. P. (2000). The emotional unconscious. In E. Eich, J. F. Kihlstrom, G. H. Bower, J. P. Forgas, & P. M. Niedenthal (Eds.), *Cognition and emotion* (pp. 30–86). New York: Oxford University Press.

Kinder, A., & Shanks, D. R. (2001). Amnesia and the declarative/nondeclarative distinction: A recurrent network model of classification, recognition, and repetition priming. *Journal of Cognitive Neuroscience, 13,* 648–669.

Kinder, A., & Shanks, D. R. (2003). Neuropsychological dissociations between priming and recognition: A single-system connectionist account. *Psychological Review, 110,* 728–744.

Kinsinger, E. A., & Schacter, D. L. (2008). Memory and emotion. In M. Lewis,

J. A. Haviland-Jones, & L. Feldman Barrett (Eds.), *Handbook of emotions* (3rd ed., pp. 601–617). New York: Guilford Press.

Kissin, B., Gottesfeld, H., & Dikes, R. (1958). Inhibition and tachistoscopic thresholds for sexually charged words. *Journal of Psychology: Interdisciplinary and Applied, 43*, 333–339.

Kiverstein, J. (2010). No bootstrapping without semantic inheritance. *Behavioral and Brain Sciences, 33*, 279–280.

Klein, D. B. (1977). *The unconscious: Invention or discovery?: A historico-critical inquiry.* Oxford, UK: Goodyear.

Klein, G. S., Spence, D. P., Holt, R. R., & Gourevitch, S. R. (1958). Preconscious influences upon conscious cognitive behavior. *Journal of Abnormal and Social Psychology, 57*, 255–266.

Klein, M. (1926). Infant analysis. *International Journal of Psycho-Analysis, 7*, 31–63.

Klein, M. (1930). The importance of symbol-formation in the development of the ego. *International Journal of Psycho-Analysis, 11*, 24.

Klein, M. (1935). A contribution to the psychogenesis of manic–depressive states. *International Journal of Psycho-Analysis, 16*, 145–174.

Klein, M. (1975). *Some theoretical conclusions regarding the emotional life of the infant: Envy and gratitude and other works 1946–1963.* London: Hogarth Press/Institute of Psycho-Analysis. (Original work published 1952)

Klinger, M. R., & Greenwald, A. G. (1994). Preferences need no inferences?: The cognitive basis of unconscious emotional effects. In P. M. Niedenthal & S. Kitayama (Eds.), *The heart's eye: Emotional influences in perception and attention* (pp. 67–85). New York: Academic Press.

Knowlton, B. J., Ramus, S. J., & Squire, L. R. (1992). Intact artificial grammar learning in amnesia: Dissociation of classification learning and explicit memory for specific instances. *Psychological Science, 3*, 172–179.

Koestner, R. F., Weinberger, J., & McClelland, D. C. (1991). An empirical investigation of the differences between non-conscious motives and conscious values. *Journal of Personality, 59*, 57–82.

Koffka, K. (1922). Perception: An introduction to the Gestalt-Theorie. *Psychological Bulletin, 19*, 531–585.

Köhler, W. (1947). *Gestalt psychology: An introduction to new concepts in modern psychology.* New York: Liveright.

Köhler, W. (1976). *The place of value in a world of facts.* Oxford, UK: Oxford University Press.

Kohut, H. (1971). *The analysis of the self: A systematic approach to the psychoanalytic treatment of narcissistic personality disorders.* Chicago: University of Chicago Press.

Kohut, H. (1977). *The restoration of the self.* Madison, CT: International Universities Press.

Kohut, H. (1980). Reflections on advances in self psychology. In A. Goldberg (Ed.), *Advances in self psychology* (pp. 473–554). New York: International Universities Press.

Kolers, P. A. (1957). Subliminal stimulation in problem-solving. *American Journal of Psychology, 70*, 437–441.

Komatsu, S. I., & Ohta, N. (1984). Priming effects in word-fragment completion for short and long retention intervals. *Japanese Psychological Research, 26,* 194–200.

Kosonogov, V. (2012). Why the mirror neurons cannot support action understanding. *Neurophysiology, 44,* 499–502.

Köveces, Z. (2000). *Metaphor and emotion: Language, culture, and body in human feeling.* Cambridge, UK: Cambridge University Press.

Köveces, Z. (2002). *Metaphor: A practical introduction.* New York: Oxford University Press.

Krass, M. (1997). The river is within us, the sea is all around us: A study of creativity and oneness motivation. *Dissertation Abstracts International, 57*(7B), 4713.

Krauss, H. H., & Ruiz, R. A. (1968). Explorations in time orientation: Future time avoidance. *Journal of Contemporary Psychotherapy, 1,* 64–66.

Krippner, S. (1978). The importance of Rosenthal's research for parapsychology. *Behavioral and Brain Sciences, 1,* 398–399.

Kuhl, J. (2000). A functional design approach to motivation and volition: The dynamics of personality systems interactions. In M. Boekaerts, P. R. Pintrich, & M. Zeidner (Eds.), *Self-regulation: Directions and challenges for future research* (pp. 111–169). New York: Academic Press.

Kuhn, T., & Bauer, R. M. (2013). Episodic and semantic memory disorders. In L. D. Ravdin & K. L. Katzen (Eds.), *Handbook on the neuropsychology of aging and dementia: Clinical handbooks in neuropsychology* (pp. 401–419). New York: Springer.

Kunst-Wilson, W. R., & Zajonc, R. B. (1980). Affective discrimination of stimuli that cannot be recognized. *Science, 207,* 557–558.

Kurland, S. H. (1954). The lack of generality in defense mechanisms as indicated in auditory perception. *Journal of Abnormal and Social Psychology, 49,* 173–177.

Kurzban, R. (2010). *Why everyone (else) is a hypocrite: Evolution and the modular mind.* Princeton, NJ: Princeton University Press.

Kurzban, R., & Aktipis, C. A. (2007). Modularity and the social mind: Are psychologists too self-ish? *Personality and Social Psychology Review, 11,* 131–149.

Lähteenmäki, M., Hyönä, J., Koivisto, M., & Nummenmaa, L. (2015). Affective processing requires awareness. *Journal of Experimental Psychology: General, 144,* 339–365.

Lai, V. T., Hagoort, P., & Casasanto, D. (2012). Affective primacy vs. cognitive primacy: Dissolving the debate. *Frontiers in Psychology, 3,* Article 243.

Lakin, J., Chartrand, T., & Arkin, R. (2008). I am too just like you: Nonconscious mimicry as an automatic behavioral response to social exclusion. *Psychological Science, 19,* 816–822.

Lakoff, G. (1987). *Women, fire, and dangerous things: What categories reveal about the mind.* Chicago: University of Chicago Press.

Lakoff, G. (2012). Explaining embodied cognition results. *Topics in Cognitive Science, 4,* 773–785.

Lakoff, G. (2014). *The all new don't think of an elephant!: Know your values and frame the debate.* White River Junction, VT: Chelsea Green.

Lakoff, G., & Johnson, M. (1980a). The metaphorical system of the human conceptual system. *Cognitive Science, 4,* 195–208.

Lakoff, G., & Johnson, M. (1980b). *The metaphors we live by.* Chicago: Chicago University Press.

Lakoff, G., & Johnson, M. (1999). *Philosophy in the flesh: The embodied mind and its challenge to Western thoughts.* New York: Basic Books.

Landau, M. J., Vess, M., Arndt, J., Rothschild, Z. K., Sullivan, D., & Atchley, R. A. (2010). Embodied metaphor and the "true" self: Priming entity expansion and protection influences intrinsic self expressions in self-perceptions and interpersonal behavior. *Journal of Experimental Social Psychology, 47*(1), 79–87.

Lansing, J. B., & Heynes, R. W. (1959). Need affiliation and frequency of four types of communication. *Journal of Abnormal and Social Psychology, 58,* 365–372.

Lashley, K. S. (1950). In search of the engram. *Society of Experimental Biology Symposium, 4,* 454–482.

Latane, B., & Darley, J. M. (1970). *The unresponsive bystander: Why doesn't he help?* New York: Appleton-Century-Crofts.

Laws, K. R., Adlington, R. L., Moreno-Martinez, F. J., & Gale, T. M. (2010). *Category-specificity: Evidence for modularity of mind.* Hauppauge, NY: Nova Science.

Lazarus, R. S. (1956). Subception: Fact or artifact?: A reply to Eriksen. *Psychological Review, 63,* 343–347.

Lazarus, R. S. (1984). On the primacy of cognition. *American Psychologist, 39,* 124–129.

Lazarus, R. S., Eriksen, C. W., & Fonda, C. P. (1951). Personality dynamics and auditory perceptual recognition. *Journal of Personality, 19*(4), 471–482.

Lazarus, R. S., & McCleary, R. (1951). Autonomic discrimination without awareness: A study of subception. *Psychological Review, 58,* 113–122.

Leander, N., Chartrand, T., & Bargh, J. (2012). You give me the chills: Embodied reactions to inappropriate amounts of behavioral mimicry. *Psychological Science, 23,* 772–779.

Leander, N., Shah, J., & Chartrand, T. (2011). The object of my protection: Shielding fundamental motives from the implicit motivational influence of others. *Journal of Experimental Social Psychology, 47,* 1078–1087.

LeDoux, J. E. (1990). Information flow from sensation to emotion: Plasticity in the neural computation of stimulus value. In M. Gabriel & J. Moore (Eds.), *Learning and computational neuroscience: Foundations of adaptive networks* (pp. 3–51). Cambridge, MA: MIT Press.

LeDoux, J. E. (1995). Emotion: Clues from the brain. *Annual Review of Psychology, 46,* 209–235.

LeDoux, J. E. (1996). *The Emotional brain: The mysterious underpinnings of emotional life.* New York: Simon & Schuster.

LeDoux, J. E. (2012). Evolution of human emotion: A view through fear. *Progress in Brain Research, 195,* 431–442.

LeDoux, J. E. (2015). *Anxious: Using the brain to understand and treat fear and anxiety.* New York: Penguin Books.

Lee, S., & Schwarz, N. (2011). Wiping the slate clean: Psychological consequences of physical cleaning. *Current Directions in Psychological Science, 20,* 307–311.

Leibniz, G. W. (1896). *New essays on human understanding* (Langley, Trans.). Cambridge, UK: Cambridge University Press. (Original work published 1704)

Leibniz, G. W. (1989). Principles of nature and grace founded on reason. In L. E. Loemker (Ed. & Trans.), *Gottfired Wilhelm Leibniz: Philosophical papers and letters* (2nd ed., pp. 636–642). Boston: Kluwer Academic. (Original work published 1714)

Leiter, E. (1982). The effects of subliminal activation of aggressive and merging fantasies in differentiated and non-differentiated schizophrenics. *Psychological Research Bulletin, 22,* 1–21.

Levine, P. (1997). *Waking the tiger: Healing trauma.* Berkeley, CA: North Atlantic Books.

Levitt, H., Korman, Y., & Angus, L. (2000). A metaphor analysis in treatments of depression: Metaphor as a marker of change. *Counseling Psychology Quarterly, 13,* 23–35.

Lewicki, P. (1986). Processing information about covariations that cannot be articulated. *Journal of Experimental Psychology, 12,* 135–146.

Lewicki, P., Czyzewska, M., & Hoffman, H. (1987). Unconscious acquisition of complex procedural knowledge. *Journal of Experimental Psychology: Learning, Memory, and Cognition, 13,* 523–530.

Lewicki, P., Hill, T., & Bizot, E. (1988). Acquisition of procedural knowledge about a pattern of stimuli that cannot be articulated. *Cognitive Psychology, 20,* 24–37.

Lewicki, P., Hill, T., & Czyzewska, M. (1992). Nonconscious acquisition of information. *American Psychologist, 47,* 796–801.

Lewicki, P., Hill, T., & Czyzewska, M. (1994). Nonconscious indirect inferences in encoding. *Journal of Experimental Psychology: General, 123,* 257–263.

Liébault, A. A. (1866). *Du Sommeil et Des Etats Analogues considérés surtout au point de sue de l'action du moral sur le physique* [*Sleep and its analogous states considered from the perspective of the action of the mind upon the body*]. Paris: Masson.

Lieberman, D. (2014). *The story of the human body: Evolution, health, and disease.* New York: Vintage Books.

Lieberman, M. (2000). Intuition: A social cognitive neuroscience approach. *Psychological Bulletin, 126,* 109–137.

Light, L. L. (1991). Memory and aging: Four hypotheses in search of data. *Annual Review of Psychology, 42,* 333–376.

Lindeman, L., & Abramson, L. (2008). The mental simulation of motor incapacity in depression. *Journal of Cognitive Psychotherapy, 22,* 228–249.

Lindner, H. (1953). Sexual responsiveness to perceptual tests in a group of sexual offenders. *Journal of Personality, 21,* 364–374.

Linehan, E., & O'Toole, J. (1982). Effect of subliminal stimulation of symbiotic fantasies on college student self-disclosure in group counseling. *Journal of Counseling Psychology, 29,* 151–157.

Linn, L. (1954). The discriminating function of the ego. *Psychoanalytic Quarterly, 23,* 38–47.

Locke, J. (1975). *An essay concerning human understanding* (P. H. Nidditch, Ed.). Oxford, UK: Clarendon Press. (Original work published 1690)

Loftus, E. F. (1997). Memories for a past that never was. *Current Directions in Psychological Science, 6,* 60–65.

Loftus, E. (2017). Eavesdropping on memory. *Annual Review of Psychology, 68,* 1–18.

Lorenz, K. (1991). *Here am I—Where are you?: The behavior of the graylag goose* (R. D. Martin, Trans.). New York: Harcourt Brace Jovanovich.

Luchins, A. S. (1950). On an approach to social perception. *Journal of Personality, 19,* 64–84.

Luyten, P., & Fonagy, P. (2015). The neurobiology of mentalizing. *Personality Disorders: Theory, Research, and Treatment, 6,* 366–379.

Mahler, M., Pine, F., & Bergman, A. (1975). On human symbiosis and the subphases of the separation–individuation process. In *The psychological birth of the human infant: Symbiosis and individuation.* New York: Basic Books.

Maia, T. V., & Cleeremans, A. (2005). Consciousness: Converging insights from connectionist modeling and neuroscience. *Trends in Cognitive Sciences, 9,* 397–404.

Malamud, W., & Linder, F. E. (1931). Dreams and their relationship to recent impressions. *Archives of Neurology and Psychiatry, 25,* 1081–1099.

Malpass, R. S., & Koehnken, G. (Eds.). (1996). *Psychological issues in eyewitness identification.* Mahwah, NJ: Erlbaum.

Mandler, G. (1980). Recognizing: The judgment of previous occurrence. *Psychological Review, 87,* 252–271.

Mandler, G., Nakamura, Y., & van Zandt, B. J. (1987). No specific effects of exposure on stimuli that cannot be recognized. *Journal of Experimental Psychology: Learning, Memory, and Cognition, 13,* 646–648.

Mann, T. (1936). *Freud und die zukunft.* Vienna: Bormann-Fischer. (Freud and the future—as cited in Ellenberger, 1970)

Manza, L., & Reber, A. S. (1997). Representing artificial grammars: Transfer across stimulus forms and modalities. In D. C. Berry (Ed.), *Debates in psychology: How implicit is implicit learning?* (pp. 73–106). New York: Oxford University Press.

Marbe, K. (1901). *Experimentell-psychologische untersuchungen über das urteil, eine einteitung in die logic.* Leipzig, Germany: Engelmann. (Experimental psychological investigations of judgment, an introduction to logic—as cited in Jaynes, 1976)

Marcel, A. J. (1983a) Conscious and unconscious perception: Experiments on visual masking and word recognition. *Cognitive Psychology, 15,* 197–237.

Marcel, A. J. (1983b). Conscious and unconscious perception: An approach to the relations between phenomenal experience and perceptual processes. *Cognitive Psychology, 15,* 238–300.

Marcel, A. J., Katz, L., & Smith, M. (1974). Laterality and reading proficiency. *Neuropsychologia, 12,* 131–139.

Marcel, A. J., & Patterson, K. E. (1978). Word recognition and production: Reciprocity in clinical and normal studies. In J. Requin (Ed.), *Attention and performance* (Vol. 7). Hillsdale, NJ: Erlbaum.

Marcus, G. (2004). *The birth of the mind.* New York: Basic Books.

Martin, A., Haxby, J., Lalonde, F., Wiggs, C., & Ungerleider, L. (1995). Discrete cortical regions associated with knowledge of color and knowledge of action. *Science, 270,* 102–105.

Martin, A., Ungerleider, L., & Haxby, J. (2000). Category specificity and the brain: The sensory/motor model of semantic representation of objects. *New Cognitive Neurosciences, 2,* 1023–1036.

Martin, A., Wiggs, C., Ungerleider, L., & Haxby, J. (1996). Neural correlates of category-specific knowledge. *Nature, 379,* 649–652.

Martin, J., Cummings, A. L., & Hallberg, E. T. (1992). Therapists' intentional use of metaphor: Memorability, clinical impact, and possible epistemic/ motivational functions. *Journal of Consulting and Clinical Psychology, 60,* 143–145.

Maslow, A. H. (1943). A theory of human motivation. *Psychological Review, 50,* 370–396.

Mathieson, F., Jordan, J., Carter, J. D., & Stubbe, M. (2015). The metaphoric dance: Co-construction of metaphor in cognitive behaviour therapy. *The Cognitive Behaviour Therapist, 8,* Article e24.

Matlock, T., Ramscar, M., & Boroditsky, L. (2005). On the experiential link between spatial and temporal language. *Cognitive Science, 29,* 655–664.

Matthews, G., & Wells, A. (2000). Attention, automaticity, and affective disorder. *Behavior Modification, 24,* 69–93.

Matthews, R. C., Buss, R. R., Stanley, W. B., Blanchard-Fields, F., Cho, J. R., & Durhan, B. (1989). Role of implicit and explicit processes in learning from examples: A synergistic effect. *Journal of Experimental Psychology: Learning, Memory, and Cognition, 15,* 1083–1100.

Mayr, E. (1960). The emergence of evolutionary novelties. In S. Tax (Ed.), *The evolution of life* (pp. 349–380). Chicago: University of Chicago Press.

McAdams, D. (1980). A thematic coding system for the intimacy motive. *Journal of Research in Personality, 14,* 413–432.

McAdams, D. (1989). *Intimacy: The need to be close.* New York: Doubleday.

McAdams, D. (1992). The intimacy motive. In C. P. Smith, J. W. Atkinson, D. C. McClelland, & J. Veroff (Eds.), *Motivation and personality: Handbook of thematic content analysis* (pp. 224–228). Cambridge, UK: Cambridge University Press.

McAdams, D., Jackson, D. P., & Kirshnit, C. (1984). Looking, laughing, and smiling in dyads as a function of intimacy motivation and reciprocity. *Journal of Personality, 52,* 261–273.

McAdams, D., & Powers, D. P. (1981). Themes of intimacy in behavior and thought. *Journal of Personality and Social Psychology, 40,* 573–587.

McAdams, D. P., & Vaillant, G. E. (1982). Intimacy motivation and psychological adjustment: A longitudinal study. *Journal of Personality Assessment, 46,* 586–593.

McAndrews, M. E., & Moscovitch, M. (1985). Rule-based and exemplar-based classification in artificial grammar learning. *Memory and Cognition, 13,* 469–475.

McBride, D. M., & Dosher, B. A. (1997). A comparison of forgetting in an implicit and explicit memory task. *Journal of Experimental Psychology: General, 126,* 371–392.

McBride, D. M., & Dosher, B. A. (1999). Forgetting rates are comparable in conscious and automatic memory: A process-dissociation study. *Journal of Experimental Psychology: Learning, Memory, and Cognition, 25,* 583–607.

McBride, D. M., Dosher, B. A., & Gage, N. M. (2001). A comparison of forgetting for conscious and automatic memory processes in word fragment completion tasks. *Journal of Memory and Language, 45,* 585–615.

McClelland, D. C. (1961). *The achieving society.* New York: Van Nostrand.

McClelland, D. C. (1972). Opinions predict opinions?: So what else is new? *Journal of Consulting and Clinical Psychology, 38,* 325–326.

McClelland, D. C. (1978). Managing motivation to expand human freedom. *American Psychologist, 33,* 201–210.

McClelland, D. C. (1984). *Motives, personality, and society: Selected papers.* New York: Praeger.

McClelland, D. C. (1985). How motives, skills, and values determine what people do. *American Psychologist, 40,* 812–825.

McClelland, D. C. (1987). *Human motivation.* New York: Cambridge University Press.

McClelland, D. C. (1989). Motivational factors in health and disease. *American Psychologist, 44,* 675–683.

McClelland, D. C., & Atkinson, J. W. (1948). Projective expression of needs: 2. The effect of different intensities of the hunger drive on thematic apperception. *Journal of Experimental Psychology, 38,* 643–658.

McClelland, D. C., Davis, W. N., Kalin, R., & Wanner, E. (1972). *The drinking man: Alcohol and human motivation.* New York: Free Press.

McClelland, D. C., & Jemmott, J. B. (1980). Power motivation, stress and physical illness. *Journal of Human Stress, 6,* 6–15.

McClelland, D. C., Koestner, R. F., & Weinberger, J. (1989). How do self attributed and implicit motives differ? *Psychological Review, 96,* 690–702.

McClelland, D. C., & Pilon, D. A. (1983). Sources of adult motives in patterns of parent behavior in early childhood. *Journal of Personality and Social Psychology, 44,* 564–574.

McClelland, D. C., & Winter, D. G. (1969). *Motivating economic achievement.* New York: Free Press.

McClelland, J. L., & Patterson, K. (2002). Rules or connections in past-tense inflections: What does the evidence rule out? *Trends in Cognitive Sciences, 6,* 465–472.

McClelland, J. L., & Rumelhart, D. E. (Eds.). (1986). *Parallel distributed processing: Explorations in the macrostructure of cognition,* (Vol. 1). Cambridge, MA: MIT Press.

McClelland, J. L., Rumelhart, D. E., & Hinton, G. E. (1986). The appeal of parallel distributed processing. In D. E. Rumelhart, J. L. McClelland, & the PDP Research Group (Eds.), *Parallel distributed processing: Explorations in the microstructure of cognition* (Vol. 1, pp. 3–44). Cambridge, MA: MIT Press.

McCusker, C., & Gettings, G. (1997). Automaticity of cognitive biases in addictive behaviours: Further evidence with gamblers. *British Journal of Clinical Psychology, 36,* 543–554.

McDougall, W. (1908). *An introduction to social psychology.* London: Methuen.

McDougall, W. (1923). *Outline of psychology.* New York: Scribners.

McGinnies, E. (1949). Emotionality and perceptual defense. *Psychological Review, 56,* 244–251.

McGinnies, E. (1950). Discussion of Howes' and Solomon's note on "Emotionality and perceptual defense." *Psychological Review, 57,* 235–240.

McGinnies, E., & Adornetto, J. (1952). Perceptual defense in normal and in schizophrenic observers. *Journal of Abnormal and Social Psychology, 47,* 833–837.

McGinnies, E., Comer, P. B., & Lacey, O. L. (1952). Visual-recognition thresholds as a function of word length and word frequency. *Journal of Experimental Psychology, 44,* 65–69.

McGinnies, E., & Sherman, H. (1952). Generalization of perceptual defense. *Journal of Abnormal and Social Psychology, 47,* 81–85.

McGurk, H., & MacDonald, J. (1976). Hearing lips and seeing voices. *Nature, 264,* 746–748.

McNally, R. (1995). Automaticity and the anxiety disorders. *Behavior Research and Therapy, 33,* 747–754.

McNamara, T. P. (2005). *Semantic priming: Perspectives from memory and word recognition.* New York: Psychology Press.

Mead, G. H. (1934). *Mind, self, and society from the standpoint of a social behaviorist* (C. W. Morris, Ed.). Chicago: University of Chicago Press.

Mearns, D., & Thorne, B. (2000). *Person-centered therapy today: New frontiers in theory and practice.* London: SAGE.

Meier, B. P., Moeller, S. K., Riemer-Peltz, M., & Robinson, M. D. (2012). Sweet taste preferences and experiences predict prosocial inferences, personalities, and behaviors. *Journal of Personality and Social Psychology, 102,* 163–174.

Meier, B. P., & Perrig, W. J. (2000). Low reliability of perceptual priming: Its impact on experimental and individual difference findings. *Quarterly Journal of Experimental Psychology: Human Experimental Psychology, 53A,* 211–233.

Meier, B. P., & Robinson, M. D. (2006). Does "feeling down" mean seeing down?: Depressive symptoms and vertical selective attention. *Journal of Research in Personality, 40,* 451–461.

Mendelsohn, E. M., & Silverman, L. H. (1982). Effects of stimulating psychodynamically relevant unconscious fantasies on schizophrenic psychopathology. *Schizophrenia Bulletin, 8,* 532–547.

Merikle, P. M. (1992). Perception without awareness: Critical issues. *American Psychologist, 47,* 792–795.

Merikle, P. M., & Reingold, E. M. (1991). Comparing direct (explicit) and indirect (implicit) measures to study unconscious memory. *Journal of Experimental Psychology: Learning, Memory, and Cognition, 17,* 224–233.

Meyer, D. E., Schvaneveldt, R. W., & Ruddy, M. G. (1975). Loci of contextual effects on visual word recognition. In P. M. A. Rabbit & S. Dornic (Eds.), *Attention and performance* (Vol. 5, pp. 98–118). London: Academic Press.

Milberg, W., & Blumstein, S. E. (1981). Lexical decision and aphasia: Evidence for semantic processing. *Brain and Language, 14,* 371–385.

Milgram, S. (1974). *Obedience to authority.* New York: Harper & Row.

Miller, G. A., Galanter, E., & Pribram, K. H. (1960). *Plans and the structure of behavior.* New York: Holt, Rinehart, & Winston.

Miller, J. (1973). *The effects of aggressive stimulation upon young adults who have experienced death of a parent during childhood and adolescence.* Unpublished doctoral dissertation, New York University (as cited in Silverman, Lachmann, & Milich, 1982).

Millward, R. B., & Reber, A. S. (1968). Event-recall in probability learning. *Journal of Learning and Verbal Behavior, 7,* 980–989.

Millward, R. B., & Reber, A. S. (1972). Probability learning: Contingent-event schedules with lags. *American Journal of Psychology, 85,* 81–98.

Milner, A. D., Goodale, M. A., & Vingrys, A. J. (2006). *The visual brain in action* (Vol. 2). Oxford, UK: Oxford University Press.

Milner, B. (1958). Psychological deficits produced by temporal lobe excision. *Research Publications of the Association for Research in Nervous and Mental Disease, 36,* 244–257.

Milner, B. (2005). The medial temporal-lobe amnesiac syndrome. *Psychiatric Clinics of North America, 28,* 599–611.

Milner, B., Corkin, S., & Teuber, H. L. (1968). Further analysis of the hippocampal amnesic syndrome: 14-year follow-up study of H. M. *Neuropsychologia, 6,* 315–334.

Mitchell, D. B. (2006). Nonconscious priming after 17 years: Invulnerable implicit memory? *Psychological Science, 17,* 925–929.

Mitchell, S. A. (1988). *Relational concepts in psychoanalysis. An integration.* Cambridge, MA: Harvard University Press.

Mitchell, S. A. (1998). Attachment theory and the psychoanalytic tradition: Reflections of human relationality. *British Journal of Psychotherapy, 15*(2), 117–193.

Mitchell, S. A. (2000). *Relationality: From attachment to intersubjectivity.* New York: Routledge.

Monteith, M. J., Ashburn-Nardo, L., Voils, C. I., & Czopp, A. M. (2002). Putting the brakes on prejudice: On the development and operation of cues for control. *Journal of Personality and Social Psychology, 83*(5), 1029–1050.

Moors, A., & De Houwer, J. (2006). Automaticity: A theoretical and conceptual analysis. *Psychological Bulletin, 132,* 297–326.

Moray, N. (1959). Attention in dichotic listening: Affective cues and the influence of instructions. *Quarterly Journal of Experimental Psychology, 11,* 56–60.

Morton, J. (1979). Facilitation in word recognition: Experiments causing change in the logogen model. In P. A. Kolers, M. Wrolstad, & H. Bouma (Eds.), *Processing of visible language* (Vol. 1, pp. 259–268). New York: Plenum Press.

Moscovitch, M. (1982). A neuropsychological approach to memory and perception in normal and pathological aging. In F. I. M. Craik & S. Trehub (Eds.), *Aging and cognitive processes* (pp. 55–78). New York: Plenum Press.

Mountcastle, V. B. (1958). Somatic functions of the nervous system. *Annual Review of Physiology, 20,* 471–508.

Mountcastle, V. B., & Henneman, E. (1952). The representation of tactile sensibility in the thalamus of the monkey. *Journal of Comparative Neurology, 97,* 409–431.

Mukamel, R., Ekstrom, A. D., Kaplan, J., Iacoboni, M., & Fried, I. (2010). Single-neuron responses in humans during execution and observation of actions. *Current Biology, 20,* 750–756.

Murch, G. M. (1965). A simple laboratory demonstration of subception. *British Journal of Psychology, 56,* 467–470.

Murch, G. M. (1967). Temporal gradients of response to subliminal stimuli. *Psychological Record, 17,* 483–492.

Murch, G. M. (1969). Responses to incidental stimuli as a function of feedback contingency. *Perception and Psychophysics, 5,* 10–12.

Murdock, B. B. (1954). Perceptual defense and threshold measurements. *Journal of Personality, 22,* 565–571.

Murdock, N., Edwards, C., & Murdock, T. (2010). Therapists' attributions for client premature termination: Are they self-serving? *Psychotherapy Theory, Research, Practice, Training, 47,* 221–234.

Murphy, S. T., & Zajonc, R. B. (1993). Affect, cognition, and awareness: Affective priming with optimal and suboptimal stimulus exposures. *Journal of Personality and Social Psychology, 64,* 723–739.

Musen, G., & Squire, L. R. (1993). Implicit learning of color–word associations using a Stroop paradigm. *Journal of Experimental Psychology: Learning, Memory, and Cognition, 19,* 789–798.

Naito, M., & Komatsu, S. (1993). Processes involved in childhood development of implicit memory. In P. Graf & M. Mason (Eds.), *Implicit memory: New directions in cognition, development, and neuropsychology* (pp. 231–260). Hillsdale, NJ: Erlbaum.

Natsoulas, T. (1965). Converging operations for perceptual defense. *Psychological Bulletin, 64,* 393–401.

Neisser, U. (1967). *Cognitive psychology*. New York: Appleton, Century, Crofts.

Neisser, U. (1981). John Dean's memory: A case study. *Cognition, 9,* 1–22.

Neuhouser, F. (1990). *Fichte's theory of subjectivity*. New York: Cambridge University Press.

Newell, A., & Simon, H. A. (1972). *Human problem solving*. Oxford, UK: Prentice-Hall.

Newell, A., & Simon, H. A. (1988). The theory of human problem solving. In A. M. Collins & E. E. Smith (Eds.), *Readings in cognitive science: A perspective from psychology and artificial intelligence* (pp. 33–51). San Mateo, CA: Morgan Kaufmann.

Newell, B. R., & Dunn, J. C. (2008). Dimensions in data: Testing psychological models using state–trace analysis. *Trends in Cognitive Sciences, 12,* 285–290.

Newirth, J. (2003). *Between emotion and cognition: The generative unconscious*. New York: Other Press.

Niedenthal, P. M. (1992). *Affect and social perception: On the psychological validity of rose-colored glasses*. New York: Guilford Press.

Niedenthal, P. M., & Alibali, M. (2009). Conceptualizing scaffolding and goals for a full account of embodied cognition. *European Journal of Social Psychology, 39,* 1268–1271.

Niedenthal, P. M., Halberstadt, J. B., & Innes-Ker, A. H. (1999). Emotional response categorization. *Psychological Review, 106,* 337–361.

Nietzsche, F. (2014). *Beyond good and evil: Prelude to a philosophy of the future* (H. Zimmern, Trans.). New York: Macmillan. (Original work published 1906)

Nisbett, R. E., & Bellows, N. (1977). Verbal reports about causal influences on social judgments: Private access versus public theories. *Journal of Personality and Social Psychology, 35,* 613–624.

Nisbett, R. E., & Wilson, T. D. (1977). Telling more than we can know: Verbal reports on mental processes. *Psychological Review, 84,* 231–259.

Nishitani, N., Schurmann, M., Amunts, K., & Hari, R. (2005). Broca's region: From action to language. *Physiology, 20,* 60–69.

Nissenfeld, S. M. (1979). *The effects of four types of subliminal stimuli on female depressives*. Unpublished doctoral dissertation, Yeshiva University.

Niu, Y., Todd, R., & Anderson, A. K. (2012). Affective salience can reverse the effects of stimulus-driven salience on eye movements in complex scenes. *Frontiers in Psychology, 3,* Article 336.

Noizet, G. (1854). *Memoire sur le somnambulisme et le magnetism animal* [Memory on somnambulism and animal magnetism]. Paris: Plon.

Norman, D. A. (1986). Reflections on cognition and parallel distributed processing. In D. E. Rumelhart, J. L. McClelland, & the PDP Research Group (Eds.), *Parallel distributed processing: Explorations in the microstructure of cognition* (Vol. 2, pp. 531–546). Cambridge, MA: MIT Press.

Norman, G. J., Norris, C. J., Gollan, J., Ito, T. A., Hawkley, L. C., Larsen, J. T., et al. (2011). Current emotion research in psychophysiology: The neurobiology of evaluative bivalence. *Emotion Review, 3,* 349–359.

Nummenmaa, L., Hyona, J., & Calvo, M. G. (2010). Semantic categorization precedes affective evaluation of visual scenes. *Journal of Experimental Psychology: General, 139,* 222–246.

Nyberg, L. (1998). Mapping episodic memory. *Behavioural Brain Research, 90,* 107–114.

O'Connor, P. A., Atkinson, J. W., & Horner, M. (1966). Motivational implications of ability grouping in schools. In J. W. Atkinson & N. T. Feather (Eds.), *A theory of achievement motivation* (pp. 231–248). New York: Wiley.

Ogden, P. (2015). *Sensorimotor psychotherapy: Interventions for trauma and attachment.* New York: Norton.

Ogden, T. H. (1992). Comments on transference and countertransference in the initial analytic meeting. *Psychoanalytic Inquiry, 12,* 225–247.

Öhman, A., & Mineka, S. (2001). Fears, phobias, and preparedness: Toward an evolved module of fear and fear learning. *Psychological Review, 108,* 483–522.

Oleszkiewicz, A., Pisanski, K., Lachowicz-Tabaczek, K., & Sorokowska, A. (2017). Voice-based assessments of trustworthiness, competence, and warmth in blind and sighted adults. *Psychonomic Bulletin and Review, 24,* 856–862.

O'Reilly, R. C. (1998). Six principles for biologically-based computational models of cortical cognition. *Trends in Cognitive Sciences, 2,* 455–462.

O'Reilly, R. C., Bhattacharyya, R., Howard, M. D., & Katz, N. (2014). Complementary learning systems. *Cognitive Science, 38,* 1229–1248.

O'Reilly, R., & Munkata, Y. (2000). *Computational explorations in cognitive science: Understanding the mind by stimulating the brain.* Cambridge, MA: MIT Press.

Osgood, C. E., Suci, C. J., & Tannenbaum, P. H. (1957). *The measurement of meaning.* Urbana: University of Illinois Press.

Ostergaard, A. L. (1999). Priming deficits in amnesia: Now you see them, now you don't. *Journal of the International Neuropsychological Society, 5,* 175–190.

Otto, M. W. (2000). Stories and metaphors in cognitive-behavior therapy. *Cognitive and Behavioral Practice, 7,* 166–172.

Packard, M. G., & Knowlton, B. J. (2002). Learning and memory functions of the basal ganglia. *Annual Review of Neuroscience, 25,* 563–593.

Paller, K. A., Acharya, A., Richardson, B. C., Plaisant, O., Shimamura, A. P., Reed, B. R., et al. (1997). Functional neuroimaging of cortical dysfunction in alcoholic Korsakoff's syndrome. *Journal of Cognitive Neuroscience, 9,* 277–293.

Paller, K. A., Hutson, C. A., Miller, B. B., & Boehm, S. G. (2003). Neural manifestations of memory with and without awareness. *Neuron, 38,* 507–516.

Palmatier, J. R., & Bornstein, P. H. (1980). Effects of subliminal stimulation of symbiotic merging fantasies on behavioral treatment of smokers. *Journal of Nervous and Mental Disease, 168,* 715–720.

Parkin, A. J. (1982). Residual learning capability in organic amnesia. *Cortex:*

A Journal Devoted to the Study of the Nervous System and Behavior, 18, 417–440.

Parkin, A. J., & Leng, N. (2014). *Neuropsyhology of the amnesic syndrome.* London: Psychology Press.

Pascal, B. (2005). *Pensees [Thoughts].* (W. F. Trotter, Trans). Stilwell, KS: Digireads. (Original work published 1670)

Payne, B. K., Burkley, M. A., & Stokes, M. B. (2008). Why do implicit and explicit attitude tests diverge?: The role of structural fit. *Journal of Personality and Social Psychology, 94,* 16–31.

Perry, C., & Laurence, J. R. (1984). Mental processing outside of awareness: The contributions of Freud and Janet. In K. S. Bowers & D. Meichenbaum (Eds.), *The unconscious reconsidered* (pp. 9–48). New York: Wiley.

Peskine, A., & Azouvi, P. (2007). Anosognosia and denial after right hemisphere stroke. In O. Godefroy & J. Bogousslavsky (Eds.), *The behavioral and cognitive neurology of stroke* (pp. 198–214). New York: Cambridge University Press.

Pessoa, L., & Adolphs, R. (2010). Emotion processing and the amygdala: From a "low road" to "many roads" of evaluating biological significance. *Nature Reviews Neuroscience, 11,* 773–783.

Pierce, C. S., & Jastrow, J. (1884). On small differences in sensation. *Memoirs of the National Academy of Science, 3,* 73–83.

Piloti, M., Meade, M. L., & Gallo, D. A. (2002). Implicit and explicit measures of memory for perceptual information in young adults, healthy older adults and patients with Alzheimer's disease. *Experimental Aging Research, 29,* 15–32.

Pine, F. (1960). Incidental stimulation: A study of preconscious transformations. *Journal of Abnormal and Social Psychology, 60,* 68–75.

Pine, F. (1961). Incidental versus focal presentation of drive related stimuli. *Journal of Abnormal and Social Psychology, 62,* 482–490.

Pine, F. (1964). The bearing of psychoanalytic theory on selected issues in research on marginal stimuli. *Journal of Nervous and Mental Disease, 138,* 205–222.

Pinker, S. (1998). Words and rules. *Lingua, 106,* 219–242.

Pinker, S. (2005). So how does the mind work? *Mind and Language, 20,* 1–24.

Pinker, S. (1997). *How the mind works.* New York: Norton.

Pinker, S., & Mehler, J. (Eds.). (1988). *Connections and symbols.* Cambridge, MA: MIT Press.

Pinker, S., & Prince, A. (1988). On language and connectionism: Analysis of a parallel distributed processing model of language acquisition. *Cognition, 28,* 73–193.

Pinker, S., & Ullman, M. (2002). The past and future of past tense. *Trends in Cognitive Science, 6,* 456–463.

Poeppel, D. (1996). A critical review of PET studies of phonological processing. *Brain and Language, 55,* 317–351.

Poldrack, R. A. (2006). Can cognitive processes be inferred from neuroimaging data? *Trends in Cognitive Science, 10,* 59–63.

Popper, K. R. (1962). *Conjectures and refutations*. New York: Basic Books.

Posner, M. I. (1973). *Cognition: An introduction*. Glenview, IL: Scott, Foresman.

Postma, A., Antonides, R., Wester, A. J., & Kessels, R. P. C. (2008). Spared unconscious influences of spatial memory in diencephalic amnesia. *Experimental Brain Research, 190*, 125–133.

Postman, L. (1953). On the problem of perceptual defense. *Psychological Review, 60*, 298–306.

Postman, L., & Bruner, J. S. (1948). Perception under stress. *Psychological Review, 55*, 314–323.

Postman, L., Bruner, J. S., & McGinnies, E. (1948). Personal values as selective factors in perception. *Journal of Abnormal and Social Psychology, 43*, 142–154.

Postman, L., Bruner, J. S., & Walk, R. D. (1951). The perception of error. *British Journal of Psychology, 42*, 1–10.

Postman, L., & Sassenrath, J. (1961). The automatic action of verbal rewards and punishments. *Journal of General Psychology, 65*, 109–136.

Postman, L., & Solomon, R. L. (1950). Perceptual sensitivity to completed and incompleted tasks. *Journal of Personality, 18*, 347–357.

Pribram, K. H. (1971). *Languages of the brain: Experimental paradoxes and principles in neuropsychology*. Englewood Cliffs, NJ: Prentice-Hall.

Prince, M. (1906). *The dissociation of personality: A biographical study in abnormal psychology*. New York: Longmans, Green and Co.

Prinz, J. J. (2006). Is the mind really modular? In R. J. Stanton (Ed.), *Contemporary debates in cognitive science* (pp. 22–36). Malden, MA: Blackwell.

Prull, M. W., Gabrieli, J. D. E., & Bunge, S. A. (2000). Age-related changes in memory: A cognitive neuroscience perspective. In F. I. M. Craik & T. A. Salthouse (Eds.), *Handbook of aging and cognition* (2nd ed., pp. 91–153). Mahwah, NJ: Erlbaum.

Pulvermuller, F. (1999). Words in the brain's language. *Behavioral and Brain Sciences, 22*, 253–336.

Quattrone, G. A. (1985). On the congruity between internal states and action. *Psychological Bulletin, 98*, 3–40.

Racker, H. (1968). *Transference and countertransference*. London: Karnac.

Ramachandran, V. S. (2000). Mirror neurons and imitation learning as the driving force behind "the great leap forward" in human evolution. *Edge*. Retrieved from *www.edge.org/3rd_culture/ramachandran/ramachandran_index.html*.

Ramachandran, V. S., & Blakeslee, S. (1998). *Phantoms in the brain: Human nature and the architecture of the mind*. London: Fourth Estate.

Ramsey, W., Stich, P., & Garon, J. (1991). Connectionism, eliminativism, and the future of folk psychology. In W. Ramsey, S. P. Stich, & D. E. Rumelhart (Eds.), *Philosophy and connectionist theory* (pp. 199–228). Hillsdale, NJ: Erlbaum.

Rao, K. R. (1978). Expectancy effects, ESP effects, and replicability. *Behavioral and Brain Sciences, 1*, 403–404.

Rapaport, D. (1960). The structure of psychoanalytic theory. *Psychological Issues, 2*(2), Monograph 6.

Rawolle, M., Schultheiss, M., & Schultheiss, O. C. (2013). Relationships between implicit motives, self-attributed motives, and personal goal commitments. *Frontiers in Psychology, 4,* Article 923.

Razran, G. (1949). Semantic and phonetographic generalizations of salivary conditioning to verbal stimuli. *Journal of Experimental Psychology, 39,* 642–652.

Reber, A. S. (1967). Implicit learning of artificial grammars. *Journal of Verbal Learning and Verbal Behavior, 6,* 855–863.

Reber, A. S. (1976). Implicit learning of synthetic languages: The role of instructional set. *Journal of Experimental Psychology: Human Learning and Memory, 2,* 88–94.

Reber, A. S. (1989). Implicit learning and tacit knowledge. *Journal of Experimental Psychology: General, 118,* 219–235.

Reber, A. S. (1992). The cognitive unconscious: An evolutionary perspective. *Consciousness and Cognition, 1,* 93–133.

Reber, A. S. (1993). *Implicit learning and tacit knowledge: An essay on the cognitive unconscious.* New York: Oxford University Press.

Reber, A. S., & Allen, R. (1978). Analogic and abstraction strategies in synthetic grammar learning: A functionalist interpretation. *Cognition, 6,* 189–221.

Reber, A. S., Kassin, S. M., Lewis, S., & Cantor, G. (1980). On the relationship between implicit and explicit modes in the learning of a complex rule structure. *Journal of Experimental Psychology: Human Learning and Memory, 6,* 492–502.

Reber, A. S., & Lewis, S. (1977). Implicit learning: An analysis of the form and structure of a body of tacit knowledge. *Cognition, 5,* 333–361.

Reber, A. S., & Millward, R. B. (1968). Event observation in probability learning. *Journal of Experimental Psychology, 77,* 317–327.

Reber, A. S., & Millward, R. B. (1971). Event tracking in probability learning. *American Journal of Psychology, 84,* 85–99.

Reber, P. J. (2008). Cognitive neuroscience of declarative and nondeclarative memory. *Advances in Psychology, 139,* 113–123.

Reber, P. J. (2013). The neural basis of implicit learning and memory: A review of neuropsychological and neuroimaging research. *Neuropsychologia, 51,* 2026–2042.

Reber, P. J., & Squire, L. R. (1999). Intact learning of artificial grammars and intact category learning by patients with Parkinson's disease. *Behavioral Neuroscience, 113,* 235–242.

Reder, L., Park, H., & Kieffaber, P. D. (2009). Memory systems do not divide on consciousness: Reinterpreting memory in terms of activation and binding. *Psychological Bulletin, 135,* 23–49.

Reed, G. S. (2017). Unconscious fantasy in context: The work of Jacob Arlow. *International Journal of Psychoanalysis, 98,* 821–830.

Reichenbach, H. (2006). *Experience and prediction: An analysis of the foundations and the structure of knowledge.* Notre Dame, IN: University of Notre Dame Press. (Original work published 1938)

Reingold, E. (1990). *Using indirect and direct measures to study unconscious processes.* Unpublished doctoral dissertation, University of Waterloo, Ontario, Canada. (Cited in Ionescu, M. D., & Erdelyi, M. H., 1992, The direct recovery of subliminal stimuli. In R. F. Bornstein & T. S. Pittman [Eds.], *Perception without awareness* [pp. 143–169]. New York: Guilford Press)

Ren, D., Tan, K., Arriaga, X. B., & Chan, K. Q. (2015). Sweet love: The effects of sweet taste experience on romantic perceptions. *Journal of Social and Personal Relationships, 32,* 905–921.

Resick, P., Monson, C., & Chard, K. (2017). *Cognitive processing therapy for PTSD: A comprehensive manual.* New York: Guilford Press.

Restak, R. M. (1994). *The modular brain.* New York: Scribner's.

Restivo, L., Vetere, G., Bontempi, B., & Ammassair-Teule, M. (2009). The formation of recent and remote memory is associated with time-dependent formation of dendritic spines in the hippocampus and anterior cingulated cortex. *Journal of Neuroscience, 29,* 8206–8214.

Ricouer, P. (1970). *Freud and philosophy* (D. Savage, Trans.) New Haven, CT: Yale University Press.

Riggs, L., McQuiggan, D. A., Anderson, A. K., & Ryan, J. D. (2010). Eye movement monitoring reveals differential influences of emotion on memory. *Frontiers in Psychology, 1,* 1–9.

Rizzolatti, G., & Craighero, L. (2004). The mirror neuron system. *Annual Review of Neuroscience, 27,* 169–192.

Rizzolatti, G., Fadiga, L., Gallese, V., & Fogassi, L. (1996). Premotor cortex and the recognition of motor actions. *Cognitive Brain Research, 3,* 131–141.

Rizzolatti, G., Fogassi, L., & Gallese, V. (2001). Neuropsychological mechanisms underlying the understanding and imitation of action. *Nature Review Neuroscience, 2,* 661–670.

Rizzolatti, G., & Sinigaglia, C. (2010). The functional role of the parieto-frontal mirror circuit: Interpretations and misinterpretations. *Natural Review Neuroscience, 11,* 264–274.

Rizzolatti, G., & Sinigaglia, C. (2015a). Curious book on mirror neurons and their myth. *American Journal of Psychology, 128,* 527–533.

Rizzolatti, G., & Sinigaglia, C. (2015b). Reply to Hickok. *American Journal of Psychology, 128,* 549–550.

Roediger, H. L., III. (1990). Implicit memory: Retention without remembering. *American Psychologist, 45,* 1043–1056.

Roediger, H. L., III, & Blaxton, T. A. (1987). Effects of varying modality, surface features, and retention interval on priming in word-fragment completion. *Memory and Cognition, 15,* 379–388.

Roediger, H. L., III, Gallo, D. A., & Geraci, L. (2002). Processing approaches to cognition: The impetus from the levels-of-processing framework. *Memory, 10,* 319–332.

Roediger, H. L., III, & McDermott, K. B. (1993). Implicit memory in normal human subjects. *Handbook of Neuropsychology, 8,* 63–131.

Rogers, C. (1959). A theory of therapy, personality and interpersonal relationships as developed in the client-centered framework. In S. Koch (Ed.), *Psychology: A study of a science: Vol. 3. Formulations of the person and the social context.* New York: McGraw-Hill.

Rogers, C. (1961). *On becoming a person.* New York: Houghton Mifflin.

Rogers, C. (1980). *A way of being.* Boston: Houghton Mifflin.

Rogers, T. T., & McClelland, J. L. (2014). Parallel distribute processing at 25: Further explorations in the microstructure of cognition. *Cognitive Science, 38,* 1024–1077.

Rokeach, M. (1973). *The nature of human values.* New York: Free Press.

Rolls. E. T. (2018). *The brain, emotion, and depression.* New York: Oxford University Press.

Rosenthal, R. (1976). *Experimenter effects in behavioral research* (Enlarged ed.). New York: Halstead Press.

Rosenthal, R., & Rosnow, R. L. (1991). *Essentials of behavioral research: Methods and data analysis* (2nd ed.). New York: McGraw-Hill.

Rosenthal, R., & Rubin, D. B. (1978). Interpersonal expectancy effects: The first 345 studies. *Behavioral and Brain Sciences, 3,* 377–386.

Ross, L. (1977). The intuitive psychologist and his shortcomings: Distortion in the attribution process. In L. Berkowitz (Ed.), *Advances in experimental social psychology* (Vol. 10, pp. 173–220). New York: Academic Press.

Rozin, P. (1976). The evolution of intelligence and access to the cognitive unconscious. In J. A. Sprague & A. N. Epstein (Eds.), *Progress in psychobiology and physiological psychology* (Vol. 6, pp. 245–280). New York: Academic Press.

Rubin, E. (1915). *Synsoplevede figurer* [*Visual figures*]. Copenhagen: Glydendalski.

Rugg, M. D., Schloerscheidt, A. M., & Mark, R. E. (1998). An electrophysiological comparison of two indices of recollection. *Journal of Memory and Language, 39,* 47–69.

Rumelhart, D. E. (1977). Toward an interactive model of reading. In S. Dornic (Ed.), *Attention and performance 6.* Hillsdale, NJ: Elrbaum.

Rumelhart, D. E., Hinton, G. E., & McClelland, J. L. (1986). A general framework for parallel distributed processing. In D. E. Rumelhart, J. L. McClelland, & the PDP Research Group (Eds.), *Parallel distributed processing: Explorations in the microstructure of cognition* (Vol. 1, pp. 45–76). Cambridge, MA: MIT Press.

Rumelhart, D. E., & McClelland, J. L. (1986). PDP models and general issues in cognitive science: Distributed representations. In D. E. Rumelhart, J. L. McClelland, & the PDP Research Group (Eds.), *Parallel distributed processing: Explorations in the microstructure of cognition* (Vol. 1, pp. 110–146). Cambridge, MA: MIT Press.

Rumelhart, D. E., McClelland, J. L., & the PDP Research Group. (1986). *Parallel distributed processing: Explorations in the microstructure of cognition: Vol. 1. Foundations* and *Vol. 2. Psychological and biological models.* Cambridge, MA: MIT Press.

Russo, J. E., & Schoemaker, P. (1989). *Decision traps.* New York: Doubleday.

Russo, R., & Parkin, A. J. (1993). Age differences in implicit memory: More apparent than real. *Memory and Cognition, 21,* 73–80.

Rutstein, E. H., & Goldberger, L. (1973). The effects of aggressive stimulation on suicidal patients: An experimental study of the psychoanalytic theory of suicide. *Psychoanalysis and Contemporary Science: An Annual of Integrative and Interdisciplinary Studies, 2,* 157–174.

Ryan, J. D., Althoff, R. R., Whitlow, S., & Cohen, N. J. (2000). Amnesia is a deficit in relational memory. *Psychological Science, 11,* 454–461.

Ryle, G. (2009). *The concept of mind.* New York: Routledge. (Original work published 1949)

Sachs, O. (1985). *The man who mistook his wife for a hat and other clinical tales.* New York: Simon & Shuster.

Saffran, J. R. (2003). Statistical language learning: Mechanisms and constraints. *Current Directions in Psychological Science, 12,* 110–114.

Saffran, J. R., Aslin, R. N., & Newport, E. L. (1996). Statistical learning by 8-month-old infants. *Science, 274,* 1926–1928.

Sagioglou, C., & Greitemeyer, T. (2014). Bitter taste causes hostility. *Personality and Social Psychology Bulletin, 40,* 1589–1597.

Sales, B. D., & Haber, R. N. (1968). A different look at perceptual defense for taboo words. *Perception and Psychophysics, 3,* 156–160.

Sanchez, D. J., & Reber, P. J. (2013). Explicit pre-training instruction does not improve implicit perceptual–motor sequence learning. *Cognition, 126,* 341–351.

Savile, A. (2000). *Leibniz.* New York: Routledge Philosophy GuideBooks.

Schacter, D. L. (1983). Feeling of knowing in episodic memory. *Journal of Experimental Psychology: Learning, Memory, and Cognition, 9,* 39–54.

Schacter, D. L. (1985). Multiple forms of memory in humans and animals. In N. Weinberger, G. Lynch, & J. McGaugh (Eds.), *Memory systems of the brain: Animal and human cognitive processes* (pp. 351–379). New York: Guilford Press.

Schacter, D. L. (1987). Implicit memory: History and current status. *Journal of Experimental Psychology: Learning, Memory, and Cognition, 13,* 501–518.

Schacter, D. L. (1990). Toward a cognitive neuropsychology of awareness: Implicit knowledge and anosognosia. *Journal of Clinical and Experimental Neuropsychology, 12,* 155–178.

Schacter, D. L. (1992). Priming and multiple memory systems: Perceptual mechanisms of implicit memory. *Journal of Cognitive Neuroscience, 4,* 244–256.

Schacter, D. L. (1994). Priming and multiple memory systems: Perceptual mechanisms of implicit memory. In D.L. Schacter & E. Tulving (Eds.), *Memory systems* (pp. 233–268). Cambridge, MA: MIT Press.

Schacter, D. L. (1996). *Searching for memory: The brain, the mind, and the past.* New York: Basic Books.

Schacter, D. L. (2001). *The seven sins of memory: How the mind forgets and remembers.* Boston: Houghton Mifflin.

Schacter, D. L., Chiu, C. Y. P., & Ochsner, K. N. (1993). Implicit memory: A selective review. *Annual Review of Neuroscience, 16,* 159–182.

Schacter, D. L., Gallo, D. A., & Kensinger, E. A. (2007). The cognitive neuroscience of implicit and false memories: Perspectives on processing specificity. In J. S. Nairne (Ed.), *The foundations of remembering: Essays in honor of Henry L. Roediger, III* (pp. 353–377). New York: Psychology Press.

Schacter, D. L., Israel, L., & Racine, C. (1999). Suppressing false recognition in younger and older adults: The distinctiveness heuristic. *Journal of Memory and Language, 40,* 1–24.

Schacter, D. L., Kaszniak, A. W., Kihlstrom, J. F., & Valdiserri, M. (1991). The relation between source memory and aging. *Psychology and Aging, 6,* 559–568.

Schacter, D. L., & Tulving, E. (1982). Memory, amnesia, and the episodic/semantic distinction. In R. L. Isaacson & N. E. Spear (Eds.), *The expression of knowledge* (pp. 33–65). New York: Plenum Press.

Schacter, D. L., Wig, G. S., & Stevens, W. D. (2007). Reductions in cortical activity during priming. *Current Opinion in Neurobiology, 17,* 171–176.

Schaffer, J. B. (1978). *Humanistic psychology.* Upper Saddle River, NJ: Prentice-Hall.

Schafer, R. A. (1980). Narration in the psychoanalytic dialogue. *Critical Inquiry, 7,* 29–53.

Schimek, J. (1975). A critical re-examination of Freud's concept of unconscious mental representation. *International Review of Psychoanalysis, 2,* 171–187.

Schimek, J. (2011). *Memory, myth, and seduction.* New York: Routledge.

Schneider, W. (1987). Connectionism: Is it a paradigm shift for psychology? *Behavior Research Methods, Instruments and Computers, 19,* 73–83.

Schneider, W., & Shiffrin, R. M. (1977). Controlled and automatic human information processing: 1. Detection, search, and attention. *Psychological Review, 84,* 1–66.

Schott, B. H., Richardon-Klaven, A., Henson, R. N. A., Becker, C., Henize, H.-J., & Duzel, E. (2006). Neuroanatomical dissociation of encoding processes related to priming and explicit memory. *Journal of Neuroscience, 26,* 792–800.

Schroeder, A. (2008). *The snowball: Warren Buffett and the business of life.* New York: Bantam Books.

Schultheiss, O. C., & Brunstein, J. C. (2001). Assessment of implicit motives with a research version of the TAT: Picture profiles, gender differences, and relations to other personality measures. *Journal of Personality Assessment, 77,* 71–86.

Schultheiss, O. C., & Brunstein, J. (2010). *Implicit motives.* New York: Oxford University Press.

Schultheiss, O. C., Jones, N. M., Davis, A. Q., & Kley, C. (2008). The role of implicit motivation in hot and cold goal pursuit: Effects on goal progress, goal rumination, and emotional well-being. *Journal of Research in Personality, 42,* 971–987.

Schultheiss, O. C., Patalakh, M., Rawolle, M., Liening, S., & MacInnes, J. J. (2011). Referential competence is associated with motivational congruence. *Journal of Research in Personality, 45,* 59–70.

Schultheiss, O. C., Patalakh, M., & Rösch, A. G. (2012). Salivary progesterone is associated with reduced coherence of attentional, cognitive, and motivational systems. *Brain and Cognition, 80,* 214–222.

Schultheiss, O. C., Rösch, A. G., Rawolle, M., Kordik, A., & Graham, S. (2010). Implicit motives: Current topics and future directions. *Advances in Motivation and Achievement, 16,* 199–233.

Schultheiss, O. C., Wirth, M. M., & Stanton, S. J. (2004). Effects of affiliation and power motivation arousal on salivary progesterone and testosterone. *Hormones and Behavior, 46,* 592–599.

Schurtman, R., Palmatier, J. R., & Martin, E. S. (1982). On the activation of symbiotic gratification fantasies as an aid in the treatment of alcoholics. *International Journal of the Addictions, 17,* 1157–1174.

Schvaneveldt, R. W., & Meyer, D. E. (1973). Retrieval and comparison processes in semantic memory. In S. Kornblum (Ed.), *Attention and performance* (Vol. 4, pp. 395–409). New York: Academic Press.

Schvaneveldt, R. W., Meyer, D., & Becker, C. (1976). Lexical ambiguity, semantic context, and visual word recognition. *Journal of Experimental Psychology: Human Perception and Performance, 2,* 243–256.

Schwartz, M. F., Marin, O. S. M., & Saffran, E. M. (1979). Dissociations of language function in dementia: A case study. *Brain and Language, 7,* 277–306.

Schyns, B., & Hansbrough, T. (2008). Why the brewery ran out of beer. *Social Psychology, 39,* 197–203.

Scott, R. B., & Dienes, Z. (2010). Knowledge applied to new domains: The unconscious succeeds where the conscious fails. *Consciousness and Cognition, 19,* 391–398.

Seamon, J. G., Brody, N., & Kauff, D. M. (1983). Affective discrimination of stimuli that are not recognized: Effects of shadowing, masking, and cerebral laterality. *Journal of Experimental Psychology: Learning, Memory, and Cognition, 9,* 544–555.

Seamon, J. G., Marsh, R. L., & Brody, N. (1984). Critical importance of exposure duration for affective discrimination of stimuli that are not recognized. *Journal of Experimental Psychology: Learning, Memory, and Cognition, 10,* 465–469.

Seamon, J. G., McKenna, P. A., & Binder, N. (1998). The mere exposure effect is differentially sensitive to different judgment tasks. *Consciousness and Cognition, 7,* 85–102.

Seamon, J. G., Williams, P. C., Crowley, M. J., Kim, I. J., Langer, S. A., Orne, P. J., et al. (1995). The mere exposure effect is based on implicit memory: Effects of stimulus type, encoding conditions, and number of exposures on recognition and affect judgments. *Journal of Experimental Psychology: Learning, Memory, and Cognition, 21,* 711–721.

Searle, J. R. (1991). Consciousness, unconsciousness and intentionality. *Philosophical Issues, 1,* 45–66.

Sedikides, C., Campbell, W. K., Reeder, G. D., & Elliot, A. J. (1998). The self-serving bias in relational context. *Journal of Personality and Social Psychology, 74,* 378–386.

Segal, H. (1964). *Introduction to the work of Melanie Klein*. London: Karnac Books.

Seger, C. A. (1994). Implicit learning. *Psychological Bulletin, 115,* 163–196.

Segerstrom, S. C., & Miller, G. E. (2004). Psychological stress and the human immune system: A meta-analytic study of 30 years of inquiry. *Psychological Bulletin, 130,* 601–630.

Seligman, M. (1970). On the generality of the laws of learning. *Psychological Review, 77,* 406–418.

Seligman, M. (1971). Phobias and preparedness. *Behavior Therapy, 2*(3), 307–321.

Shallice, T., & Saffian, E. (1986). Lexical processing in the absence of explicit word identification: Evidence from a letter-by-letter reader. *Cognitive Neuropsychology, 3,* 429–458.

Shane, M., & Shane, E. (1993). Self psychology after Kohut: One theory or many? *Journal of the American Psychoanalytic Association, 41,* 777–797.

Shanks, D. R., & John, M. F. (1994). Characteristics of dissociable human learning systems. *Behavioral Brain Science, 17,* 367–447.

Shapiro, T. (1983). The unconscious still occupies us. *Psychoanalytical Study of the Child, 38,* 547–567.

Shapiro, T., & Inderbitzin, L. B. (1989). Unconscious fantasy. *Journal of the American Psychoanalytic Association, 37,* 823–835.

Sharot, T., & Yonelinas, A. P. (2008). Differential time-dependent effects of emotion on recollective experience and memory for contextual information. *Cognition, 106,* 538–547.

Shelley, B. P. (2016). Footprints of Phineas Gage: Historical beginnings on the origins of brain and behavior and the birth of cerebral localizationism. *Archives of Medicine and Health Sciences, 4,* 280–286.

Shevrin, H., Bond, J. A., Brakel, L. A., Hertel, R. K., & Williams, W. J. (1996). *Conscious and unconscious processes*. New York: Guilford Press.

Shevrin, H., & Dickman, S. (1980) The psychological unconscious: A necessary assumption for all psychological theory? *American Psychologist, 35,* 421–434.

Shiffrin, R. M., & Geisler, W. S. (1973). Visual recognition in a theory of information processing. In R. Solso (Ed.), *The Loyola Symposium: Contemporary issues in cognitive psychology* (pp. 53–101). Washington, DC: Halsted Press.

Shiffrin, R. M., & Schneider, W. (1977). Controlled and automatic human information processing: II. Perceptual learning, automatic attending and a general theory. *Psychological Review, 84,* 127–190.

Shimamura, A. (1995). Memory and frontal lobe function. In M. Gazzaniga (Ed.), *The cognitive neurosciences* (pp. 803–813). Cambridge, MA: MIT Press.

Sidis, B. (Ed.). (1902). *Psychological researches: Studies in mental dissociation*. London: W. Rider & Son.

Siegel, P., & Weinberger, J. (1998). Capturing the "mommy and I are one" merger fantasy: The oneness motive. In R. Bornstein & J. Masling (Eds.),

Empirical studies of psychoanalytic theories (pp. 71–98). Washington, DC: APA Press.

Siegel, P., & Weinberger, J. (2012). Less is more: The effects of very brief versus clearly visible exposure. *Emotion, 12,* 394–402.

Silverman, L. H. (1976). Psychoanalytic theory: The reports of my death are greatly exaggerated. *American Psychologist, 31,* 621–637.

Silverman, L. H. (1983). The subliminal psychodynamic method: Overview and comprehensive listing of studies. In J. Masling (Ed.), *Empirical studies of psychoanalytic theory* (Vol. 1, pp. 69–103). Mahwah, NJ: Erlbaum.

Silverman, L. H., Bronstein, A., & Mendelsohn, E. (1976). The further use of the subliminal psychodynamic method for the experimental study of the clinical theory of psychoanalysis: On the specificity of the relationship between symptoms and unconscious conflicts. *Psychotherapy: Theory, Research and Practice, 13,* 2–16.

Silverman, L. H., Frank, S. G., & Dachinger, P. (1974). A psychoanalytic reinterpretation of the effectiveness of systematic desensitization: Experimental data bearing on the role of merging fantasies. *Journal of Abnormal Psychology, 83,* 313–318.

Silverman, L. H., Klinger, H., Lustbader, L., Farrell, J., & Martin, A. D. (1972). The effects of subliminal drive stimulation on the speech of stutterers. *Journal of Nervous and Mental Disease, 155,* 14–21.

Silverman, L. H., Lachman, F., & Milich, R. (1982). *The search for oneness.* New York: International Universities Press.

Silverman, L. H., Martin, A., Ungaro, R., & Mendelsohn, E. (1978). Effect of subliminal stimulation of symbiotic fantasies on behavior modification treatment of obesity. *Journal of Consulting and Clinical Psychology, 46,* 432–441.

Silverman, L. H., Ross, D. L., Adler, J. M., & Lustig, D. A. (1978). Simple research paradigm for demonstrating subliminal psychodynamic activation: Effects of Oedipal stimuli on dart-throwing accuracy in college males. *Journal of Abnormal Psychology, 87,* 341–357.

Silverman, L. H., Spiro, R. H., Weissberg, J. S., & Candell, P. (1969). The effects of aggressive activation and the need to merge on pathological thinking in schizophrenia. *Journal of Nervous and Mental Disease, 148,* 39–51.

Silverman, L. H., & Weinberger, J. (1985). Mommy and I are one: Implications for psychotherapy. *American Psychologist, 40,* 1296–1308.

Simon, H. A. (1962). The architecture of complexity. *Proceedings of the American Philosophical Society, 106,* 467–482.

Simon, H. A., & Newell, A. (1971). Human problem solving: The state of the theory in 1970. *American Psychologist, 26,* 145–159.

Simpson, D. (2005). Phrenology and the neurosciences: Contributions of F. J. Gall and J. G. Spurzheim. *ANZ Journal of Surgery, 75,* 475–482.

Singer, C. (1959). *A short history of scientific ideas to 1900.* London: Oxford University Press.

Singer, T., Seymour, B., O'Doherty, J., Kaube, H., Dolan, R. J., & Frith, C. D.

(2004). Empathy for pain involves the affective but not sensory components of pain. *Science, 303,* 1157–1162.

Skinner, B. (1953). *Science and human behavior.* New York: Free Press.

Skinner, B. (1974). *About behaviorism.* New York: Knopf.

Smith, C. E. (1992). *Motivation and personality: Handbook of thematic content analysis.* New York: Cambridge University Press.

Smith, E. D., Jonides, J., & Koeppe, R. A. (1996). Dissociating verbal and spatial working memory using PET. *Cerebral Cortex, 6,* 11–20.

Smith, E. D., & Kosslyn, S. (2007). *Cognitive psychology: Mind and brain.* Upper Saddle River, NJ: Pearson/Prentice-Hall.

Smith, E. E., & Miller, F. (1978). Limits on the perception of cognitive processes: Reply to Nisbett and Wilson. *Psychological Review, 85,* 355–362.

Smith, E. R. (1996). What do connectionism and social psychology offer each other? *Journal of Personality and Social Psychology, 70,* 893–912.

Smith, G. J., & Henriksson, M. (1955). The effect on an established percept of a perceptual process beyond awareness. *Nordisk Psykologi, 7,* 170–179.

Smith, G. J., Spence, D. P., & Klein, G. S. (1959). Subliminal effects of verbal stimuli. *Journal of Abnormal and Social Psychology, 59,* 167–177.

Smith, J., Siegert, R. J., & McDowall, J. (2001). Preserved implicit learning on both the serial reaction time and artificial grammar in patients with Parkinson's disease. *Brain and Cognition, 45,* 378–391.

Sohlberg, S., Arvidsson, M., & Birgegard, A. (1997). Stroop and mood/memory measures in the study of unconscious "oneness." *Perceptual and Motor Skills, 85,* 81–82.

Sohlberg, S., & Birgegard, A. (2003). Persistent complex subliminal activation effects: First experimental observations. *Journal of Personality and Social Psychology, 85,* 302–316.

Sohlberg, S., Birgegard, A., Czartoryski, W., Overfelt, K., & Strombom, Y. (2000). Symbiotic oneness and defensive autonomy: Yet another experiment demystifying Silverman's findings using "Mommy and I are one." *Journal of Research in Personality, 34,* 108–126.

Sohlberg, S., Claesson, K., & Birgegard, A. (2003). Memories of mother, complementarity and shame: Predicting response to subliminal stimulation with "Mommy and I are one." *Scandinavian Journal of Psychology, 44,* 339–346.

Spangler, W. D. (1992). Validity of questionnaire and TAT measures of need for achievement: Two meta-analyses. *Psychological Bulletin, 112,* 140–154.

Spence, D. P. (1961). The multiple effects of subliminal stimuli. *Journal of Personality, 29,* 40–53.

Spence, D. P. (1964). Conscious and preconscious influences on recall: Another example of the restricting effects of awareness. *Journal of Abnormal and Social Psychology, 68,* 92–99.

Spence, D. P., & Bressler, J. (1962). Subliminal activation of conceptual associates: A study of rational preconscious thinking. *Journal of Personality, 30,* 89–105.

Spence, D. P., & Ehrenberg, B. (1964). Effects of oral deprivation on responses to subliminal and supraliminal verbal food stimuli. *Journal of Abnormal and Social Psychology, 69,* 10–18.

Spence, D. P., & Gordon, C. M. (1967). Activation and measurement of an early oral fantasy: An exploratory study. *Journal of the American Psychoanalytic Association, 15,* 99–129.

Spence, D. P., & Holland, S. (1962). The restricting effects of awareness: Paradox and an explanation. *Journal of Abnormal and Social Psychology, 64,* 163–174.

Sperber, D. (1996). *Explaining culture: A naturalistic approach.* Oxford, UK: Basil Blackwell.

Sperry, R. W. (1968). Hemisphere de-connection and unity in conscious awareness. *American Psychologist, 23,* 723–733.

Spinoza, B. (2015). *Ethics.* (R. H. M. Elwes, Trans.). Denham Springs, LA: Cavalier Classics. (Original work published 1677)

Spruyt, A., Gast, A., & Moors, A. (2011). The sequential priming paradigm: A primer. In K. C. Klauer, A. Voss, & C. Stahl (Eds.), *Cognitive methods in social psychology* (pp. 48–77). New York: Guilford Press.

Squire, L. R. (1986). Mechanisms of memory. *Science, 232,* 1612–1619.

Squire, L. R. (1987). *Memory and brain.* New York: Oxford University Press.

Squire, L. R. (1992). Memory and the hippocampus: A synthesis from findings with rats, monkeys, and humans. *Psychological Review, 99,* 195–231.

Squire, L. R. (2004). Memory systems of the brain: A brief history and current perspective. *Neurobiology of Learning and Memory, 82,* 171–177.

Squire, L. R. (2009). Memory and brain systems: 1969–2009. *Journal of Neuroscience, 29,* 12711–12716.

Squire, L. R., & Dede, A. J. O. (2015). Conscious and unconscious memory systems. *Cold Spring Harbor Perspectives in Biology, 7,* 1–14.

Squire, L. R., & Wixted, J. T. (2016). Remembering. In S. Groes (Ed.), *Memory in the twenty-first century: New critical perspectives from the arts, humanities, and science* (pp. 251–262). Hampshire, UK: Palgrave-Macmillan.

Squire, L. R., & Zola-Morgan, S. (1988). Memory: Brain systems and behavior. *Trends in Neuroscience, 11,* 170–175.

Squire, L. R., & Zola-Morgan, S. (1991). The medial temporal lobe memory system. *Science, 253,* 1380–1386.

Stadler, M. A., & Frensch, P. A. (Eds.). (1998). *Handbook of implicit learning.* Thousand Oaks, CA: SAGE.

Starr, A., & Phillips, L. (1970). Verbal and motor memory in the amnestic syndrome. *Neuropsychologia, 8,* 75–88.

Stein, K. B. (1953). Perceptual defense and perceptual sensitization under neutral and involved conditions. *Journal of Personality, 21,* 467–478.

Steinert, C., Hoffman, M., Kruse, J., & Leichsenring, F. (2014a, January). The prospective long-term course of adult depression in general practice and the community: A systematic literature review. *Journal of Affective Disorders, 152–155,* 65–75.

Steinert, C., Hoffman, M., Kruse, J., & Leichsenring, F. (2014b). Relapse rates after psychotherapy for depression—stable long-term effects?: A meta-analysis. *Journal of Affective Disorders, 168*(15), 107–118.

Stern, D. B. (1983). Unformulated experience. *Contemporary Psychoanalysis, 19,* 71–99.

Stern, D. B. (1997). *Unformulated experience: From dissociation to imagination in psychoanalysis.* Hillsdale, NJ: Analytic Press.

Stern, D. N. (1985). *The interpersonal world of the infant: A view from psychoanalysis and developmental psychology.* New York: Basic Books.

Stevens, S. S. (1957). On the psychophysical law. *Psychological Review, 64,* 153–181.

Stolorow, R. D., & Atwood, G. E. (1989). The unconscious and unconscious fantasy: An intersubjective–developmental perspective. *Psychoanalytic Inquiries, 9,* 364–374.

Stolorow, R. D., Atwood, G. E., & Branchaft, B. (1994). *The intersubjective perspective.* Lanham, MD: Rowman & Littlefield.

Stolorow, R., Brandchaft, B., & Atwood, G. (1987). *Psychoanalytic treatment: "An intersubjective approach."* Hillsdale. NJ: Analytic Press.

Storbeck, J., & Robinson, M. D. (2004). Preferences and inferences in encoding visual objects: A systematic comparison of semantic and affective priming. *Personality and Social Psychology Bulletin, 30,* 81–93.

Storbeck, J., Robinson, M. D., & McCourt, M. E. (2006). Semantic processing precedes affect retrieval: The neurological case for cognitive primacy in visual processing. *Review of General Psychology, 10,* 41–55.

Storey, S., & Workman, L. (2013). The effects of temperature priming on cooperation in the iterated Prisoner's Dilemma. *Evolutionary Psychology, 11,* 52–67.

Stott, R., Mansell, W., Salkovskis, P., Lavender, A., & Cartwright-Hatton, S. (2010). *Oxford guide to metaphors in CBT: Building cognitive bridges.* London: Oxford University Press.

Stoycheva, V., Weinberger, J., & Singer, E. (2014). The place of the normative unconscious in psychoanalytic theory and practice. *Psychoanalytic Psychology, 31,* 100–118.

Strack, F., & Deutsch, R. (2015). The duality of everyday life: Dual-process and dual-system models in social psychology. In M. Mikulincer & P. Shaver (Eds.), *APA handbook of personality and social psychology: Vol. 1. Attitudes and social cognition* (pp. 891–927). Washington, DC: American Psychological Association.

Sullivan, H. S. (1964). *The fusion of psychiatry and social science.* New York: Norton.

Sun, R. (Ed.). (2008). *The Cambridge handbook of computational psychology.* New York: Cambridge University Press.

Swets, J. A., Tanner, W. P., & Birdsall, T. G. (1955). The evidence for a decision-making theory of visual detection. *Electronic Defense Group, University of Michigan Technological report, No. 40.*

Swets, J. A., Tanner, W. P., & Birdsall, T. G. (1961). Decision processes in perception. *Psychological Review, 68,* 301–340.

Tamietto, M., Castelli, L., Vighetti, S., Perozzo, P., Geminiani, G., Weiskrantz, L., et al. (2009). Unseen facial and bodily expressions trigger fast emotional reactions. *Proceedings of the National Academy of Sciences of the USA, 106,* 1761–1766.

Tamietto, M., & de Gelder, B. (2010). Neural bases of the non-conscious perception of emotional signals. *Nature Reviews Neuroscience, 11,* 697–709.

Tanner, W. P., Jr. (1955). On the design of psychophysical experiments. In H. Quastler (Ed.), *Information theory in psychology* (pp. 403–414). Glencoe, IL: Free Press.

Tanner, W. P., Jr., & Swets, J. A. (1954). A decision-making theory of visual detection. *Psychological Review, 61,* 401–409.

Tay, D., & Jordan, J. (2015). Metaphor and the notion of control in trauma talk. *Text and Talk, 35,* 553–573.

Teachman, B., Joormann, J., Steinman, S., & Gotlib, I. (2012). Automaticity in anxiety disorders and major depressive disorder. *Clinical Psychology Review, 32,* 575–603.

Tellegen, A. (1982). *Content categories: Absorption items* (rev.). Unpublished manuscript, University of Minnesota.

Terhune, K. W. (1968). Motives, situation, and interpersonal conflict within Prisoner's Dilemma. *Journal of Personality and Social Psychology, 8,* 1–24.

Thagard, P. (2005). *Mind: Introduction to cognitive science* (2nd ed.). Cambridge, MA: MIT Press.

Thibaut, J., & Riecken, H. (1955). Some determinants and consequences of the perception of social causality. *Journal of Personality, 24,* 113–133.

Thomson, D. R., Milliken, B., & Smilek, D. (2010). Long-term conceptual implicit memory: A decade of evidence. *Memory and Cognition, 38,* 42–46.

Tinbergen, N. (1951). *The study of instinct.* New York: Clarendon Press/Oxford University Press.

Titchener, E. B. (1908). *Lectures on the elementary psychology of feeling and attention.* New York: Macmillan Books.

Titchener, E. B. (1972). *Systematic psychology.* Ithaca, NY: Cornell University Press. (Original work published 1929)

Todd, R. M., Cunningham, W. A., Anderson, A. K., & Thompson, E. (2012). Affect-biased attention as emotion regulation. *Trends in Cognitive Science, 16,* 365–372.

Todorov, A., Mandisodza, A. N., Goren, A., & Hall, C. C. (2005). Inferences of competence from faces predict election outcomes. *Science, 308,* 1623–1626.

Tolman, E. C. (1949). *Purposive behavior in animals and men.* Berkeley: University of California Press.

Tooby, J., & Cosmides, L. (1992). The psychological foundations of culture. In J. H. Barkow, L. Cosmides, & J. Tooby (Eds.), *The adapted mind: Evolutionary psychology and the generation of culture* (pp. 19–136). Oxford, UK: Oxford University Press.

Tooby, J., & Cosmides, L. (1995). Mapping the evolved functional organization of mind and brain. In M. Gazzaniga (Ed.), *The cognitive neurosciences* (pp. 1185–1197). Cambridge, MA: MIT Press.

Tranel, D., & Damasio, A. R. (1985). Knowledge without awareness: An autonomic index of facial recognition by prosopagnosics. *Science, 228,* 1453–1454.

Treisman, A. M. (1960). Contextual cues in selective listening. *Quarterly Journal of Experimental Psychology, 12,* 242–248.

Treisman, A. M. (1964). Monitoring and storage of irrelevant messages in selective attention. *Journal of Verbal Learning and Verbal Behavior, 3,* 449–459.

Treisman, A. M. (1969). Strategies and models of selective attention. *Psychological Review, 76,* 282–299.

Trevouledes, D. (2003). *The relationship between hypnotic susceptibility and oneness motivation.* Unpublished doctoral dissertation, Adelphi University.

Trimble, R., & Eriksen, C. W. (1966). "Subliminal cues" and the Müller-type illusion. *Perception and Psychophysics, 1,* 401–404.

Tulving, E. (1972). Episodic and semantic memory. In E. Tulving & W. Donaldson (Eds.), *Organization of memory* (pp. 381–403). New York: Academic Press.

Tulving, E., & Schacter, D. L. (1990). Priming and human memory systems. *Science, 247,* 301–306.

Tulving, E., Schacter, D. L., & Stark, H. A. (1982). Priming effects in word-fragment completion are independent of recognition memory. *Journal of Experimental Psychology: Learning, Memory, and Cognition, 8,* 336–342.

Turk-Browne, N. B., Yi, D. J., & Chun, M. M. (2006). Linking implicit and explicit memory: Common encoding factors and share representations. *Neuron, 49,* 917–929.

Tversky, A., & Kahneman, D. (1973). Availability: A heuristic for judging frequency and probability. *Cognitive Psychology, 5,* 207–232.

Tversky, A., & Kahneman, D. (1974). Judgment under uncertainty: Heuristics and biases. *Science, 184,* 1124–1131.

Tversky, A., & Kahneman, D. (1981). The framing of decisions and the psychology of choice. *Science, 211,* 453–458.

Uleman, J., & Bargh, J. (1989). *Unintended thought.* New York: Guilford Press.

van Gaal, S., & Lamme, V. A. F. (2012). Unconscious high-level information processing: Implication for neurobiological theories of consciousness. *The Neuroscientist, 18,* 287–301.

van Gelder, T. (1991). What is the "D" in "PDP"?: A survey of the concept of distribution. In W. Ramsey, S. P. Stich, & D. E. Rumelhart (Eds.), *Philosophy and connectionist theory* (pp. 33–59). Hillsdale, NJ: Erlbaum.

Varga, M. (1973). *An experimental study of aspects of the psychoanalytic study of elation.* Unpublished doctoral dissertation, New York University.

Verneau, M., van der Kamp, J., Savelsbergh, G. J. P., & de Looze, M. P. (2014). Age and time effects on implicit and explicit learning. *Experimental Aging Research, 40,* 477–511.

Veroff, J. (1969). Social comparison and the development of achievement motivation. In C. P. Smith (Ed.), *Achievement related motives in children* (pp. 46–101). New York: Russel Sage.

Vivona, J. M. (2009). Embodied language in neuroscience and psychoanalysis. *Journal of the American Psychoanalytic Association, 57,* 1327–1360.

Von Hartmann, E. (1884). *Philosophy of the unconscious.* (W. C. Coupland, trans.) London: Trübner.

Von Helmholtz, H. (1962). *Treatise on physiological optics* (J. P. C. Southall, Trans.). New York: Dover. (Original work published 1859)

Vuilleumier, P. (2005). How brains beware: Neural mechanisms of emotional attention. *Trends in Cognitive Science, 9,* 585–594.

Walker, E. L., & Heyns, R. W. (1962). *An anatomy for conformity.* Englewood Cliffs, NJ: Prentice-Hall.

Wang, Z., Xu, B., & Zhou, H.-J. (2014). Social cycling and conditional responses in the Rock-Paper-Scissors game. *Scientific Reports, 4,* Article number 5,830.

Wardlaw, K. A., & Kroll, N. E. A. (1976). Automatic responses to shock associated words in a non-attended message: A failure to replicate. *Journal of Experimental Psychology: Human Perception and Performance, 2,* 357–360.

Warrington, E. K., & Weiskrantz, L. (1968). New method of testing long-term retention with special reference to amnesic patients. *Nature, 217,* 972–974.

Warrington, E. K., & Weiskrantz, L. (1970). Amnesia: Consolidation or retrieval? *Nature, 228,* 628–630.

Warrington, E. K., & Weiskrantz, L. (1978). Further analysis of the prior learning effect in amnesic patients. *Neuropsychologia, 16,* 169–177.

Watson, J. (1913). Psychology as the behaviorist views it. *Psychological Review, 20,* 158–177.

Watson, J. (1919). *Psychology from the standpoint of a behaviorist.* Philadelphia: J. B. Lippincott.

Watt, H. J. (1905). Experimentelle beiträge zur einer theorie des denkens. *Archives für Geschichte der Psychologie, 4,* 289–436. (Experimental contribution to a theory of thinking. *Journal of Anatomy and Physiology, 40,* 257–266—as cited in Jaynes, 1976)

Wegner, D. M. (1989). *White bears and other unwanted thoughts: Suppression, obsession, and the psychology of mental control.* New York: Penguin Press.

Wegner, D. (1994). Ironic processes of mental control. *Psychological Review, 101,* 34–52.

Weinberger, J. (1986). Comment on Robert Fudin's paper "Subliminal psychodynamic activation: Mommy and I are not yet one." *Perceptual and Motor Skills, 63,* 1232–1234.

Weinberger, J. (1987). Lloyd Silverman (1930–1986): A personal appreciation. *Psychological Reports, 60,* 429–430.

Weinberger, J. (1989). Response to Balay and Shevrin: Constructive critique or misguided attack? *American Psychologist, 44,* 1417–1419.

Weinberger, J. (1992). Validating and demystifying subliminal psychodynamic activation. In R. F. Bornstein & T. S. Pittman (Eds.), *Perception without awareness* (pp. 170–190). New York: Guilford Press.

Weinberger, J. (1994). Conclusions. In F. Heatherton & J. Weinberger (Eds.), *Can personality change?* (pp. 333–350). Washington, DC: APA Books.

Weinberger, J. (1995). Common factors aren't so common: The common factors dilemma. *Clinical Psychology: Science and Practice, 2,* 45–69.

Weinberger, J. (2000). William James and the unconscious: Redressing a century-old misunderstanding. *Psychological Science, 6,* 439–445.

Weinberger, J. (2014). Common factors are not so common and specific factors are not so specified: Toward an inclusive integration of psychotherapy research. *Psychotherapy, 51,* 514–518.

Weinberger, J., Bonner, E., & Barra, M. (1999, April). *Reliability and validity of the oneness motive.* Paper presented at the meeting of the American Psychological Association, Boston, MA.

Weinberger, J., & Eig, A. (1999). Expectancies: The ignored common factor in psychotherapy. In I. Kirsch (Ed.), *How expectancies shape experience* (pp. 357–382). Washington, DC: APA Books.

Weinberger, J., & Hardaway, R. (1990). Separating science from myth in subliminal psychodynamic activation. *Clinical Psychology Review 10,* 727–756.

Weinberger, J., Kelner, S., & McClelland, D. (1997). The effect of subliminal symbiotic stimulation on free-response and self-report mood. *Journal of Nervous and Mental Disease, 185,* 599–605.

Weinberger, J., & Levy, K. N. (2005). Psychoanalysis and psychology. In E. S. Person, A. Cooper, & G. Gabbard (Eds.), *Textbook of psychoanalysis* (pp. 463–478). Washington, DC: Psychiatric Press.

Weinberger, J., & McClelland, D. (1990). Cognitive versus traditional motivational models: Irreconcilable or complimentary? In R. Sorrentino & J. Higgins (Eds.), *Handbook of motivation and cognition* (Vol. 2, pp. 562–597). New York: Guilford Press.

Weinberger, J., & Rasco, C. (2007). Empirically supported common factors. In S. G. Hoffman & J. Weinberger (Eds.), *The art and science of psychotherapy* (pp. 103–129). New York: Routledge.

Weinberger, J., Siefert, C., & Haggerty, G. (2010). Implicit processes in social and clinical psychology. In J. E. Maddux & J. P. Tangney (Eds.), *Social psychological foundations of clinical psychology* (pp. 461–475). New York: Guilford Press.

Weinberger, J., Siegel, P., & DeCamello, A. (2000). On integrating psychoanalysis and cognitive science. *Psychoanalysis and Contemporary Thought, 23,* 147–175.

Weinberger, J., Siegel, P., Siefert, C., & Drwal, J. (2011). What you cannot see can help you: The effect of exposure to unreportable stimuli on approach behavior. *Consciousness and Cognition, 20,* 173–180.

Weinberger, J., & Silverman, L. H. (1987). Subliminal psychodynamic activation: An experimental approach to testing psychoanalytic propositions. In R. Hogan & W. Jones (Eds.). *Perspectives in personality: Theory, measurement, and interpersonal dynamics* (Vol. 2, pp. 251–288). Greenwich, CT: JAI Press.

Weinberger, J., & Smith, B. (2011). Investigating merger: Subliminal psychodynamic activation and oneness motivation research. *Journal of the American Psychoanalytic Association, 59,* 553–570.

Weinberger, J., & Weiss, J. (1997). Psychoanalytic and cognitive conceptions of the unconscious. In D. J. Stein (Ed.), *Cognitive science and the unconscious* (pp. 23–54). Washington, DC: American Psychiatric Press.

Weiner, B. (1986). *An attributional theory of motivation and emotion.* New York: Springer Verlag.

Weiner, B. (2000). Intrapersonal and interpersonal theories of motivation from an attributional perspective. *Educational Psychology Review, 12,* 1–14.

Weiskrantz, L. (1980). Varieties of residual experience. *Quarterly Journal of Experimental Psychology, 32,* 365–386.

Weiskrantz, L. (1983). Evidence and scotomata. *Behavioral and Brain Sciences, 3,* 464–467.

Weiskrantz, L. (1986). *Blindsight: A case study and implications.* New York: Oxford University Press.

Weiskrantz, L., Warrington, E. K., Sanders, M. D., & Marshall, J. (1974). Visual capacity in the hemianopic field following a restricted occipital ablation. *Brain, 97,* 709–728.

Welch, M. J. (1984). Using metaphor in psychotherapy. *Journal of Psychosocial Nursing, 22,* 13–18.

Wentura, D., & Degner, J. (2010). A practical guide to sequential priming and related tasks. In B. Gawronski & B. K. Payne (Eds.), *Handbook of implicit social cognition* (pp. 95–116). New York: Guilford Press.

Wernicke, C. (1989). Neurology: Recent contributions on aphasia. *Cognitive Neuropsychology, 6,* 547–569. (Original work published 1885)

Westen, D. (1998). The scientific legacy of Sigmund Freud: Toward a psychodynamically informed psychological science. *Psychological Bulletin, 124,* 333–371.

Westen, D., & Gabbard, G. (2002). Developments in cognitive neuroscience: 2. Implications for theories of transference. *Journal of the American Psychoanalytic Association, 50,* 648–655.

Westen, D., Novotny, C., & Thompson-Brenner, H. (2004). The empirical status of empirically-supported therapies: Assumptions, findings, and reporting in controlled clinical trials. *Psychological Bulletin, 130,* 631–663.

Wheeler, M., Stuss, D., & Tulving, E. (1995). Frontal lobe damage produces episodic memory impairment. *Journal of the International Neuropsychological Society, 1,* 525–536.

Whitmarsh, S., Udden, J., Barendregt, H., & Petersson, K. (2013). Mindfulness reduces habitual responding based on implicit knowledge: Evidence from artificial grammar learning. *Consciousness and Cognition, 22,* 833–845.

Whittaker, E. M., Gilchrist, J. C., & Fischer, J. W. (1952). Perceptual defense or response suppression? *Journal of Abnormal and Social Psychology, 47,* 732–733.

Whyte, L. (1960). *The unconscious before Freud.* New York: Basic Books.

Wicker, B., Keysers, C., Plailly, J., Royet J. P., Gallese, V., & Rizzolatti, G. (2003). Both of us disgusted in my insula: The common neural basis of seeing and feeling disgust. *Neuron, 40,* 655–664.

Widgery, A. G. (1950). Classical German idealism, the philosophy of Schopenhauer and neo-Kantianism. In V. Fern (Ed.), *A history of philosophical systems* (pp. 291–306). New York: Philosophical Library.

Williams, J., Watts, F. N., MacLeod, C., & Mathews, A. (1988). *Cognitive psychology and emotional disorders.* Chichester, UK: Wiley.

Williams, L., & Bargh, J. (2008a). Experiencing personal warmth promotes personal warmth. *Science, 322,* 606–607.

Williams, L., & Bargh, J. (2008b). Keeping one's distance: The influence of spatial distance cues on affect and evaluation. *Psychological Science, 19,* 302–308.

Williams, L. E., Huang, J. Y., & Bargh, J. A. (2009). The scaffolded mind: Higher mental processes are grounded in early experience of the physical world. *European Journal of Social Psychology, 39,* 1257–1267.

Willis, J., & Todorov, A. (2006). First impressions: Making up your mind after a 100-ms exposure to a face. *Psychological Science, 17,* 592–598.

Wilson, A. E., & Ross, M. (2001). From chump to champ: People's appraisals of their earlier and present selves. *Journal of Personality and Social Psychology, 80,* 572–584.

Wilson, T. D., Houston, C. E., Etling, K. M., & Brekke, N. (1996). A new look at anchoring effects: Basic anchoring and its antecedents. *Journal of Experimental Psychology: General, 125,* 387–402.

Wilson, T. D., Lindsey, S., & Schooler, T. (2000). A model of dual attitudes. *Psychological Review, 107,* 101–126.

Wilson, W. R. (1979). Feeling more than we can know: Exposure effects without learning. *Journal of Personality and Social Psychology, 37,* 811–821.

Winkielman, P., Niedenthal, P., Wielgosz, J., Eelen, J., & Kavanagh, L. C. (2015). Embodiment of cognition and emotion. *APA handbook of personality and social psychology, 1,* 151–175.

Winter, D. G. (1973). *The power motive.* New York: Free Press.

Winter, D. G. (1987). Enhancement of an enemy's power motivation as a dynamic of conflict escalation. *Journal of Personality and Social Psychology, 52,* 41–46.

Winter, D. G. (1991). A motivational model of leadership: Predicting long-term management success from TAT measures of power motivation and responsibility. *Leadership Quarterly, 2,* 67–80.

Winter, D. G. (1992). Power motivation revisited. In C. P Smith, J. W. Atkinson, D. C. McClelland, & J. Veroff (Eds.), *Motivation and personality: Handbook of thematic content analysis* (pp. 301–310). New York: Cambridge University Press.

Winter, D. G. (1998). Toward a science of personality psychology: David McClelland's development of empirically derived TAT measures. *History of Psychology, 1,* 130–153.

Winter, D. G. (1999). Linking personality and "scientific" psychology: The development of empirically derived Thematic Apperception Test measures.

In L. Gieser & M. I. Stein (Eds.), *Evocative images: The Thematic Apperception Test and the art of projection* (pp. 107–124). Washington, DC: American Psychological Association.

Winter, D. G. (2003). Personality and political behavior. In D. O. Sears, L. Huddy, & R. Jervis (Eds.), *Oxford handbook of political psychology* (pp. 110–145). New York: Oxford University Press.

Winter, D. G. (2005). Things I've learned about personality from studying political leaders at a distance. *Journal of Personality, 73,* 557–584.

Winter, D. G. (2010). Why achievement motivation predicts success in business but failure in politics: The importance of personal control. *Journal of Personality, 78,* 1637–1667.

Winter, D. G., John, O. P., Stewart, A. J., Klohnen, E. C., & Duncan, L. E. (1998). Traits and motives: Toward an integration of two traditions in personality research. *Psychological Review, 105,* 230–250.

Wirth, M. M., & Schultheiss, O. C. (2006). Effects of affiliation arousal (hope of closeness) and affiliation stress (fear of rejection) on progesterone and cortisol. *Hormones and Behavior, 50,* 786–795.

Wirth, M. M., Welsh, K. M., & Schultheiss, O. C. (2006). Salivary cortisol changes in humans after winning or losing a dominance contest depend on implicit power motivation. *Hormones and Behavior, 49,* 346–352.

Woollams, A. M., Taylor, J. R., Karayanidis, F., & Henson, R. N. (2008). Event-related potentials associated with masked priming of test cues reveal multiple potential contributions to a recognition memory. *Journal of Cognitive Neuroscience, 20,* 1114–1129.

Worrell, L., & Worrell, J. (1966). An experimental and theoretical note on conscious and preconscious influences on recall. *Journal of Personality and Social Psychology, 3,* 119–123.

Yoon, K. L., Hong, S. W., Joormann, J., & Kang, P. (2009). Perception of facial expressions of emotion during binocular rivalry. *Emotion, 9,* 172–182.

Young, R. M. (1990). The mind–body problem. In R. C. Olby, G. N. Cantor, J. R. R. Christie, & M. J. S. Hodge (Eds.), *Companion to the history of modern science* (pp. 702–711). New York: Routledge.

Zajonc, R. (1968). Attitudinal effects of mere exposure. *Journal of Personality and Social Psychology, 9,* 1–27.

Zajonc, R. (1980). Feeling and thinking: Preferences need no inferences. *American Psychologist, 35,* 151–175.

Zajonc, R. (1984). On the primacy of affect. *American Psychologist, 39,* 117–123.

Zajonc, R. (2000). Feeling and thinking: Closing the debate over the independence of affect. In J. P. Forgas (Ed.), *Feeling and thinking: The role of affect in social cognition: Studies in emotion and social interaction, second series* (pp. 31–58). New York: Cambridge University Press.

Zajonc, R. (2001). Mere exposure: A gateway to the subliminal. *Current Directions in Psychological Science, 10,* 224–228.

Zbozinek, T. D., & Craske, M. G. (2017). Positive affect predicts less reacquisition of fear: Relevance for long-term outcomes of exposure therapy. *Cognition and Emotion, 31,* 712–725.

Zeddies, T. (2000). Within, outside, and in between. *Psychoanalytic Psychology, 17*, 467–487.

Zhong, C. B., & Leonardelli, G. (2008). Cold and lonely: Does social exclusion literally feel cold? *Psychological Science, 19*, 838–842.

Zhong, C. B., & Liljenquist, K. (2006). Washing away your sins: Threatened morality and physical cleansing. *Science, 313*, 1451–1452.

Zigler, E., & Yospe, L. (1960). Perceptual defense and the problem of response suppression. *Journal of Personality, 28*, 220–239.

Zimbardo, P. G. (1969). *The cognitive control of motivation.* Glenview, IL: Scott, Foresman.

Zimbardo, P. G., Cohen, A. R., Weisenberg, M., Dworkin, L., & Firestone, I. (1966). Control of pain motivation by cognitive dissonance. *Science, 151*, 217–219.

Zimbardo, P. G., Weissenberg, M., Firestone, I., & Levy, B. (1965). Communicator effectiveness in producing public conformity and private attitude change. *Journal of Personality, 33*, 233–255.

Zuckerman, M. (1960). The effects of subliminal and supraliminal suggestion on verbal productivity. *Journal of Abnormal and Social Psychology, 60*, 404–411.

Zuckerman, M., Koestner, R., Collela, M. J., & Alton, A. O. (1984). Anchoring in the detection of deception and leakage. *Journal of Personality and Social Psychology, 47*, 301–311.

Index